FUNDAMENTALS *of*
SPECIAL
RADIOGRAPHIC
PROCEDURES

FUNDAMENTALS *of* SPECIAL RADIOGRAPHIC PROCEDURES

FIFTH EDITION

ALBERT M. SNOPEK, BS, RT (R)(CV)(M)(QM)

Chairman
Radiologic Technology Department
Middlesex County College
Edison, New Jersey

with over 375 illustrations

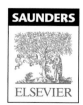

SAUNDERS

ELSEVIER

SAUNDERS
ELSEVIER

11830 Westline Industrial Drive
St. Louis, Missouri 63146

FUNDAMENTALS OF SPECIAL RADIOGRAPHIC PROCEDURES,
FIFTH EDITION

ISBN 13: 978-0-7216-0632-3
ISBN 10: 0-7216-0632-6

ISBN 13: 978-0-7216-0632-3
ISBN 10: 0-7216-0632-6

Executive Editor: Jeanne Wilke
Managing Editor: Mindy Hutchinson
Senior Developmental Editor: Linda Woodard
Developmental Editor: Christina Pryor
Publishing Services Manager: Patricia Tannian
Project Manager: John Casey
Senior Book Designer: Teresa McBryan

Printed in United States of America
Last digit is the print number: 9 8 7 6 5 4 3 2 1

Reviewers

Angela Dopkowski Anderson, MA, RT(R)(CT)(QM)
Radiography Program Director
Prince George's Community College
Largo, Maryland

William C. Arentz, BS, RT(R) (CV)
CV Lab Tech
St. Joseph Medical Center
Reading, Pennsylvania

Mary Jo Bergman, MEd, MS, RN, RT(R)
Program Director
Merit Care Health System
Fargo, North Dakota

Joseph R. Bittengle, MEd, RT(R)(ARRT)
Chairman
University of Arkansas for Medical Sciences
Little Rock, Arkansas

Bobbie Burks, ASRT, ARRT, AERS, OSRT
Ohio Department of Health
Radiologic Technology
Professor of Radiology
Owens Community College
Toledo, Ohio

Michael P. Covone, MEd, RT(R), CT
Assistant Professor
Pennsylvania College of Technology
Williamsport, Pennsylvania

Schlena Dowell, RTR(M)(CV)
Interventional Radiology Supervisor
Hospital
Milwaukee, Wisconsin

Karen A. Frazier, MS, RT(R)
Program Director
Columbus Regional Hospital
School of Radiologic Technology
Columbus, Indiana

Sharyn D. Gibson, EdD, RT(R)
Head of the Department of Radiologic Sciences
Armstrong Atlantic State University
Savannah, Georgia

Jeanne S. Kelleher, RT(R), MS
Department Chairperson of Medical Imaging
Hudson Valley Community College
Troy, New York

Evans Lespinasse, MS, RT(R)(M)
Assistant Professor
New York City College of Technology of the City University of New York
Brooklyn, New York

Jeannean Hall Rollins, MRC, RT(R)(CV)
Associate Professor
Radiology Sciences
Arkansas State University
Jonesboro, Arkansas

Writing a book is an adventure. To begin with, it is a toy and an amusement; then it becomes a mistress, and then it becomes a master, and then a tyrant. The last phase is that just as you are about to be reconciled to your servitude, you kill the monster, and fling him out to the public.

WINSTON CHURCHILL

Preface

The fifth edition of this textbook went through many different conceptual phases before evolving into its final form. Although the term "special procedures" has become somewhat obsolete, the procedures can still be considered "special" because they signify an advanced level of knowledge, technique, and equipment. The studies that are performed under this heading have evolved from the realm of diagnosis to that of diagnosis and intervention. The American Registry of Radiologic Technology in recognition of this trend has changed the original advanced-level certification from "Cardiovascular—Interventional" into two specialty advanced levels: vascular interventional and cardiac interventional technology.

Much of the primary diagnosis is now accomplished utilizing one or more of the specialty modalities, such as computed tomography, magnetic resonance imaging, nuclear medicine, and diagnostic ultrasound. Before or as a part of the actual therapeutic intervention, angiography is usually performed to confirm or localize the suspected pathology. Although angiography has become commonplace in the realm of diagnostic examinations, the procedures are still performed under what are considered to be "specialized" conditions, utilizing equipment that differs considerably from that found in the normal radiographic/fluorographic room.

Several reviewers of the manuscript indicated that the text should maintain the information relevant to second-year radiography students in an advanced imaging (Special Procedures) course. This involved keeping information in the text regarding some of the "special procedures" that were still being performed and retaining the discussions on the ancillary diagnostic modalities. Other reviewers suggested that the focus of the text be primarily directed toward providing material required for preparation for the advanced-level certification(s) and that the extraneous information should be excluded.

I wanted the focus of the book to be broad enough to encompass both tasks: to serve as a preparatory text for the advanced-level certification, as well as a book that would be useful in an advanced imaging course in a radiologic technology curriculum. This became a challenge. After several revisions of the project, I realized that the performance of both diagnostic and interventional examinations requires special skills and advanced knowledge that are the same for both types of procedures. I grouped the discussions of common material into specific chapters including basic pharmacology, expanded patient care, contrast media, image capture, and common principles of angiography rather than repeat these concepts for each procedure category. The specific procedures that are performed are covered in separate chapters and are grouped according to the various systems.

The introduction to the other modalities—CT, MRI, ultrasound, and nuclear medicine—were added, expanded, or updated to provide only a rudimentary discussion of each specialty. The four "special procedures" that were included are studies that are still relevant in the radiologic community and had specific reference in the research. Chapters on vascular, cardiac, and nonvascular interventions have also been included, as have discussions of procedures confined to specific anatomical regions, such as cardiac, thoracic, genitourinary, visceral neurological, and peripheral.

Special procedure radiography has always been dynamic. Changes in equipment, procedures, and techniques occur rapidly. Keeping up with these changes and constantly adjusting the manuscript for currency was difficult. Many of the changes were the result of reviewers' comments, which were greatly appreciated. The innovations in equipment came fast and furious from company representatives even until the final deadline for submission of the manuscript. Chapter objectives and study questions have been added to make the text more compatible from an educator's perspective. The answers to the study questions are included at the end of the book. As in previous editions, an understanding of the physical principles of radiography and basic radiographic positioning is a prerequisite for use of this text.

The suggested readings at the end of each chapter have been included for those who wish to expand their understanding. I anticipate that this new edition will remain a helpful educational tool for students and a reference source for practicing radiographers seeking information about the basics of diagnostic and interventional special procedures and the ancillary modalities such as digital radiography, CT, MRI, and nuclear medicine.

I would like to say to the students who will be using this text that the material is complex and at times may seem overwhelming. This is to be expected, since the basic technology that we learn as beginning students is rapidly being replaced by more complex systems and concepts. The field of radiology is changing, and with the changes comes the requirement for a higher level of knowledge on the part of the radiographer. As a program director and instructor I have seen these changes accelerate the transformation of our profession from "on-the-job" training into the sophisticated complex profession that it has become. The level of understanding and knowledge required to meet our responsibilities has also increased. This text represents the transition from basic radiography into the realm of advanced imaging. As students and practitioners we must remember that there will always be more to learn.

Evolve

Evolve is an interactive learning environment designed to work in coordination with the fifth edition of *Fundamentals of Special Radiographic Procedures*. All of the images included in the textbook are available in jpeg and PowerPoint formats on Evolve. Instructors may use Evolve to provide an Internet-based course component that reinforces and expands the concepts presented in class. Evolve may be used to publish the class syllabus, outlines, and lecture notes; set up "virtual office hours" and e-mail communication; share important dates and information through the online class calendar; and encourage student participation through chat rooms and discussion boards. Evolve allows instructors to post exams and manage their grade books online. For more information, visit http://evolve.elsevier.com/Snopek/ or contact an Elsevier sales representative.

Acknowledgments

I would like to especially thank the individuals who made the completion of the fifth edition of this textbook possible. Representatives from the various manufacturers of the specialized equipment were extremely helpful in providing information about the latest improvements to their products. The following people graciously shared product information and provided many illustrations that were incorporated into the book: Mr. Charles Van Deursen, Siemens, Inc., Ms. Kris Faber, Baxter Healthcare, Ms. Beth Fred, Tyco Healthcare, Ms. Dawn Harley, Becton Dickinson, Ms. Eileen Heizyk, Kodak, Mr. David Kent, Medrad Corporation, Mr. Bill Koll, Varian/Interay, Jaqueline Medwad, Cooper Surgical, Ms. Katherine Merrigan, EZEM, John Ouelette, GE Healthcare, and Mr. Jason Rudy, RADI Medical US.

Certain individuals have been invaluable resources, enabling me to bring this text to life. From Siemens, Inc., I would like to extend a special thank you to Mr. Erik Busch, who graciously helped me with my many requests for information and art. Special thanks should also go to Ms. Christina Pryor, who acted as my trail boss in getting the manuscript from its rough stage through production. Her vigilance, suggestions, "gentle" prodding, and understanding made the task a pleasant experience.

Albert M. Snopek, BS, RT(R), (CV), (M), (QM)
Edison, NJ

Contents

1 Design Elements for Advanced Procedures

CHAPTER OBJECTIVES

After completing this chapter, the reader will be able to perform the following:

- Identify the differences between diagnostic and interventional procedures
- Define the principles of room design for advanced procedures and additional design considerations
- List and describe the requirements for the x-ray generator and the x-ray tube
- Define the concept of heat units and describe the effect of accumulated heat units during advanced procedures
- Identify the formula for heat units
- Identify the rectification constant factors that are applied to the heat units formula
- Explain the line focus principle and its application in x-ray tube design

CHAPTER OUTLINE

DIAGNOSIS VERSUS TREATMENT

ADVANCED PROCEDURE ROOM AND SUITE DESIGN

INTERVENTIONAL RADIOGRAPHY ROOM AND SUITE DESIGN

ADDITIONAL DESIGN CONSIDERATIONS

    X-Ray Generator Requirements

    X-Ray Tube Requirements

SUMMARY

Special procedure radiography had its beginnings soon after the discovery of x-radiation by Roentgen. It was noted that the introduction of certain substances into various organs of the body provided an amazing demonstration of their anatomic features. In the early 1900s, special procedure radiography was limited to such areas as the gallbladder, gastrointestinal tract, and genitourinary tract. As more complicated procedures were developed, these early procedures became the routine diagnostic contrast procedures performed daily in modern radiology departments.

DIAGNOSIS VERSUS TREATMENT

A special procedure can be defined as a radiographic method of demonstrating certain anatomic features that lack natural contrast with surrounding structures by the instillation of a substance to produce structural contrast. This definition encompasses all contrast studies done today. Most of these procedures are considered routine and can be performed without specialized radiographic equipment.

Modern diagnostic and interventional procedures have been segmented into two areas, cardiac and vascular. Each area is broken down into diagnostic and therapeutic (interventional) studies. **Diagnostic procedures,** as their name implies, are performed to identify a particular pathologic process. These procedures are also used to localize certain vessels or tumors prior to the performance of therapeutic procedures. When the object of the procedure is related to the vascular system the general term angiography is used. If the subject vessel is an artery, the study is called an arteriogram. Venography refers to advanced studies of the venous system.

Interventional procedures are performed to treat the pathologic process. The American Registry of Radiologic Technology (AART) (www.ARRT.org) has segmented this specialty into those studies considered to be vascular interventions and those pertaining to the heart (cardiac interventions). Each of these subdivisions encompasses different techniques, equipment, and knowledge and can be considered as separate and distinct disciplines.

ADVANCED PROCEDURE ROOM AND SUITE DESIGN

Interventional radiology is a complex specialty providing minimally invasive treatments for a wide variety of vascular and cardiac diseases. As the techniques become more complex, the equipment required also becomes specialized, and consideration must be given to the design of the special studies suite and the specialized equipment required for the procedures.

In addition to specialized equipment, these advanced procedures require a highly specialized team of individuals to execute the techniques required to successfully obtain the most accurate diagnostic information and to provide an intervention, if necessary. The radiographer is an integral part of this team and is responsible for understanding some basic pharmacology, the operation of the equipment, making the preparations for the procedure, monitoring the patient, and assisting the physician during the examination.

Modern advanced diagnostic and interventional procedures require a special room (or rooms) equipped to perform these examinations. The room or suite is generally dedicated to the performance of these advanced procedures, and its size, location, and construction should be given special consideration when this area is planned. The advanced level radiographer will not always have a role in planning the construction and design of the special procedures suite, but it is helpful to have a basic understanding of the requirements for a dedicated suite.

Unlike the routine diagnostic radiographic room, the advanced procedure suite must serve various purposes. The procedure room must be designed so that it can be used for minor surgery as well as for the advanced diagnostic procedures that will be performed. Standard equipment such as cardiac monitoring devices, emergency supplies, and certain specialty measurement instruments should also be available.

The numbers of advanced studies have increased in recent years. Generally speaking these studies encompass nonvascular, vascular, and cardiac procedures. A larger number of diagnoses are being performed utilizing magnetic resonance imaging and computed tomography, which is less invasive than diagnostic angiography. That being said, diagnostic angiography is still performed on a routine basis. Some design differences in the vascular and cardiac suites are required to accommodate the different types of procedures.

Before discussing equipment, consideration should be given to the planning or layout of the advanced procedure suite. In addition to a team of personnel, a wide variety of specialized equipment is necessary for diagnostic and interventional radiography. At times, the procedures may pose a risk to the patient, and severe, if not fatal, reactions may occur. These considerations require a room that is considerably larger than a routine radiographic room. The room should be a minimum of 400 ft² (37.16 m²); more complex advanced radiographic rooms can approach 600 ft² (55.74 m²). (This does not take into consideration the control, monitoring, preparation, and dressing rooms.)

The control room must be larger than a simple control booth found in routine radiographic rooms. The additional space is required to accommodate the specialized equipment. The control room should be adjacent to or in the special procedure suite and should be designed to permit an unobstructed view of the entire suite. Protection from radiation hazards is mandatory, yet rapid access to the suite in emergency situations must be assured. In general, the special procedure control room should be a minimum of 100 to 150 ft^2 to provide ample room for the placement and operation of the equipment. In the cardiac catheterization suites, the control room should be large enough to house the equipment required for cardiac monitoring and testing. The amount and type of monitoring equipment available to the institution ultimately determines the actual size of the control area. An unobstructed view of the radiographic room and free communication with the other major areas in the advanced procedure suite are also necessary design requirements.

The preparation (prep) room is an important addition to the special procedure suite providing necessary storage space for the smaller pieces of equipment that are essential to the examinations. The prep room can also be designed and equipped to function as a scrub room, if necessary. In larger teaching and research institutions, the prep room should contain a work area that may be used for making the catheters required during the procedure. Although this is not common practice in most institutions, it is still practiced when newer procedures or techniques are developed.

Smaller hospitals use disposable catheters almost exclusively, which diminishes the importance of this area. If nondisposable tools and equipment are used, the prep area should have facilities for cleaning this equipment adequately after the procedure before it is repackaged for sterilization. In summary, the prep room should provide ample work space to allow the technologist to prepare and clean the equipment before and after the procedure.

If a large number of special procedures are done on an outpatient basis, dressing and waiting rooms should be provided adjacent to the suite for the comfort and convenience of the patient. A consultation area should also be provided to allow for the patient and the family to privately discuss the specifics of the procedure with the physician. Figures 1-1 and 1-2 illustrate some possible special procedure suite layouts for vascular and cardiac catheterization procedures.

INTERVENTIONAL RADIOGRAPHY ROOM AND SUITE DESIGN

The need for a dedicated interventional radiography room is determined by the numbers and types of procedures performed. Vascular interventional procedures are usually performed in the general special procedure suite. The design and equipment make it ideal for use during diagnostic angiography as well as for interventional radiographic procedures.

Nonvascular interventional studies may also be performed in the angiography suite, but the room design is usually too sophisticated for this type of radiography, which does not require the elaborate

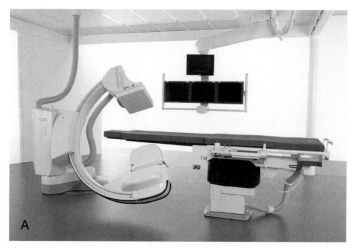

FIGURE 1-1.   A, Dedicated cardiac interventional equipment.   *Continued*

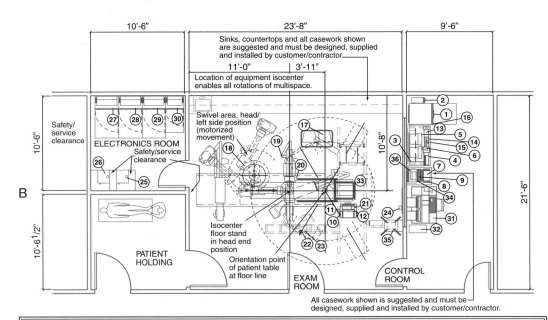

No	Description	SMS SYM	Weight (lbs)	BTU/hr to air	Dimensions (in) W	D	H	Remarks
1	Image system	(IS)	205	3,072	27	32	28 1/4	Mtd. on casters
2	UPS for image system (option)	(−)	42	102	6 3/4	17 1/4	8 1/2	Mtd. on floor/shelf
3	Control room distributor	(CRX)	64	342	41 1/2	8 1/4	16 1/8	Mtd. on wall
4	Keyboard	(−)	2.2	342	17 1/2	6 1/8	2 1/8	Mtd. under counter or on console
5	44-cm monitor	(−)	49	512	16	18	16	On counter or console
6	19" color monitor	(−)	49	512	18 1/2	18 1/2	19	On counter or console
7	Video recorder (option)	(−)	27	342	10 1/2	14 1/2	5 1/2	On shelf below counter
8	VCR interface (option)	(−)	9	342	17 1/2	8 1/4	1 3/4	On shelf below counter
9	Monitor M44-2M (option)	(−)	33	342	16	11 1/2	15 1/4	On counter or console
10	Examination control console (ECC)	(−)	7	---	14 1/2	8 3/4	3 1/2	On table or trolley
11	Control module patient table	(−)	2.2	---	3 1/2	6 1/4	3 1/4	On table or trolley
12	Control module floor stand and collimator	(−)	4.5	---	8 1/2	6 1/4	3 1/4	On table or trolley
13	2nd examination control console (ECC) (option)	(−)	7	---	14 1/2	8 3/4	3 1/2	On counter or console
14	2nd control module patient table (option)	(−)	2.2	---	3 1/2	6 1/4	3 1/4	On counter or console
15	2nd control module floor stand and collimator (option)	(−)	4.5	---	8 1/2	6 1/4	3 1/4	On counter or console
16	Control console (option)	(−)	132	---	54 3/4	31 1/2	28 1/4	Floor mounted
17	MTS-H6 54-cm monitor ceiling suspension	(D)	1,210	2,730	167 1/8	27 7/8	50 7/8	Ceiling suspended
18	Floor stand including mounting plate	(P1)	1,466	683	---	---	---	C-arm floor mounted
19	Ceiling stand including longitudinal rails	(P2)	1,248	683	---	---	---	C-arm ceiling mounted
20	Patient table (peri table)	(T)	1,063	683	---	---	---	Table floor mounted
21	Trolley for control modules	(TRC)	59	---	23	21	40	Mounted on casters
22	Upper body radiation shield (option)	(SU)	258	---	---	---	---	Track mounted
23	Ceiling mtd. mavig surgical light (option)	(−)	143	---	---	---	---	
24	Injector wall terminal box (option)	(WO)	11	---	12 3/4	4	10 1/2	Exam room
25	Kluver cooling unit (plane A)	(CU1)	93	8,192	18 3/4	15 1/2	18 3/4	Floor or shelf mounted
26	Kluver cooling unit (plane B)	(CU2)	93	8,192	18 3/4	15 1/2	18 3/4	Floor or shelf mounted
27	Polydoros M (power unit 1)	(PU1)	772	3,413	31 1/2	17 1/8	87	Floor mounted
28	Polydoros M (power unit 2)	(PU2)	772	3,413	31 1/2	17 1/8	87	Floor mounted
29	Cable cabinet (option)	(−)	265	---	31 1/2	17 1/8	87	Floor mounted
30	System control cabinet	(SC)	518	3,072	23 1/2	17 1/8	87	Floor mounted
31	Cathcor–C – patient monitoring (option)	(CRE)	277	2,048	33 1/2	22 7/8	30 3/8	Compact version
32	Cathcor U.P.S. system (option)	(UPS)	86	2,901	10	12	22	Under counter
33	Cathcor remote input box (option)	(IB)	10	---	18	7	3	Mounted at table
34	Cathcor laser printer (option)	(LP)	45.6	2,730	15 3/8	19 3/8	13 1/2	Under counter on shelf
35	Medrad injector on mobile pedestal (option)	(IN1)	90	---	---	---	---	See mfg requirements
36	Medrad control room console (option)	(IN2)	43	---	19	10 1/2	12 3/4	See mfg requirements

AXIOM ARTIS BC EQUIPMENT LEGEND

FIGURE 1-1, cont'd   B, Schematic layout of a dedicated cardiac interventional suite setup.

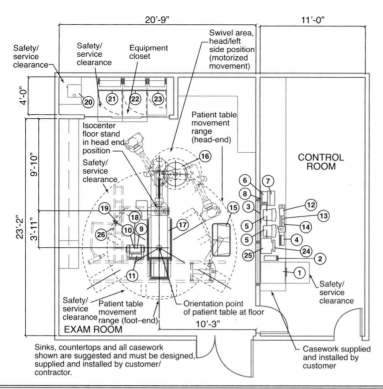

No	Description	SMS SYM	Weight (lbs)	BTU/hr to air	Dimensions (in) W	D	H	Remarks
①	Image system	(IS)	192	2,390	27	32	28 1/4	Mtd. on casters
②	UPS for image system (option)	(−)	42	102	6 3/4	17 1/4	8 1/2	Mtd. on floor/shelf
③	Control room distributor	(CRX)	64	342	41 1/2	8 1/4	16 1/8	Mtd. on wall
④	Keyboard	(−)	2.2	342	17 1/2	6 1/8	2 1/8	Mtd. under counter or on console
⑤	44cm monitor	(−)	49	512	16	18	16	On counter or console
⑥	Video recorder	(−)	27	342	10 1/2	14 1/2	5 1/2	On shelf below counter
⑦	VCR interface	(−)	9	342	17 1/2	8 1/4	1 3/4	On shelf below counter
⑧	Monitor M44-2M (monitor for VCR)	(−)	33	342	16	11 1/2	15 1/4	On counter or console
⑨	Examination control console (ECC)	(−)	7	---	14 1/2	8 3/4	3 1/2	On table or trolley
⑩	Control module patient table	(−)	2.2	---	3 1/2	6 1/4	3 1/4	On table or trolley
⑪	Control module floor stand and collimator	(−)	4.5	---	8 1/2	6 1/4	3 1/4	On table or trolley
⑫	2nd examination control console (ECC)	(−)	7	---	14 1/2	8 3/4	3 1/2	On counter or console
⑬	2nd control module patient table	(−)	2.2	---	3 1/2	6 1/4	3 1/4	On counter or console
⑭	2nd control floor stand and collimator	(−)	4.5	---	8 1/2	6 1/4	3 1/4	On counter or console
⑮	MTS–H2 2–54cm monitor ceiling suspension	(D)	567	921	167 1/8	27 7/8	50 7/8	Ceiling suspended
⑯	Floor stand including mounting plate	(P1)	1,466	683	---	---	---	C-arm floor mounted
⑰	Patient table (basic)	(T)	997	683	---	---	---	Table floor mounted
⑱	Trolley for control modules	(TRC)	59	---	23	21	40	Mounted on casters
⑲	Upper body radiation shield	(SU)	258	---	---	---	---	Track mounted
⑳	Kluver cooling unit	(CU)	93	8,192	18 3/4	15 1/2	18 3/4	Floor or shelf mounted
㉑	Polydoros M (power unit 1)	(PU1)	772	3,143	31 1/2	17 1/8	87	Floor mounted
㉒	Cable cabinet (option)	(−)	265	---	31 1/2	17 1/8	87	Floor mounted
㉓	System control cabinet	(SC)	518	3,072	23 1/2	17 1/8	87	Floor mounted
㉔	Medrad injector remote panel	(IN1)	5	---	14 1/2	7 3/8	3 1/4	See mfg requirements
㉕	Medrad control room console	(IN2)	43	---	19	10 1/2	12 3/4	See mfg requirements
㉖	Medrad injector on ceiling counterpoise	(IN3)	79	---	---	---	---	See mfg requirements

AXIOM ARTIS FCIFA EQUIPMENT LEGEND

FIGURE 1-2.   A, Schematic layout of a vascular interventional room.

Continued

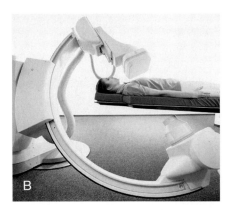

FIGURE 1-2, cont'd. B, Dedicated vascular interventional equipment.

recording equipment necessary for vascular studies. The nonvascular interventional procedures need a slightly more sophisticated room design than is provided by a general fluoroscopic room.

As the number of interventional examinations increases, especially in the larger hospitals, dedicated interventional radiography rooms will become necessary to prevent the disruption of the normal work flow in either a special-purpose fluoroscopic room or a special procedure suite. The design of the interventional radiography room is very similar to that of the advanced procedure suite discussed previously. Vascular interventional procedures can be performed in the angiography suite, and unless the number of these procedures interferes with the normal work flow of these rooms, a dedicated room will not be necessary. The nonvascular interventional room will require some modification of the basic special procedure room design.

Basic interventional radiography room design considerations may be summarized as follows:

Radiographic room
- 400 to 600 ft² (37.16 to 55.74 m²) minimum size
- Doorways, 4 ft (1.2 m) minimum width
- Patient holding and monitoring area, 96 ft² (8.91 m²) minimum size
- Adequate radiation protection
- Image illuminators for review of films or digital grayscale monitors
- Vertical wall-mounted chest changer
- Ceiling-mounted cathode ray tube (CRT) monitors
- Biplane fluoroscopic and radiographic capabilities desirable
- 90° to 90° floating top table
- Three-phase generator, 800 to 1000 mA capacity

Control room
- 50 to 75 ft² (4.645 to 6.9677 m²) minimum size
- Optimal view of procedural area
- Adequate radiation protection

Laboratory and/or work areas
- 50 to 75 ft² (4.64 to 6.96 m²) minimum size, size dependent on equipment
- Image illuminators and/or digital workstations equipped with color and grayscale monitors
- Storage cabinets
- Laboratory table with staining facilities for bacteriologic and pathologic specimens
- Scrub basin

The interventional radiography room should be close to the special procedure area as well as to the ultrasonography and computed tomography (CT) rooms. Room size should be comparable to that of the basic angiography suite, a minimum of 400 to 600 ft^2 (37.16 to 55.74 m^2). Doorways should be at least 4 ft (1.2 m) wide to accommodate stretchers, beds, and any extra-wide equipment that may be necessary.

Adjacent to the interventional suite should be a patient holding and monitoring area that will be used to hold patients before and after the procedure as well as to house any preprocedural or post-procedural monitoring equipment. The room should comfortably allow for a minimum of two isolated stretchers or beds. An appropriate room size is about 100 ft^2 (9.29 m^2). It should be equipped with a centralized supply of oxygen and vital sign monitors.

The control room area is equal in size and capacity to that used for general angiography, affording the occupants optimum viewing of the procedure as well as maximum radiation protection.

Ideally, a laboratory and workroom should be part of the interventional suite. The size of this room will depend on the type of equipment used. Space should be provided for a laboratory table with facilities to process cytologic samples obtained by needle aspiration or brush biopsy. This area can also be used as a viewing room, storage center, and scrub room, if size and design permit.

The design and construction of dedicated vascular and nonvascular interventional radiography suites will depend on the amount of funding allotted to the project, the types of procedures performed, and the personal preferences of the staff involved in the design process.

ADDITIONAL DESIGN CONSIDERATIONS

If film radiography is being utilized, the film processing can be done in the general radiographic darkroom. In some institutions in which the special procedure or interventional radiography suite is located far from a darkroom facility, it may be necessary to provide a darkroom adjacent to the suite for the rapid development of the radiographs. This may also be desirable when the case load is great enough to conflict with the processing requirements of the routine diagnostic department. Currently state-of-the-art radiography is performed digitally and will not require film to acquire and archive the images produced during the study. However, hard copy images are often requested, and these will require some type of processing system. Wet or dry laser processor as well as dye sublimation systems are available for creating hard copy images from the digital copy.

The advanced diagnostic or interventional radiography room must be constructed with its ultimate operation in mind. Electric wiring should be arranged so that the floors are virtually free of any type of obstruction that may be hazardous to the patient or personnel during the procedure or in an emergency situation. The power supply and wiring requirements for any particular special procedure room will vary with the equipment used. If new installations are planned, consultation with the manufacturers of desired equipment will be essential. If some procedures are to be done in areas in which combustible or explosive substances are used for general anesthesia, the wiring should adhere to specific codes governing electric connections in hazardous locations. The National Fire Code★ (National Fire Prevention Association Handbook No. 99 — Standards for Health Care Facilities) lists the requirements for installation and use of permanent and mobile x-ray apparatus in hazardous locations at health care facilities.

The construction of the room should allow for ease of cleaning after a procedure. Because many special procedures require surgical techniques, the physical construction of the floors and walls should be the same as that of an operating room. These surfaces should be tiled or finished with a smooth material to permit proper cleaning.

If new facilities are planned, provision should be made for equipping the room with a centralized supply of oxygen. Outlets should be strategically placed so that oxygen may be easily and quickly supplied to the patient.

The specialized equipment necessary for the suite will vary according to the types of procedures to be done, the personal preferences of the radiologist, and the budget of the institution. Certain essential

---

★National Fire Codes: NFPA 99, Standard for Health Care Facilities, National Fire Prevention Association, Quincy, MA, 2002.

pieces of equipment, however, are found in all modern special procedure rooms; these include the x-ray generator, controls, and tube; a system to record the events of the procedure; and some type of automatic injector. The equipment for each of these categories is manufactured by many companies, and all offer a selection of features suitable for large or small budgets. The ultimate choice of equipment should be made on the basis of the type and amount of special procedures to be performed. If optional features are not absolutely essential to the operation of the suite, they should be avoided if cost is a major consideration. However, it is unwise to compromise on the purchase of essential equipment. Image recording systems and automatic injectors used during special procedures are discussed in Chapters 2 and 3.

X-Ray Generator

The type of x-ray generator chosen should offer high performance with minimum ratings of 500 mA. In special procedure suites in which a great deal of vascular radiography is done, minimum ratings of 700 to 1500 mA should be considered because of the short exposure frequency required by vascular studies. Multiphase generators are required in these cases because they permit higher ratings (shorter exposure times) than the conventional single-phase equipment. In departments in which much interventional radiography is performed, a constant potential generator is advantageous. This type of generator has capabilities for ratings up to 3000 mA and exposure times as short as 0.001 s. Major consideration should be given to the constant potential generator because it produces essentially monochromatic or homogeneous x-radiation, which effectively reduces the radiation dosage to the patient, and because its extremely short exposure times facilitate rapid sequence filming at rates above eight exposures per second, thus expanding the possibilities and uses of cineradiography.

The generator should be capable of generating 80 to 100 kW of power. This will enable the use of very short exposure times and high milliamperage to reduce or eliminate motion artifacts during rapid multi-imaging series.

The choice of a generator for special procedure radiography depends on the type and number of procedures being done. It is important to utilize an optimum kVp with a high mA and short exposure time. This will maximize the contrast produced on the final images while providing a practical radiation dose to the patient. In all cases, however, the unit should supply a minimum rating of 500 mA if a nominal number of vascular procedures are performed and 1500 mA if a large number of varied cardiovascular studies are done.

High frequency generators with mid to high frequency inverters are recommended because the closed feedback loop provides excellent reproducibility and linearity of the tube current (mA) and tube potential (kVp). Some of the advantages of the use of this type of generator include: shorter exposure times, virtually no ripple thereby providing an almost constant potential, and reduction of line voltage fluctuations due to the immediate conversion of the AC current to DC; closed feedback looping provides for automatic calibration of the tube current, and the kVp calibration is easier and more stable. High frequency (constant potential) generators are also smaller in size and more economical to produce.

X-Ray Tube Requirements

The x-ray tube chosen for special procedure radiography must be capable of providing the detail necessary for adequate diagnosis yet must withstand the increased heat generated from rapid sequence exposures. In routine diagnostic radiography, it is rare for the tube rating to be exceeded during one procedure. During a cineangiographic or angiographic procedure, however, it can easily occur, especially when a high exposure per second frequency is used. It is necessary for the technologist to adhere to the manufacturer's suggested exposure ratings, and for this reason, a tube rating chart should be posted in the special procedure suite. Cooling charts should also be available to the technologist.

BOX 1-1	*Constant Factors for Heat Unit Calculation*
Type of Generation	**Factor**
Single-phase	1
Three-phase (6-pulse)	1.35
Three-phase (12-pulse)	1.41
High frequency	1.45

Heat units are the product of the multiplication of peak kilovoltage by milliamperage by seconds. This basic formula for heat units remains constant for all types of generators; however, multiphase generators will produce a greater number of heat units than single-phase machines. Therefore, the total number of heat units must be multiplied by a constant factor when multiphase generators are used. These factors are listed in Box 1-1. The formula is:

$$HU = kV \text{ peak} \times mA \times s \times C$$

where HU is heat units, kV peak is peak kilovoltage, s is time (in seconds), and C is a constant factor specific to the type of generator used.

The Varian G1582TRI/G1582BI/G1582BI-G rotating anode x-ray tube can easily be used for radiography, cineradiography, and digital and analog (film screen) angiography (Fig. 1-3). This tube insert can be used for digital radiography, film/screen angiography, and cineradiography as well as general radiographic procedures. The "tri" version of the tube insert has three focal spot sizes, 0.3, 0.6 and 1.0 mm, that can be accessed. It has a heat loading capacity of 1072 kilojoules (1.5 MHU). This tube also offers a rhenium-tungsten target with a superior heat load rating.

Because the tube can be used for a variety of procedures it is important that the proper tube rating chart be used to determine the maximum rating for the study being performed (Fig. 1-4). X-ray tube rating charts for radiography, angiography, and cineradiography are supplied by the manufacturer and should be referred to when determining a specific imaging protocol.

Unlike radiographic studies, angiography and cineangiography require that a series of exposures be made in rapid succession to demonstrate the contrast agent movement through the vascular system. The angiographic tube rating chart will help the technologist to determine the maximum amount of kilowatts or the maximum exposure time for a particular imaging series. When cineradiographic tube rating charts are used, the maximum amount of time the cine run can last and the maximum allowable kW of the cine pulse can be determined.

It is assumed that the reader has a working knowledge regarding the use of x-ray tube rating charts when used for radiography. A short discussion of their use in cineradiography and angiography follows.

Serial Angiographic Tube Rating Charts

During serial angiography a large number of exposures are made in a relatively short period of time. A large heat load is administered to the anode, which cannot be quickly dispersed. Angiographic tube rating charts relate peak kilovolts and milliamperage to determine the maximum kilowatts allowed for each exposure in a series or the maximum number of exposures that can be made for any given series.

Figure 1-5 is a sample angiographic tube rating chart for the Varian A182/A282 series tube. This chart can be used to determine the maximum kilowatts or exposure time for each exposure in the series.

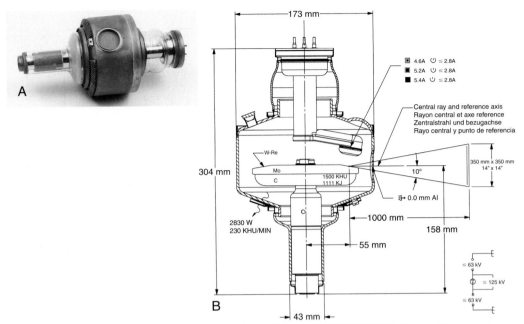

FIGURE 1-3. **A,** Illustration of the Varian G1582TRI/G1582BI/G1582BI-G rotating anode x-ray tube **B,** Schematic diagram of the G1582TRI/G1582BI/G1582BI-G rotating anode x-ray tube.

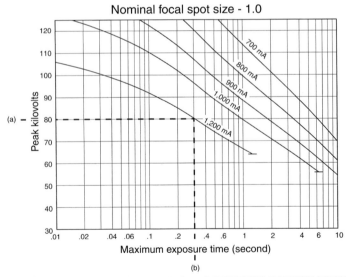

FIGURE 1-4. Sample tube rating chart for the Varian G1582TRI/G1582BI/G1582BI-G rotating anode x-ray tube series tube inserts. Maximum exposure time is found by drawing a line between the desired peak kilovoltage and milliamperes (*a*). A vertical line (*b*) drawn to intersect this point also crosses the maximum exposure time that can be used for a single exposure.

Tube load (kW) as a function of the exposure time of the individual radiographs of the series

Exposure rate per second	0.010	0.020	0.030	0.040	0.050	0.060	0.080	0.100	0.120	0.140	0.160	0.180	0.200	0.225	0.250	NUMBER OF EXPOSURES IN SERIES
1	104.9	100.7	97.5	94.9	92.6	90.5	86.9	83.7	81.0	78.5	76.2	74.1	72.2	70.0	68.0	
2	104.4	99.6	96.1	93.1	90.4	88.1	84.0	80.4	77.3	74.6	72.1	69.8	67.7	65.4	63.2	
3	103.8	98.6	94.7	91.4	88.5	85.9	81.4	77.5	74.2	71.2	68.6	66.2				
4	103.4	97.8	93.6	90.0	86.8	84.0	79.1	74.9	71.4	68.3						10
8	101.8	95.1	89.8	85.4	81.6	78.3										
15	99.8	91.7	85.4	80.1												
30	97.3	87.4														
1	104.2	99.3	95.5	92.4	89.6	87.1	82.7	79.0	75.7	72.7	70.1	67.7	65.4	62.9	60.6	
2	103.5	98.0	93.8	90.2	87.1	84.3	79.4	75.3	71.7	68.5	65.7	63.1	60.8	58.1	55.8	
3	102.8	96.8	92.1	88.2	84.8	81.7	76.5	72.0	68.2	64.9	62.0	59.3				
4	102.2	96.7	90.7	86.6	82.8	79.5	73.9	69.2	65.2	61.8						20
8	100.1	92.2	86.0	80.9	76.5	72.7										
15	97.3	87.5	80.1	74.1												
30	93.1	81.0														
1	102.8	96.8	92.1	88.1	84.7	81.6	76.2	71.6	67.7	64.3	61.2	58.4	55.9	53.2	50.7	
2	101.9	95.3	90.1	85.8	82.0	78.6	72.8	68.0	63.8	60.3	57.1	54.3	51.8	49.0	46.5	
3	101.1	93.9	88.3	83.6	79.5	75.9	69.8	64.8	60.5	56.9	53.7	50.9				
4	100.4	92.7	86.7	81.7	77.4	73.6	67.2	61.9	57.6	53.9						40
8	97.9	88.6	81.4	75.5	70.5	66.3										
15	94.4	83.0	74.5	67.8												
30	88.9	74.9														
1	101.5	94.5	89.0	84.4	80.4	76.9	70.8	65.8	61.5	57.8	54.5	49.6	44.7	39.7	35.7	
2	100.6	93.0	87.0	82.1	77.8	74.0	67.6	62.4	58.0	54.2	51.0	48.1	44.7	39.7	35.7	
3	99.7	91.5	85.2	79.9	75.3	71.4	64.8	59.4	54.9	51.2	47.9	45.1				
4	99.0	90.3	83.5	78.0	73.2	69.1	62.2	56.8	52.3	48.5						60
8	96.3	85.9	78.0	71.7	66.4	61.9										
15	92.4	79.9	70.9	63.8												
30	86.3	71.2														
1	100.2	92.4	86.2	81.1	76.7	72.8	66.2	60.9	55.8	47.9	41.9	37.2	33.5	29.8	26.8	
2	99.3	90.8	84.2	78.8	74.1	70.0	63.3	57.8	53.3	47.9	41.9	37.2	33.5	29.8	26.8	
3	98.4	89.4	82.4	76.6	71.7	67.5	60.6	55.1	50.5	46.7	41.9	37.2				
4	97.6	88.1	80.7	74.7	69.7	65.3	58.2	52.6	48.1	44.4						80
8	94.8	83.6	75.2	68.5	63.0	58.4										
15	90.8	77.5	68.0	60.8												
30	84.2	68.5														
1	99.0	90.3	83.6	78.0	73.3	69.1	62.3	53.6	44.7	38.3	33.5	29.8	26.8	23.8	21.4	
2	98.1	88.8	81.7	75.8	70.8	66.6	59.5	53.6	44.7	38.3	33.5	29.8	26.8	23.8	21.4	
3	97.2	87.3	79.8	73.7	68.6	64.2	57.0	51.4	44.7	38.3	33.5	29.8				
4	96.4	86.0	78.2	71.9	66.6	62.1	54.8	49.2	44.7	38.3						100
8	93.5	81.5	72.7	65.8	60.2	55.5										
15	89.3	75.4	65.6	58.2												
30	82.6	66.3														
1	96.2	85.7	77.8	71.4	66.0	59.6	44.7	35.7	29.8	25.5	22.3	19.9	17.9	15.9	14.3	
2	95.2	84.2	76.0	69.3	63.9	59.3	44.7	35.7	29.8	25.5	22.3	19.9	17.9	15.9	14.3	
3	94.3	82.8	74.2	67.4	61.9	57.3	44.7	35.7	29.8	25.5	22.3	19.9				
4	93.5	81.5	72.7	65.8	60.1	55.5	44.7	35.7	29.8	25.5						150
8	90.5	77.1	67.5	60.2	54.4	49.7										
15	86.2	71.0	60.8	53.2												
30	79.2	62.0														

FIGURE 1-5.   A, Sample angiographic tube rating chart for the Varian A182/A282 series tube insert. This chart can be used to determine the maximum allowed kilowatts per exposure in a series.

The **maximum amount of kilowatts (kW)** allowed per exposure is determined using the following steps:

1. Determine the number of exposures in the series (**a**). It is important not to underestimate the number.
2. Determine the exposure rate (number of exposures per second) (**b**).
3. The point at which the exposure rate per second (**b**) and the exposure time (**c**) intersect indicates the maximum amount of kilowatts (kVp × mA) allowed per exposure.

The **maximum exposure time** is determined by:

1. Choosing the number of exposures in the series (**a**)
2. Determining the exposure rate (number of exposures per second) (**b**)
3. Calculating the maximum kW tube load
4. The point at which the maximum kW tube load for the chosen parameters intersects the exposure time (**c**) represents the maximum time that can be used for each of the radiographs in the series.

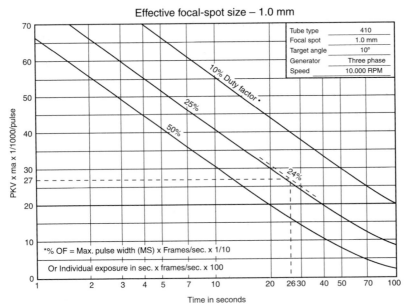

FIGURE 1-6. Sample percent duty factor curves illustrating how to determine the maximum length of time the tube can be run during cineangiography.

Cineangiographic Tube Rating Charts

Cineangiographic tube rating charts differ from those used for angiographic tubes. Cineangiographic tube rating charts are primarily used to determine the maximum amount of time the tube can be used under certain conditions. These charts are sometimes called percent duty factor curves (Fig. 1-6).

The **percent duty factor (%DF)** can be calculated using the following formula:

$$\%DF = \frac{[\text{Maximum pulse duration (ms)}]\,[\text{Frames per second}]}{10}$$

Each chart is constructed with the power level (kVp × mA × 1/1000) on the y-axis. The **peak pulse power level (P)** is expressed in kilowatts and can be calculated for any combination of factors using the following formula:

$$P\,(\text{kW}) = \frac{(\text{kVp})\,(\text{mA})}{1000}$$

Given the following factors and using the foregoing formulae and the percent duty factor curve for the Varian G1582-150/180 HZ, 1.0-mm rotating anode tube, the length of time that the tube can be run can be determined.

Focal spot size	1.0 mm
Maximum pulse duration	4 ms
Frames per second	60 fps
Peak voltage	90 kVp
Tube current	300 mA

For these factors the percent duty factor (%DF) is calculated as follows:

$$\%DF = \frac{(4\text{ ms})\,(60\text{ fps})}{10}$$

$$\%DF = \frac{240}{10}$$

$$\%DF = 24$$

It is now necessary to calculate the peak pulse power (P) for the exposure factors listed:

$$P\ (kW) = \frac{(90\ kVp)\ (300\ mA)}{1000}$$

$$P\ (kW) = \frac{27{,}000}{1000}$$

$$P = 27\ kW$$

At the point at which 70 kW crosses a 24% duty factor line, the tube can be run for a maximum of 20 s.

Line Focus Principle

Maximum detail must be obtained during vascular special procedures to affect a diagnosis. Because detail depends on focal spot size, the smallest possible focal spot should be used. Of course, the smaller the focal spot, the greater the restriction on the individual exposure values that can be used. One method used by tube manufacturers to increase the tube rating for a particular tube is to use a decreasing target angle, thereby maintaining the actual focal spot size but decreasing the effective focal spot size (Fig. 1-7). A problem inherent in this method of increasing tube ratings is that at steeper target angles, film coverage becomes critical (Fig. 1-8). The chart shows that if 14- × 14-in (35- × 35-cm) coverage is important, the **source–image receptor distance (SIRD)** has to be increased over the standard 40 in when the 7-degree anode angle tube is used. This tube, however, is useful for work requiring a radiographic field size of less than 10 × 12 in (25 × 30 cm) at a 40-in SIRD. Such a tube could have considerable use for cineradiography, and image intensification, in which smaller field sizes are used continually.

The film coverage can be calculated for any combination of target angle and SIRD with the following formula[1]:

$$C = D_{fs-f} \times \tan TA \times 2$$

where C is the dimension of one side of a square coverage pattern (in), D is SIRD (in) (focal spot to image receptor distance), and tan TA is the tangent of the target angle. (Box 1-2 lists the tangents for various target angles.)

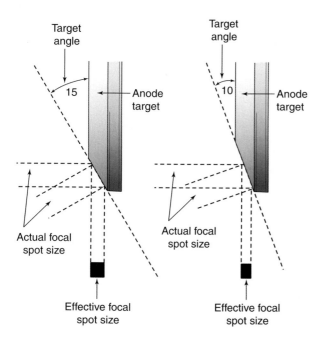

FIGURE 1-7. Target angle versus focal spot size. As the angle of the target face decreases, the effective focal spot size is reduced. This permits increased tube loading with a corresponding change in filament size. In both situations, the actual focal spot size remains unchanged.

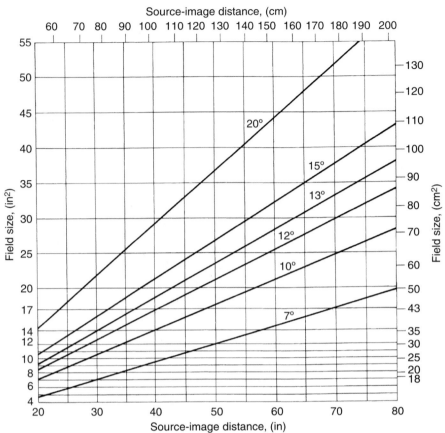

FIGURE 1-8. Target angle versus film coverage. This chart illustrates the effect produced by decreasing the target angle. As the target angle becomes steeper, the area of film coverage at a specific source-image receptor distance (SIRD) is decreased. For example, the film coverage for a tube possessing a 10-degree target angle is 14 × 14 in at an SIRD of 40 in, whereas that for a tube with a 7-degree target angle is less than 10 × 10 in at the same SIRD.

BOX 1-2	*Tangents for Various Target Angles*
Target Angle	**Tangent**
7°	0.12278
10°	0.17633
12°	0.21256
16°	0.28674

The formula can easily be applied to any combination of tube angle and SIRD. For example, using a rotating anode tube with a 10-degree target angle at an SIRD of 40 in, the dimension of one side of the square coverage pattern could be calculated as follows:

$$C = 40 \times 0.17633 \times 2$$
$$C = 14.1064 \text{ in}$$

Therefore, the maximum amount of coverage on the film would be 14 × 14 in. Figure 1-9 lists coverage for a variety of SIRD and target angles.

Source-to-image distance		Dimension "c" for various target angles (in)			
(in)	(cm)	7°	10°	12°	16°
100	254.0	24.6	35.3	42.5	57.4
80	203.2	19.7	28.2	34.0	45.9
72	182.9	17.7	25.4	30.6	41.3
60	152.4	14.7	21.2	25.5	34.4
48	121.9	11.8	16.9	20.4	27.5
44	111.7	10.8	15.5	18.7	25.2
42	106.7	10.3	14.8	17.9	24.1
40	101.6	9.8	14.1	17.0	22.9
38	96.5	9.3	13.4	16.2	21.8
34	86.4	8.4	12.0	14.5	19.5
30	76.2	7.4	10.6	12.8	17.2

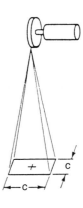

FIGURE 1-9.   Film coverage for various target angles and source-image receptor distances.

Some other factors influencing tube ratings are the size, thickness, and speed of rotation of the target. The special procedure x-ray tube should allow a combination of these factors to produce the high tube ratings necessary for vascular radiography.

The ultimate choice of an x-ray tube for the special procedure suite will depend on the types of procedures to be done and the equipment with which it will be used.

SUMMARY

Special procedure rooms should be given careful consideration when they are being planned. The rooms should be larger than routine diagnostic radiographic rooms to provide the special procedure team with ample space in which to function effectively during the examination or in an emergency. The increased room size is also required to house the specialized equipment necessary for the examinations. Additional areas should be planned adjacent to the radiographic area to provide work and storage areas to facilitate preparation for the procedure. A dressing room should be provided for the convenience of outpatients.

The essential equipment for a special procedure suite includes the generator, console, x-ray tube, and recording and automatic injection devices. These should be chosen on the basis of the types of procedures to be done, physician preference, and budget requirements. Compromises should not be made on the purchase of essential equipment, but optional features should be chosen on the basis of procedural requirements.

REFERENCE

1.   Information Bulletin 3283 Rev B, Varian X-Ray Tube Products, Salt Lake City, Utah, 2002.

SUGGESTED READINGS

Bashore TM, Bates ER, Berger PB, Clark DA, Cusma JT, Dehrner EJ, Kern MJ, Laskey WK, O'Laughlin MP, Oesterle J, Popma JJ: Cardiac catheterization. Laboratory standards. A Report of the College of Cardiology Task

Force on Clinical Expert Consensus Document on Cardiac Catheterization Laboratory Standards. *J Am Coll Cardiol* 37:2170–214, 2001.

HBN–6, Facilities for Diagnostic Imaging and Interventional Radiology—Design and Briefing, 2001, accessed at http://www.nhsestates.gov.uk/download/publications_guidance/es_diagnostic_imaging.pdf.

Selman J: *The Fundamentals of Imaging Physics and Radiobiology,* 9th ed. Springfield, IL, 2000, CC Thomas.

Siegel E, Reiner B: Radiology reading room design: the next generation. *Appl Radiol* 31(4):12–16, 2002.

STUDY QUESTIONS

1. An advanced diagnostic radiographic room should have a minimum of:
   a. 200 square feet
   b. 250 square feet
   c. 300 square feet
   d. 400 square feet

2. Biplane image recorders are used to:
   a. image more than one study at a time
   b. capture the image in more than one plane utilizing a single injection of contrast agent
   c. enable the patient to be positioned in a variety of positions during the study
   d. provide a backup to ensure that the image is not missed owing to a faulty image receptor

3. The codes governing electrical connections in hazardous locations are provided by the:
   a. ASRT Handbook for hospital facilities
   b. NCRP Handbook # 99 for advanced procedure suites and operating room
   c. NFPA 99 Standard for health care facilities
   d. JCAHO Safety Handbook for radiographic installations

4. The constant factor "C" that is used in the calculation of heat units when a high-frequency generator is employed is:
   a. 1.25
   b. 1.35
   c. 1.41
   d. 1.45

5. The percent duty factor curve is generally used to determine x-ray tube ratings for:
   a. cineangiography
   b. interventional angiography
   c. diagnostic angiography
   d. general radiography

6. Which of the following formulas is used to calculate peak pulse power level?
   a. $\dfrac{[\text{Maximum pulse duration (ms)}] \, [\text{Frames per second}]}{10}$
   b. $\dfrac{(kVp)\,(mA)}{1000}$
   c. $D_{fs-f} \times \tan TA \times 2$
   d. $kV\ peak \times mA \times s \times C$

7. X-ray tube manufacturers can increase the heat loading of the x-ray tube and increase detail by:
   a. increasing the target angle and decreasing the actual focal spot size
   b. decreasing the target angle and maintaining the actual focal spot size
   c. decreasing the actual focal spot size and maintaining the same target angle
   d. increasing the actual focal spot size and having no angle on the anode

STUDY QUESTIONS (*cont'd*)

8. The patient holding area should be a minimum of _____ and have capacity for a minimum of _____ patients.
   a. 50, 1
   b. 65, 2
   c. 75, 2
   d. 96, 2

9. In the formula $C = D_{fs-f} \times \tan TA \times 2$ the SID is represented by which of the following?
   a. $\tan TA$
   b. D_{fs-f}
   c. C
   d. none of the above

10. Doorways to the advanced procedures suite should be a minimum width of:
   a. 2 foot 6 inches
   b. 3 foot 0 inches
   c. 3 foot 6 inches
   d. 4 foot 0 inches

2 Image Capture—Analog and Digital

CHAPTER OBJECTIVES

After completing this chapter, the reader will be able to perform the following:

- Describe the history of image recording in advanced procedures
- Define the roll and cut film changers from a historical perspective
- Describe biplanar radiography
- Identify the various indirect methods of recording the radiographic images
- Define the basic concepts of analog versus digital imaging
- Identify the use of flat panel detector systems
- List and describe the principles underlying radiographic subtraction

CHAPTER OUTLINE

DIRECT IMAGING SYSTEMS

    Rapid Serial Changers—An Historical Perspective
    Biplane Radiography

INDIRECT IMAGING SYSTEMS

    Image Intensification

IMAGE OUTPUT

    DICOM Standard
    Hard Copy Image Output

LASER IMAGING SYSTEMS

DIGITAL IMAGING

    Analog versus Digital—Basic Concepts
    Image Processing

IMAGE SUBTRACTION—HOW TO SEE MORE WITH LESS

    Basic Subtraction Principles

SUMMARY

During special procedures, as with conventional radiography, there must be a system to capture the images produced during the studies, store the images for processing, and display the images during the procedure as well as providing a permanent copy for archiving and future analysis. The images must also be portable so that they can be viewed by several different medical specialists for diagnosis.

In conventional radiography, the image is recorded on x-ray film, which is then processed, viewed, and filed to provide permanent storage and communication capabilities. Generally speaking, the images produced by conventional radiographic methods are "passive" and are not meant to demonstrate motion or changes in the anatomic part during the procedure. These images are usually archived on film and can be physically transported for viewing at remote locations. Their main disadvantage is that the films can degrade over time and can also be lost or damaged.

Conventional fluoroscopy can capture the images on x-ray film, cine film, or magnetic media while displaying the images of the study on a display monitor for viewing in real time during the procedure. The advantages of this system are that changes can be recorded as they happen, analyzed during the procedure, and also kept for future use. The images produced by conventional fluoroscopy also share the disadvantages of those produced by conventional radiography.

In general, advanced procedures are dynamic studies. They are designed to demonstrate physiologic sequences, such as the passage of a bolus of contrast medium through a portion of the vascular system. These sequences last only a few seconds, and if any abnormality is present, it might be visible for only a fraction of a second. The images have been produced by means of serial exposures which are captured, stored, processed, and presented for viewing. Several types of systems have been used to archive these images—conventional film/screen images from rapid serial changers, storage on magnetic recording devices, laser optical devices (videodisc), large-format serial spot filming devices, cinefluorography, and digital image storage devices.

Radiographic systems have been designed with one or more of these recording media incorporated into the design. Analog imaging systems were the systems of choice for many institutions, primarily because of the expense of digital systems. In recent years, however, as older equipment is being replaced, digital imaging systems are becoming more prevalent, especially in the advanced procedure suites. The use of image sharing systems such as PACS (picture archiving and communication systems) is also becoming commonplace in the imaging department. Older analog systems are giving way to the newer CR (computed radiography) and DR (digital radiography) systems.

A historical review of some of the analog image capture devices that have been used in the past and present is presented. It is anticipated that within the next 5 years digital radiographic systems and flat panel technology will replace these systems in the advanced radiography suite.

DIRECT IMAGING SYSTEMS

Rapid Serial Film Changers—An Historical Perspective

As their name implies, rapid serial film changers were used to record a sequential series of images that occurred during the special procedure. Images that were captured via analog techniques were recorded on radiographic film and were processed in the usual manner to provide the finished image. These types of systems produced a series of static images representing the changes that developed during the procedure. The images produced represented glimpses of the process over a period of time. The disadvantage to this type of system was that the dynamic nature of the pathologic or physiologic process could not be demonstrated.

Rapid serial changers were produced by a variety of manufacturers. However, all systems had several elements in common. A short discussion of the basic operational features of rapid serial changers is presented primarily from the historical point of view.

Rapid serial film changers were produced in one of two types—those that transported cut film and those that transported roll film.

Roll Film Changers

Roll film changers are obsolete and are considered here only in a historical perspective. The operation of a rapid serial roll film changer can be compared with that of a movie projector. Roll film changers had four major parts: (1) changer and mounting stand; (2) supply magazine; (3) receiving magazine; and (4) program selector.

1. **Film changer and mounting stand assembly.** This was the drive portion of the roll film changer. It housed the mechanism necessary to transport the film from the supply magazine to the receiving magazine.
2. **Supply magazine.** This served to hold the unexposed roll of film.

3. **Receiving magazine.** This could be transported to the darkroom under normal lighting conditions without the risk of exposure of the film by light.

4. **Program selector.** This was the heart of the variable speed film changers. It operated the film changer during single or serial exposures and established the film rate (number of films per second) and the duration of each phase.

Cut Film Changers

Rapid serial cut film changers rapidly transported single sheets of film of a specific size. The 14- × 14-in (35.6- × 35.6-cm) and the 10- × 12-in (25- × 30-cm) sizes were most often used. These units were available as single-plane changers; however, two units on different mounting stands were often combined for biplane operation.

The cut film changer was similar to a roll film changer in that it also contained four major components: (1) changer and mounting stand assembly; (2) supply magazine; (3) receiving cassette; and (4) program selector.

- **Film changer and mounting stand assembly.** The cut film changer, unlike the roll film changer, transported film by means of roller systems. This type of changer was similar to an automatic processor in some respects.

- **Mounting stand.** The two basic mounting stands were made for horizontal or vertical changers. These changers were also attached to the image intensifier on the C-arm or as built-in models in a radiographic table. When the units were attached to a C-arm, conversion from fluoroscopy to serial radiography was easily accomplished in a minimal amount of time.

- **Supply magazine.** The supply, or loading, magazine was a stainless-steel box that was easily carried to and from the darkroom.

- **Receiving cassette.** The receiving cassette, a stainless-steel container with a light-tight lid, served as a carrying case for the exposed films that were sent through the changer.

- **Program selector** The program selectors for both roll and cut film changers operated in a similar manner. The display panel listed all the information necessary for a specific program, even listing errors that needed to be corrected before beginning the procedure.

An automatic cut film changer was also available for peripheral angiography, with an exposure frequency of two exposures per second. An interesting feature of this unit was the central radio transparent opening, through which fluoroscopy could be used to position the patient and place the catheter. Its operation was similar to that of the cut film changer previously described.

Basic Operational Considerations

All of the rapid serial changers discussed operated in a similar manner (Fig. 2-1). They moved the imaging material into place for the exposure and then removed it to a storage location. In other words, with all rapid serial changers there was a period of time during which the film or cassette was in motion **(transport time)** and a period of time during which no motion occurred and the film was in position for the exposure **(stationary period).** The radiograph had to be produced during the stationary period. The stationary period for each of the types of rapid serial changers was different; however, it was usually less than 50% of the **total film cycle time** (transport time + stationary period). Certain inherent electronic delays prevented the entire stationary period from being used to make the exposure. These were the zero time and phase-in time.

- **Zero time** was the delay caused by the operational time of the relays and contacts in the x-ray exposure control. This delay was constant for any particular apparatus and was preset by the manufacturer

- **Phase-in time** was related to the point at which the exposure contact was closed in relation to the cycle of the line voltage. This cycle is usually shown as a sine wave, and the exposure could be initiated only when the cycle of the line voltage passed through zero. This delay varied from no delay to a maximum delay of one cycle of line frequency. The maximum phase-in time for single-phase equipment was $1/60$ s and for three-phase units, $1/360$ s.

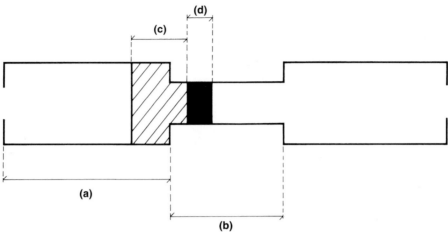

FIGURE 2-1. A typical film cycle period. (*a*) Transport time; (*b*) stationary period; (*c*) zero time; (*d*) phase-in time.

The actual amount of phase-in time varied with each exposure and could not be predetermined. However, the maximum exposure time that could be used for a particular system was calculated by deducting the greatest phase-in time delay from the stationary period. Table 2-1 illustrates the maximum phase-in time delays for single-phase and three-phase units.

Biplane Radiography

A discussion of image capture would not be complete without consideration of biplane operation. The term **biplane** as applied to rapid sequence radiography is defined as simultaneous radiography in two planes (Fig. 2-2).

When rapid sequence changers are used for biplane radiography, certain technical difficulties arise. The most important factor, scatter, necessitates the use of special crossed grids in the vertical changer. This grid should absorb the scatter radiation produced in a biplane setup that strikes the vertical changer. This causes an increase in the density of the film in the horizontal changer. These factors should be considered when choosing the technical parameters for biplane operation. If single-plane study is required on the same patient, an adjustment in technique will be necessary to compensate for this effect.

We can see, therefore, that during biplane studies, it is necessary to use different exposure factors in each of the two planes. This is possible only if the x-ray tubes are supplied with separate generators, thus providing flexibility of technical factors for each tube. If, however, the x-ray tubes are connected in parallel on one generator, the selection of these factors will be severely compromised, and technical adjustments for the increased scatter radiation to one plane will be limited.

TABLE 2-1   *Maximum Phase-in Time*

Type of Unit	Maximum Phase-in Time (s)	Calculation of Maximum Phase-in Time*	Maximum Phase-in Time (ms)
Single Phase	1/60	1000/60	16.67
Three Phase	1/360	1000/360	2.78

*1 s = 1000 ms.

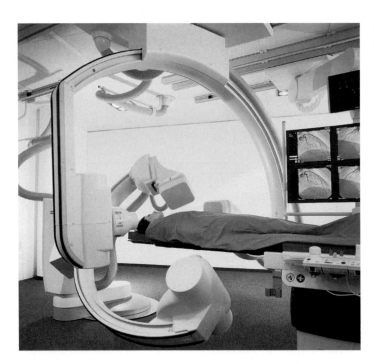

FIGURE 2-2. An example of a biplane system.

INDIRECT IMAGING SYSTEMS

Rapid serial radiographic systems produce the image through the direct interaction of the x-radiation with the screen/film system. Indirect imaging systems, however, record the image using the information produced at the output phosphor of an image intensification device. Indirect imaging systems include videotape recorders, videodisc recorders, digital recording systems, serial spot filming devices, and cinefluorographic systems. Videotape, videodisc, and digital recording systems use an electronic signal to produce the image, whereas the serial spot filming devices and cinefluorographic units (photofluorographic systems) capture the image directly from the output phosphor of the image intensifier. Digital imaging systems are replacing spot film devices and cinefluorography systems. However, the devices used in the indirect imaging systems discussed in this chapter are still in use and in some cases are still being sold as generic add-ins by some retailers. A brief discussion of their operation is included.

Knowledge of the operation of the image intensification system is essential to understanding the principles of the indirect imaging recording devices. Several changes have been made in image intensification design to improve the quality of the images produced; however, the basic process and materials have not changed. A brief review of the principles of image intensification follows.

Image Intensification

An image intensifier (II) is used to increase the brightness of the image. This is accomplished with the II tube (Fig. 2–3). The input side of the II tube is coated with a phosphor layer, usually cesium iodide, that produces the image as a direct result of the action of the remnant radiation. Photoemissive material is coated on the substrate opposite the phosphor layer; this material converts the visible light image into an electron image. The electrons making up the image are accelerated across the II tube by an electron lens system and focused to strike the output side of the tube.

The output side of the II tube is also coated with a phosphor, which converts the electron image to a smaller, corresponding light image. The image at the output side of the II tube is brighter. This results from the process of reducing the size of the image and the acceleration of the electrons.

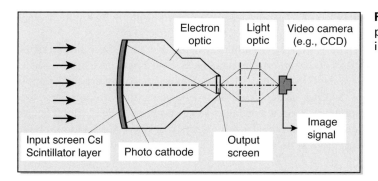

FIGURE 2-3. The functional principles underlying an image intensification system.

A television camera, either high resolution **charge-coupled device** (**CCD**) video camera or pickup tube, is attached directly to the output side of the II tube via a special lens system or fiberoptic disc. The CCD is an integrated light-sensitive circuit (chip) that can store and display the data of an image. The image is produced as separate picture elements (pixels), which exhibit electrical charges of varying intensities. The intensities are related to a corresponding "color" of the visible spectrum. Charge-coupled devices are found in digital cameras. The advantage to this type of system is that images can be produced in low light situations without the loss of resolution. The images produced can be transmitted to a television monitor as well as other types of recording devices. The use of an image distribution device will also allow the attachment of a serial spot filming device, a cinefluorographic unit, or both, to the system.

IMAGE OUTPUT

DICOM Standard

The data collected through the image capture systems can be made available globally and should be readily accessible. Originally, there were several different proprietary standards, and the information could not be shared by the systems that were in use. This limited the value of the data to a specific institution and its diagnostic imaging department. In order to accomplish global sharing of information, there was a need for some type of standard in medical imaging for the archiving and communications of medical images and information. The need also existed for a common database that could be accessed and searched easily.

The American College of Radiology (ACR) and the National Electronics Manufacturers Association (NEMA) recognized this with the advent of computed tomography and formed a consortium to develop a standard for file formats that could be understood by equipment and systems manufactured by different companies. The format was termed the **Digital Imaging and Communications in Medicine Standard**, or **DICOM**. In 1983 the ACR and NEMA formulated a standard[1] that would:

- Promote the communication of digital imaging information, regardless of the manufacturer of the device
- Facilitate the development and expansion of picture archiving and communication systems that could communicate with other systems of hospital information
- Allow the development of diagnostic information databases that could be searched by a wide variety of devices in different geographical areas

The original standard was published in 1985, and it proposed a specific type of interface, special software commands, and consistent data formats. Since the original standard was published, it has undergone several revisions that include several enhancements to the original version. NEMA views the DICOM standard as an evolving set of guidelines. The DICOM standard is directed at providing a platform for the interoperability of various devices and systems primarily in the area of diagnostic medical imaging. The specific guidelines and specifications of the DICOM standard are beyond the scope of this text. They are available from the National Electrical Manufacturers Association and can be found on their website—(http://www.nema.org).

Previously, magnetic videodisc systems were used to indirectly record the images produced during the study using a rigid disc coated with an emulsion similar to magnetic tape. These have been replaced by recordable CD-ROM devices that use the CD Medical DICOM 3 international format. An example of this type of system is the Siemens ACOM, an archiving and review station with accompanying ACOM.PC software (Fig. 2-4). The computer system is a relatively small computer system, which houses the DICOM software. The information from this system can be sent to a PACS workstation, or the images can be archived either on the hard drive or on CD-ROM.

Hard Copy Image Output

Hard copy images produced in the state of the art digital equipment results from the conversion of a digital image into its analog counterpart. This process is accomplished using a digital to analog conversion (DAC) system and usually a laser or dye sublimation printer.

Older systems used film to capture the image, and the cameras were usually attached to the image intensifiers (II). The image capture systems discussed next may be used in certain areas and warrant a brief discussion of the principles of their operation.

Photofluorographic Systems

This category includes the serial spot filming device and the cinefluorographic camera. It should be noted that the spot film devices are not necessary in the current "state of the art" equipment, digital systems. These components were attached to the II by an image distribution unit. This unit contains a beam–splitting mirror for diverting the optical image onto the lens of the photofluorographic device. The serial spot filming and cinefluorographic camera record the image from the output phosphor of the II in the same way; that is, the light image from the output phosphor creates the image on the photofluorographic film.

Serial Spot Film Cameras. This type of unit is also called a *large-format, spot film,* or *rapid sequence* camera. Such cameras may be referred to by the size of film they use. The current film size formats were 70, 90, 100, and 105 mm; the most commonly used film formats were 100 and 105 mm. Spot film cameras are capable of recording from 1 to 12 pictures (frames) per second (fps) and can use either roll or cut film depending on the manufacturer and model.

The serial spot filming devices do not contain a shutter. The image is produced on the II by using a pulsed x-ray beam. When the beam is on, an image is recorded; when the beam is off, no image is produced on the output phosphor and therefore no image is recorded in the camera.

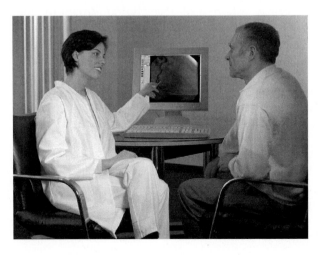

FIGURE 2-4. Siemens ACOM review station for image replay direct from the computer system or from a CD-ROM.

The major difference between the photofluorographic and serial spot film systems is the finished product. The serial spot filming units produce images that are separated by a specific time interval and demonstrate the changes in the anatomy and pathology as a sequence of static events. These are usually cut from the roll of film and are viewed in sequential order.

Cinefluorographic Systems. The cine camera is similar in construction to a movie camera. The device contains (1) lens system; (2) supply spool; (3) motor-driven film transport mechanism; (4) take-up spool; and (5) rotating shutter. Film sizes for the cine camera are 16 and 35 mm. The larger format is more popular because it produces a better-quality image.

The operation of the cine camera is also similar to that of a home movie camera. The film is passed in front of an aperture (hole) in synchronization with the shutter system; therefore, the film is in motion when the shutter is closed and stationary when the shutter is open. The image on the output phosphor of the II tube is produced by a pulsed x-ray beam. The pulsed format reduces the radiation dose to the patient, decreases the heat loading of the x-ray tube, and helps reduce motion artifacts, allowing very short exposure times.

The motor used to drive the transport mechanism is capable of varying speed settings. The speed of the motor will govern the number of frames per second that are exposed. The range of frames per second can be from 8 to 200 depending on the film size used. Cinefluorography is usually accomplished at frame rates in excess of 16 fps to produce the effect of motion when the final images of the study are projected for viewing.

Cineradiographic film must be properly matched with the emission spectrum of the output phosphor of the II. The type of film used is either orthochromatic (yellow or green-blue sensitive) or panchromatic (orange, red, green, yellow, and violet sensitive). Film processing can be accomplished with a specialized processor that can handle film sizes ranging from 35 to 105 mm.

Cinefluorographic units are used during cardiac catheterization to record the sequences in the coronary vasculature. They can be used in a single-plane setup or, if a C-arm is used, as a biplane system.

Multiformat Cameras. The systems discussed above all relied upon the photography of an image either on an intensifying screen, cathode ray tube (CRT), television, or oscilloscope. In all of the cases the image was captured, stored, and displayed or converted into a hard copy image. The quality of the image produced depended upon the components of the image recording system. This is a well-known principle in general radiography. The image is degraded by a variety of factors in the system. Among them were the CRT brightness, phosphor graininess, distortion, and artifacts as well as the optical systems themselves. The image output devices discussed earlier produced a single image on a single frame or film. The desire to place more images on a single film as in CT and ultrasound studies led to the development of the multiformat camera.

Initial systems used various methods to produce the images. These included motorized optics and multiple lenses to produce the images. By varying the distances of the lenses and the film, it became possible to change the size of the images produced. Many advances were introduced to improve on the quality of the output produced by these cameras. These included better optics, the use of flat screen monitors. and improved phosphors. Eastman Kodak produces several types of single-emulsion radiographic film for use with the multiformat camera. Figure 2-5 illustrates the sensitometric properties of three of Eastman Kodak's multiformat films. Note that there is a suitable variety of film speeds and average gradients among the films. These are all sensitive to the higher wavelength green light and are compatible with most CRT monitors. These cameras are still employed in many institutions and find their greatest use in ultrasound and nuclear medicine.

LASER IMAGING SYSTEMS

Digital images are easily stored and shared through the PACS; however, there is still a need in all of the modalities using digital imaging for hard copy images. This is accomplished through the use of laser imaging systems. Laser imagers record the digital image on special radiographic film. A special infrared

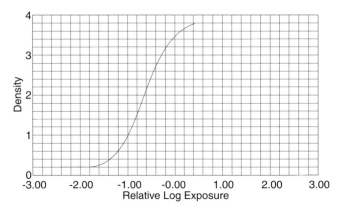

FIGURE 2-5. Sensitometric properties of Kodak Ektascan B/RA films for use in multiformat cameras.

single-emulsion film is scanned by the laser, which then transfers the digitized densities to the film emulsion as various shades of gray. In current 12-bit systems it is possible to produce 4096 shades of gray. This allows the laser printing system to reproduce the image without the loss of information or the introduction of artifacts.

Laser imaging systems can be either "wet" or "dry" systems. The "wet" laser imager is connected directly to a film processor, and the film can be processed in the usual manner utilizing processor chemistry. These systems have the disadvantage that the film must be handled in total darkness. Laser imaging film used in "wet" systems is sensitive to light and will respond in the same way as conventional film if exposed to light. The image is produced on the film by exposing it to a laser light beam that transfers the digital signal into a visible image having a number of gray levels. When the film has been completely exposed, it is sent to a film processor, and the latent image produced by the laser light is processed into a visible image by means of processor chemistry.

Laser imaging systems are also available in a "dry imaging" format. This type of system makes use of thermal imaging to produce lasting hard copy prints of digital studies. These systems are much smaller than the "wet" laser systems and have the advantage that the film can be loaded easily in daylight. Dry laser imaging also affords the practitioner the ability to produce images up to 4096 gray levels but also color printing as well as grayscale paper images.

Laser imaging systems can be interfaced with several modalities such as computed tomography (CT), magnetic resonance imaging (MRI), or digital radiography units, making them versatile as well as affording the institution a potential cost savings in operating costs.

DIGITAL IMAGING

Analog versus Digital—Basic Concepts

In order to begin to understand the concept of digital imaging, we must first understand the difference between the terms **analog** and **digital**. An image is a representation of some object or thing. Both analog and digital methods arrive at the representation of the item in different ways. In both cases the image cannot be seen until it is processed in some manner. Analog images are generally processed utilizing the chemical systems that we are all familiar with. Digital images on the other hand must be manipulated by a software program and then displayed on some type of output device. Discussion of analog representations will refer to the finished (processed) product.

The term **analog** is generally associated with two concepts: ambiguity and continuity. These terms may seem foreign when applied to radiography, but their use is based on the fact that radiographs are two-dimensional images that can be measured by using a variety of methods. These measurements can be taken at any point across the image. The reproducibility of these measurements is dependent upon the equipment/method being used and the person doing the measurement. In most cases the measurements will differ. Precision is difficult to achieve, and variations of the measurements will exist. The measurements can be taken across the film in a continuous manner. Thus, measurements can be available in any pattern and at any point.

This concept can be further illustrated by a painting, which is a two-dimensional representation of an artist's perception of an object or an idea. It is continuous in that the artist continuously applies the paint until the painting is complete. Once done, measurements can be taken to analyze the image. One can look at any or all of the following features: specific colors, thickness of paint layers, length of brushstrokes, and so forth. Another artist may attempt to copy the painting, but variations will exist in the finished product owing to the imprecision introduced in the measurements. The same can be applied to the world of music. In order to play a tune, one note must continuously follow another until the end of the tune is reached. Also, the music will sound pleasant if the transition from each note to the next is smooth. If we assume that several different musicians are going to play the same sequence of notes, the same tune, it more than likely will sound different. This is because the instruments may differ in tone or their individual tuning or the musician may play the notes in a more rapid or slower tempo. The reproducibility of something that is analog is imprecise, and the copy will not sound or look the same. In other words the term "analog" refers to a continuous representation in which measurement and reproducibility are imprecise.

The term **digital**, as its name implies, is related to numbers or digits. It is represented by a series of values in some sort of table format. This number table is often referred to as an **array**. The values consist of unconnected and distinct parts and are related to a finite number of states. Digital images, unlike the analog counterpart, are not continuous but move from one individually distinct value to another. There is no continuous transition to a next state. In the digital world, movement involves the jumping from one state to another in an isolated (discrete) manner.

A digital image is invisible until it is manipulated and revealed through the use of some sort of output device. The number table, or array, has no meaning for us until the information has been synthesized through the use of a computer program, or **algorithm**. Once processed by the algorithm the values can be sent to an output device such as a printer or display monitor. The quality of the final image is dependent upon the quality of the output device as well as other operator-selected factors. Digital images can be copied without a loss of quality. They also can be manipulated to make the image more useful.

In both analog and digital radiography the production of the "aerial" image is similar. The patient is exposed to a certain set of exposure factors, and the remnant radiation forms an invisible image in the space between the patient and the image receptor. Once the aerial image has been produced, it can be considered as data that can be captured, stored, processed, displayed, and distributed. These functions are accomplished by people and equipment systems. These equipment systems can present the output as analog or digital images by means of conventional radiography, computed radiography, or digital radiography.

Digital radiography differs from conventional radiography and fluoroscopy in the manner of data capture and processing. In conventional radiography, the data (attenuated radiation that passes through the patient) is collected as a latent image on a film-based material that is subsequently processed via chemical means to produce an image. This image is usually viewed by passing light through the processed film. Conventional fluoroscopy and analog image intensifiers collect the data with an electronic image receptor, intensifies the image, and displays it as a television image. The image can then be stored on a variety of devices for future retrieval and study.

Computed radiography is similar to conventional radiography in that image receptors equipped with photostimulable phosphor plates are used. These image receptors look like their counterparts (cassettes) from conventional radiography. The image plate is not affected by light and provides the storage medium for the data prior to processing and display. To continue the comparison with conventional radiography, the image stored on the plate in a computed radiography cassette can also be referred to as the latent image.

Digital image intensifiers work in the same manner as the conventional systems with the exception that the imaging chain is linked to a CCD (charge-coupled device) that collects the light produced at the output window of the image intensifier, converting it into a charge that subsequently emits a signal that results in a digital image. Digital image intensification systems are being replaced by flat panel detector technology. The major difference between the systems is in the imaging chain. In the flat panel system the aerial image strikes the detector and is converted into an electrical signal. Flat panel technology can produce the digital signal by two different methods—direct or indirect conversion (Fig. 2-6).

Flat panel digital systems are based on solid state integrated circuitry in the same manner as the digital camera. The primary difference between the two is the field or detector size. Large detector sizes sufficient for radiographic applications were made possible by means of the thin film transistor array (TFT). Taking another note from the current technology, the TFT systems are similar to those found in laptop computers. The flat panel is constructed similar to a sandwich with the readout electronic layer on the bottom, the charge collector electrodes in the middle, and a top layer of light or x-ray sensitive material.

The TFT layer is composed of a thin layer of silicon in an amorphous state. This simply means that it is shapeless or ill defined. On the surface, however, the silicon is imprinted with an ordered array of transistors. These are arranged in a gridlike fashion, and each section of the grid is attached to the photodiode or photoconductor to make up an individual pixel (picture element) (Fig. 2-7). The top of the system is composed of some type of scintillator material. This material is either gadolinium oxysulfide or cesium iodide. Cesium iodide has certain advantages over the gadolinium. It has a greater conversion efficiency, and as it is made it forms columns that function to channel the light produced in a much more focused fashion (Fig. 2-8). The middle of the sandwich is the photodiode. This is the element that converts the light produced by the scintillator into a charge. Flat panel detectors are designed as either indirect or direct conversion systems.

In the indirect system the top layer is composed of a scintillator material coupled with a photodiode. The scintillator will produce light when stimulated by x-ray. The light is then converted to an electric charge by the photodiode, which is read out by the TFT layer.

The direct system consists of an x-ray sensitive photoconductor coupled with the TFT layer. In this case the charge is generated by the photoconductor and directly read out by the TFT array.

In the direct digital method the x-ray quanta are converted into electrical charges that are deposited on the pixel electrodes. An analog to digital converter then changes the electric charges into a digital signal. The indirect digital system converts the aerial image into the digital signal in two steps: the conversion of the remnant radiation into light within a scintillator and the conversion of the light into an electrical signal by means of a photodiode on the pixel surface.

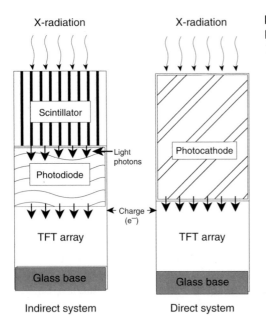

FIGURE 2-6. Simple schematic of the difference between an indirect and direct flat panel system. *TFT,* Thin film transistor.

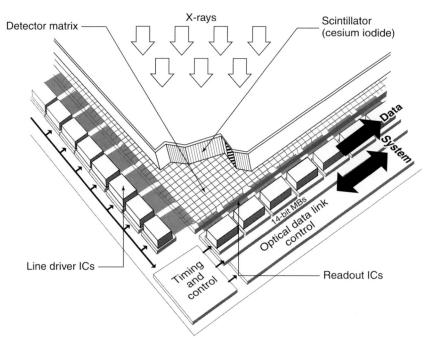

FIGURE 2-7. Diagram of a flat panel system showing the readout integrated circuitry (IC), scintillator, and detector matrix.

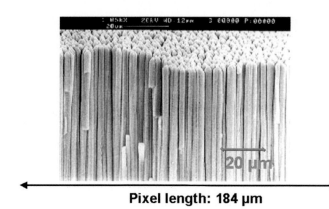

Pixel length: 184 µm

FIGURE 2-8. Closeup view of a portion of a cesium iodide scintillator showing its columnar structure.

The process by which the system collects the information is beyond the scope of this text. The advantages of flat panel technology are its size and weight when compared to current conventional image intensification and film screen radiographic systems. These factors will determine the application possibilities of the flat panel systems in the coming years.

Regardless of the manner in which the data from the aerial image is collected, it is initially referred to as **analog data**. The analog information is converted into **digital data**, processed, and stored in a computer system. It can be retrieved at a later time, reconverted to analog data, and viewed by means of an electronic device that displays the image. Digital radiography has several advantages over conventional radiography and fluoroscopy; these are summarized in Box 2-1.

The physical principles of radiography that are used during this phase are the same as those that would be used during conventional radiography. In this phase, the radiation passes through the patient and is attenuated, and the resultant radiation is picked up by a detector system. The image capture can be from digitized fluoroscopic images, direct digital imaging, computed radiography, flat panel detector systems. and digitized conventional images. If the image is collected from fluoroscopic images, the light image from the intensifier tube is focused and strikes the tube of a video camera. At this point, the image is still considered a latent image and is represented by a matrix of electric charges. The output from the video camera is also transferred to the second component, the image processing center, as a timed sequence of electrical pulses (the analog data). To understand this process, it is important to realize that the analog data (image) are measured in a point-by-point fashion in the image processing center. A radiographic image consists of many different density levels. The image processor looks at the image as if a rectangular grid (matrix) were placed over it. This grid divides the image into many squares, which represent discrete picture elements (pixels). Some common image matrix sizes are 256 × 256, 512 × 512, 1024 × 1024, and 4096 × 4096 pixels. Given a standard field size, the larger the number of pixels in the matrix, the greater the resolution and the smaller the size of each pixel, yielding greater spatial resolution.

Image Processing

When the video output (analog data) reaches this stage, the signal may be amplified. There are two methods available for the amplification of the output signal—logarithmic amplification and linear amplification. The former method is used most often, with amplification of the data being proportional to the strength of the signal itself. It is usually used for carotid and vertebral studies. Linear amplification is used when the anatomy under study is of a uniform tissue density. This type of amplification is most often used for studies of the abdominal area.

In the next step of the process, the analog data signals are passed through an analog-to-digital (A/D) converter (Fig. 2-9). The intensity of the analog signal of each pixel is measured, and a numerical value is then assigned. This number represents the average density (analog signal) within the individual pixel areas. The A/D converter digitizes the analog information; that is, it transfers the analog signal into a digital number. The digital data (numerical values) are represented by binary numbers shown as an array, and the image consists of a matrix, a specific group of numbers arranged in rows

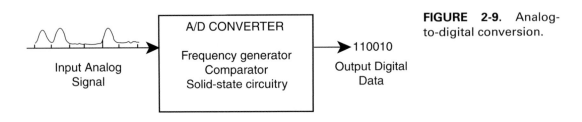

FIGURE 2-9. Analog-to-digital conversion.

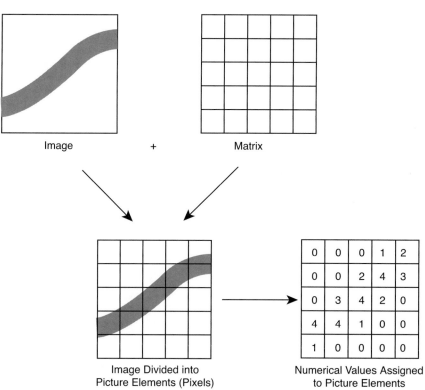

Image   +   Matrix

Image Divided into
Picture Elements (Pixels)

Numerical Values Assigned
to Picture Elements

FIGURE 2-10.   Transfer of the analog grid into a digital number.

and columns. The elements of the matrix are called pixels or picture elements. Figure 2-10 illustrates how the digital image is displayed in the matrix as well as the array of numbers that are used to define the image.

Analog-to–digital converters (ADCs) can allow from 256 (2^8, or 8 bits) to 4096 (2^{12}, or 12 bits) gray levels for each image point (pixel). A **bit** is a contraction of the term **binary digit**.

The binary number system is made up of only 0s and 1s. It differs from the decimal system in that its base is 2. The decimal system has a base of 10 and is represented by the numbers 0, 1, 2, 3, 4, 5, 6, 7, 8, and 9. In the decimal system, numbers are formed using these digits multiplied by a power of 10.

Table 2-2 illustrates the differences between the binary number and decimal systems. It can be seen from the examples in Table 2-2 that binary numbers can be very long. To facilitate reading these numbers, other systems were developed based on the binary system—the octal system and the hexadecimal system. Each of these is a variation of the binary system using groups of binary numbers to represent larger numbers.

Table 2-3 illustrates the relationship between the binary number system and the other systems available for computer use. As mentioned, each binary digit is called a bit. The term **byte** refers to a group of one or more bits; however, it is normally used to identify a group of 8 bits, which is also known as an 8-bit code. For this information to be useful to the computer, it must be represented by a binary number system code.

The human eye can distinguish only 32 shades (gray levels) at one time. The gray levels can be manipulated for optimal demonstration of different structures in the image. Displaying a segment of the total pixel value range at a time and displaying these values in shades of gray from black to white is termed **windowing**. The window level corresponds to the midpoint of the chosen gray scale as represented on the master scale. Any pixel either above or below the range will exhibit no contrast. In other words contrast will be evident only within the selected window.

TABLE 2-2 *Relationship Between the Decimal and Binary Systems**

Decimal System			Binary System							
100	10	1	128	64	32	16	8	4	2	1
		1	0	0	0	0	0	0	0	1
		2	0	0	0	0	0	0	1	0
		3	0	0	0	0	0	0	1	1
		4	0	0	0	0	0	1	0	0
		5	0	0	0	0	0	1	0	1
		6	0	0	0	0	0	1	1	0
		7	0	0	0	0	0	1	1	1
		8	0	0	0	0	1	0	0	0
		9	0	0	0	0	1	0	0	1
	1	0	0	0	0	0	1	0	1	0
	1	1	0	0	0	0	1	0	1	1
	1	5	0	0	0	0	1	1	1	1
	2	0	0	0	0	1	0	1	0	0
	3	0	0	0	0	1	1	1	1	0
	4	0	0	0	1	0	1	0	0	0
	5	0	0	0	1	1	1	1	0	0
	7	5	0	1	0	0	1	0	1	1
1	0	0	0	1	1	0	0	1	0	0
1	5	0	1	0	0	1	0	1	1	0
2	0	0	1	1	0	0	1	0	0	0
2	5	0	1	1	1	1	1	0	1	0
2	5	5	1	1	1	1	1	1	1	1

*Base 10 in the decimal system uses the digits 0, 1, 2, 3, 4, 5, 6, 7, 8, and 9; base 2 in the binary system uses the digits 0 and 1.

TABLE 2-3 *Relationships Between the Various Number Systems Used for Computers*

Decimal	Binary	Octal	Hexadecimal
150	10010110	001, 101, 000	1111, 000
	150	1 5 0	F 0
		150	15 0
Base 10	Base 2	Groups of three digits are represented by one octal digit	Groups of four binary digits are represented by one hexadecimal digit
Ten digits are represented: 0, 1, 2, 3, 4, 5, 6, 7, 8, 9	Two digits are represented: 0, 1	Eight digits are represented: 0, 1, 2, 3, 4, 5, 6, 7	Sixteen digits are represented: 0, 1, 2, 3, 4, 5, 6, 7, 8, 9, 10 (A), 11 (B), 12 (C), 13 (D), 14 (E), 15 (F)

After the analog-to-digital conversion (digitization) has taken place, the information is entered into the memory system. In most digital subtraction units, two memory systems are used, with the digitized image stored in one of the two memories. The second memory holds the images taken during the passage of the contrast medium. The information from the memories can then be integrated, and the images are manipulated in the computer. The resulting images can be stored in a short-term storage system as either digital or analog data. If the images are to be kept for any length of time, long-term storage capabilities are essential.

IMAGE SUBTRACTION—HOW TO SEE MORE WITH LESS

Image subtraction is routinely accomplished in today's state of the art digital systems, and the principles underlying it are hidden in the software algorithms that make it possible. The purpose of this output technique is to provide a clear visualization of information on a radiograph by removing the images of nonessential structures. The technique does not add any information to the radiograph but makes the diagnostically important images more visible. Subtraction is actually an image of the *differences* between two similar images.

Simple subtraction techniques have become obsolete as a result of the modern imaging systems. Subtraction is now accomplished during the procedure by the computer. It is a technique that is now taken for granted, and in some cases the underlying principles are not clearly recognized. An understanding of the principles of simple subtraction can dispel the mystery of digital subtraction.

Subtraction is used primarily during advanced imaging procedures, especially those utilizing a contrast agent. The images produced during these studies usually show confusing bone shadows superimposed over contrast-filled vessels. The presence of all of this information on the radiograph makes small opacified vessels virtually invisible. Subtraction eliminates the nonessential shadows and allows the contrast-filled vessels to stand out against a relatively "clean" (homogeneous) background.

The basic principles of simple subtraction are discussed to provide both a historical and technical familiarity with the process.

Basic Subtraction Principles

The process of digital subtraction is somewhat similar to simple subtraction. Digital subtraction is accomplished automatically and has become a routine process in the manipulation of the digitally captured images. The process described here is now accomplished quickly and accurately in the state of the art systems; however, the underlying principle remains the same as in simple subtraction.

To perform simple subtraction, at least two separate radiographs of the same anatomic region are required. One, the **scout film**, contains all of the information normally available radiographically concerning that specific region. The second film, in this case the **angiogram film**, contains all of the information found in the scout film plus that found in the contrast-filled vessels. One other specific criterion is necessary to perform a perfect subtraction: there must be no change of position (or motion) by the patient between exposures of the scout and angiogram films. This factor is all but eliminated in real-time subtraction.

Simple subtraction was accomplished using the following five steps (Fig. 2-11):
- Expose a base film.
- Prepare a positive reverse tone subtraction (diapositive) mask.
- Produce the angiogram films.
- Superimpose the mask and angiogram films.
- Make the final subtraction print.

Preparation of the Reverse Tone Subtraction Mask

A diapositive mask is an exact copy of the base film, with the densities exactly reversed. This is the basis for the theory behind the subtraction methods. It is well known that details are visible on a radiograph because of contrast. Contrast is defined as the difference between densities in adjacent areas. In other words, details are visible because there are density differences on a radiograph. A film that possesses only one density does not show an image. The diapositive mask, which is a reversed image of the scout film, produces a radiograph of a single density when superimposed over the scout film. Because there is no contrast, there is no image.

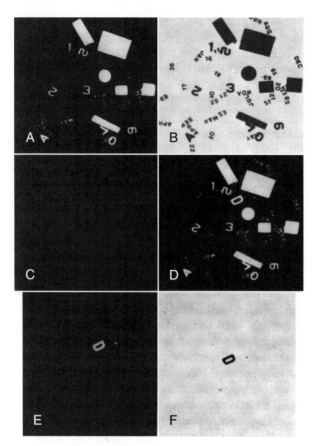

FIGURE 2-11. Flow representation of the subtraction technique. **A,** The base, or scout, film, is usually the initial film of a series. **B,** The mask is produced by making a reversed image of the density differences found on the scout film. **C,** The mask superimposed over the scout film. When this is done, there should be no resultant density differences seen, and a black image of a single density should then be produced. **D,** The angiogram film containing the same information present on the scout film plus some added information. **E,** The mask and the angiogram films superimposed. All information that is the same on both films is obliterated (the same effect produced in **C**) while the added information is enhanced. **F,** The final permanent print of the image produced by the superimposition of the mask and the angiogram film.

When the reverse tone (diapositive) subtraction mask is superimposed over an angiogram film, any information that was the same as that recorded on the base film will be canceled out. Only the structures filled with contrast medium should exhibit radiographic contrast. These structures should stand out and be clearly seen without confusing shadows.

The preparation of the reverse tone (diapositive mask) is the most critical step in the subtraction procedure. If the mask is not properly prepared, the final subtraction prints will be of poor quality.

This principle is illustrated as follows. Assume that a particular scout film possesses the following densities:

	Area A	Area B	Area C
Scout film	0.6	1.2	2.0

To produce a reverse tone (diapositive mask), it is important to produce reversed density differences that correspond exactly to the density differences on the scout film. In other words:

	Area A	Density Difference Between Area A & Area B	Area B	Density Difference Between Area B & Area C	Area C
Scout film	0.6	+0.6	1.2	+0.8	2.0
Reverse tone mask	1.9	-0.6	1.3	-0.8	0.5

Superimposition of Diapositive Mask and Scout Film

When the scout film and reverse tone (diapositive) mask are superimposed, the resultant densities should be equal:

	Area A	Area B	Area C
Scout film	0.6	1.2	2.0
Reverse tone mask	<u>1.9</u>	<u>1.3</u>	<u>0.5</u>
Scout film plus diapositive mask	2.5	2.5	2.5

Superimposition of Diapositive Mask and Angiogram Film

Because the angiogram film is made using the same exposure factors as the scout film, the density differences of areas A, B, and C should equal those on the scout film. Also on the angiogram film is the density of area D, the contrast-filled vessels. If the angiogram film is superimposed over the diapositive mask, it can be readily seen that the only contrast that exists is between the contrast-filled vessels (area D) and the densities from areas A, B, and C. The contrast-filled vessels stand out clearly against the homogeneous background.

	Area A	Area B	Area C	Area D
Reverse tone mask	1.9	1.3	0.5	0.0
Angiogram film	<u>0.6</u>	<u>1.2</u>	<u>2.0</u>	<u>0.3</u>
Reverse tone plus angiogram film	2.5	2.5	2.5	0.3

It is important that the film used to prepare the diapositive mask produce a negative complementary to that of the scout film. In other words, it must neither exaggerate nor lessen the density differences. This property is a function of the film gamma (G), a sensitometric measurement that corresponds to the maximum slope, or gradient, of the characteristic curve of the film. This gamma is calculated by the use of a characteristic curve and by the following formula:

$$\text{Gamma} = \frac{D_2 - D_1}{\log E_2 - \log E_1}$$

where log E is the logarithmic value of the relative exposure and D is density.

Film used for subtraction must have a gamma of 1 (Fig. 2-12). The subtraction films available are designed to yield a gamma of 1 when processed automatically. In general, subtraction films possess only one emulsion side, which should be remembered when preparing the diapositive mask. It is essential that the emulsion side of the subtraction film be placed in close contact with the scout film when making the diapositive mask.

If a permanent record of the superimposed diapositive mask and angiogram film is required, a copy of the superimposed films can easily be made.

Subtraction can be performed by radiographic, photographic, electronic, and computer-assisted (digital) methods.

Digital Subtraction

Digital radiography has the same type of limitation as conventional radiography when it comes to the image. Because tomographic principles are not applied to digital radiography in general, there is some superimposition of details in the image. As in conventional radiography, the

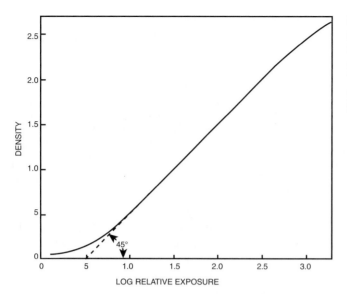

FIGURE 2-12. A sensitometric curve of du Pont Cronex subtraction film, showing that the curve forms a 45-degree angle with the base line. This produces a gamma of 1, a property necessary for all film used to make subtraction prints.

superimposition can obscure details and compromise the diagnostic value of the procedure. Digital radiography uses the principle of subtraction to achieve an image without superimposition. When applied to advanced radiography angiographic procedures, it is referred to as digital subtraction angiography (DSA).

DSA is more than just a technical method of producing a diagnostic film; it is a computer-assisted diagnostic procedure.

DSA depends on the use of certain image acquisition system components for successful results. The major components include a high-performance generator system (with capabilities in the 1000- to 1300-mA range), a high-quality image intensifier, a high-quality video camera, and an electronic computer system capable of processing and storing data. DSA uses an analog to digital converter to translate the attenuated x-ray beam (analog information) into binary numbers (digital information), which can be manipulated and stored as required by the physician. These components are usually matched to provide the highest quality image possible. DSA may be described in terms of the procedure, image processing, and image storage.

Before the digitized subtracted image can be displayed on a cathode ray tube (CRT) screen or stored as analog data, it must be passed through a digital-to-analog converter (DAC). This process is similar to that occurring in the analog-to-digital converter (ADC), but in this case the solid-state electronics generate an output voltage proportional to the digital number. The resultant electrical pulses are then converted into the light and dark patterns of the image on the television monitor.

Medical Aspects. DSA was accomplished by both the intravenous and intra-arterial methods of introducing the contrast agent into the patient. Originally, a somewhat modified technique of the basic intravenous method for contrast injection was used exclusively. The use of the intravenous injection presented several advantages over catheter angiography—the procedure could be performed on an outpatient basis, thus avoiding the cost of a hospital stay, and complications and pain that can result from the placement of catheters could be avoided. The procedure promised to be less of a risk and much less expensive than catheter angiography.

The intravenous digital subtraction method had several disadvantages. Among these were the constant problem of both voluntary and involuntary motion artifacts, superimposition of vessels caused by the generalized opacification from the intravenous injection, limitations on the study imposed by diminished cardiac output in certain patients, and the disadvantages of the large volume of contrast agent required for intravenous injection. The ability of the system components to detect lower levels of contrast made intravenous DSA a relatively safe and cost-effective technique.

Intra-arterial concentrations of 40 to 50% are required to produce satisfactory contrast images during standard angiographic procedures. Generally speaking, concentrations of less than 5% are not visible, even when routine subtraction techniques are used. Digital subtraction enables contrast agent concentrations as low as 1 to 3% to be visualized when they are administered intravenously. The amount of contrast agent that will produce satisfactory digital subtraction angiograms is generally about 0.70 ml/kg body weight. For example, a person weighing 150 lb (68.04 kg) would require approximately 48 ml of contrast agent to provide the necessary arterial contrast. An automatic injection device is required to deliver the contrast agent bolus. The intravenous injection procedure can be modified by first loading approximately 40 ml of saline solution into the syringe and then loading the appropriate amount of contrast agent. This layering of saline solution and contrast agent allows the contrast medium to be pushed through the venous system as a bolus to allow the maximum concentration to be delivered to the arterial system. Intravenous injections can also be made with a catheter placed in the superior vena cava. Another modification to the injection method is the use of the Angiocatheter type of venous catheter, which reduces the possibility of contrast agent extravasation.

A variety of advances in intra-arterial catheter techniques have changed the approach to DSA. Intra-arterial catheter insertion is now being done on a same-day basis. After the procedure, the patient is returned to the ambulatory surgery department for recovery and is usually released the same day. The primary reason, however, for the change to intra-arterial injection was the consistency of the results and the dramatic increase in the quality of the images produced.

The improved image quality resulted from the reduction or elimination of many of the disadvantages of the intravenous injection method. Motion artifacts were limited because the contrast agent was delivered to the site under study and imaging could proceed without delay. Lower doses of the contrast agent (15 to 20 ml for arterial DSA and 40 to 50 ml for intravenous DSA) coupled with use of the nonionic contrast agents reduced the incidence of many of the symptoms experienced by the patient. This made the study more comfortable, which further reduced involuntary motion. The smaller doses and direct delivery also diminished the dependence on cardiac output to deliver a sufficient bolus for opacification of the anatomy. The arterial injections are also made with smaller catheters (usually 4F or 5F), which diminishes the incidence of postcatheterization bleeding. One added advantage of the intra-arterial method was that conventional angiography could be used interchangeably with DSA. This allowed the performance of the conventional procedure without the need for a return visit or additional catheterization if the study could not be performed using the DSA method.

Image Storage. The images resulting from the subtraction process can be stored in a short-term storage system as either digital or analog information. This type of storage can be considered primary storage, which occurs in the memory unit of the computer. If another procedure is performed, the short-term stored information is replaced by the newly generated data. The long-term storage of data requires that secondary storage systems be available.

Equipment. The computer hardware and system designs used for DSA vary with the individual manufacturers of the components. The x-ray tube should be specifically designed for digital subtraction, especially in a dedicated DSA suite; however, standard angiographic tubes will function adequately during DSA under normal use.

The tube should have a high thermal capacity anode as well as dual focal spot capabilities. The larger focal spot will be used during DSA, because this is a low-resolution procedure. The small focal spot can be used for fluoroscopy, cineangiography, and some magnification work.

The x-ray generator should be a three-phase or high-frequency system. It should be linked with the computer to provide test exposures that are then computer adjusted to optimize the final exposure factors and provide the correct amount of light output from the image intensifier. The generator should be able to provide pulsed as well as continuous fluorography. If possible, the generator should be able to control the radiation dose (*photon flux*) according to the amount of contrast agent used. This is useful when DSA is performed on a patient whose tolerance to large doses of contrast agent is low. In such cases, the x-ray exposure could be increased and a smaller amount of contrast agent used, with satisfactory results.

The image intensifier input screen is usually a cesium iodide (CsI) scintillator that serves to convert the x-rays into light. As in conventional image intensification systems, the input scintillator directs the light to a photocathode layer, which converts the light into electrons. The electrons are drawn to the output screen that contains a phosphor, which converts the electrons back into a light image. Because of the high kinetic energy of the electrons, each one is capable of producing 1000 light photons, thereby increasing the brightness of the original image. The image intensification system should operate without loss of contrast at an exposure rate of 1 to 2 mR per image.

The television camera is the next link in the digital subtraction system. The image intensifier must also have some type of filtration or aperture system to control the light level striking the television camera and to allow for the change of photon flux provided by the generator. Signal-to-noise ratio (SNR) is a critical factor in this component of the system. Generally, noise as it applies electronically refers to anything that serves to hide the signal being measured. The SNR is the ratio of the signal voltage to the noise voltage. Table 2-4 illustrates the SNRs of different radiographic systems. A television system should be chosen that provides the highest SNR possible to control the intrinsic system noise.

Another component in the television link is the monitor itself. Conventional television monitors have a format of 525 lines (rasters) for a single frame of video information. There are two methods by which the video information is displayed on the television monitor—the interlaced scan and the progressive scan. The interlaced scan mode reads out the video information in two separate scanning fields, with each containing half of the total 525 raster lines of the television tube. The completed video picture, also called a frame, is read out onto two separate scanning fields, with each containing $262\frac{1}{2}$ raster lines. When the two $262\frac{1}{2}$ raster line fields are interlaced, they form one complete frame comprising 525 raster lines.

The progressive scan reads out the entire frame of video information on the single 525-line field. Using the progressive system decreases the possibilities of motion artifacts occurring and allows for what is called the "snapshot" mode in digital fluoroscopy. The snapshot mode separates the x-ray exposure from the camera readout. The exposure is made with the television system blanked out, and the resultant image is stored on the face of the pickup tube. The information is read and then can be digitized. The advantage of using this type of mode is that the exposure time can be very short, which has the effect of stopping any motion. It is disadvantageous in that the rapid acquisition of information is compromised. In considering the components for this segment of the system, it would be useful to have both scan modes available—the progressive scan mode for snapshot digital fluorography and the interlaced mode for regular fluoroscopic applications.

Imaging Capabilities. All digital subtraction units available today provide for real-time subtraction. This means that the subtracted images can be displayed for viewing while the procedure is still being performed. The images can be produced by pulsed digital fluorography (serial imaging) or continuous digital fluorography (dynamic imaging). Figure 2-13 provides typical examples of digital subtraction images.

Pulsed digital fluorography is similar to conventional serial radiography. It is often used when image acquisition rates range from one to eight images per second.

Continuous digital fluorography is similar to cineradiography, with image acquisition occurring at a rate of 30 frames per second. This type of imaging is used for visualizing dynamic or rapidly changing processes. A disadvantage of the continuous digital fluorography method is the decrease in resolution of

TABLE 2-4 *Summary of Signal-to-Noise Ratios of Various Radiographic Systems*

System	Signal-to-Noise Ratio
Standard radiography	100:1
Standard fluoroscopy	200:1
Dedicated digital fluoroscopy	1000:1

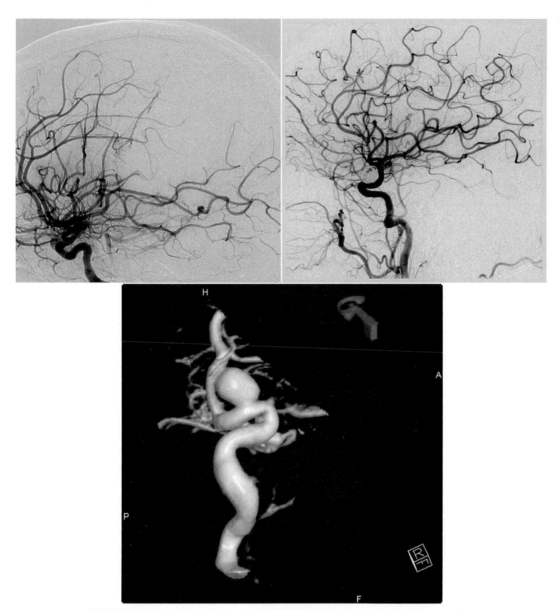

FIGURE 2-13.   Several examples of digital subtraction angiography.

the image compared with images produced by the pulsed digital method. There also is a decrease in exposure times when this type of imaging is used.

There are three methods of performing subtraction in digital radiography—temporal (mask mode) subtraction, energy subtraction, and hybrid subtraction.

Temporal subtraction requires that an image be recorded before the introduction of the contrast agent. This image is referred to as the **mask**. Images recorded after the introduction of the contrast agent are then subtracted from the mask; that is, all of the information that was present on the mask is eliminated from subsequent images, leaving only the images of the opacified vessels. Temporal subtraction can be performed in different modes depending on how the images are collected. The various modes of temporal subtraction are serial mask mode, continuous mode, time interval difference, and postprocessing subtraction. Table 2-5 lists the differences among these methods.

TABLE 2-5 *Comparison of the Various Modes of Temporal Subtraction*

Mode	Method of Acquisition	Use
Serial mask	1. X-ray beam is pulse. 2. Preinjection mask image is recorded. 3. Contrast is injected. 4. Postinjection images are subtracted from mask at a rate of about one or two per second. 5. Images are stored.	Carotid arteriography Peripheral arteriography Visceral arteriography Renal arteriography
Continuous	1. X-ray beam is continuous, similar to conventional fluoroscopy but with higher mA values. 2. Preinjection mask image is recorded. 3. Contrast is injected. 4. Fluoroscopic images are continuously subtracted from the mask. 5. Images are stored.	Pulmonary arteriography Assessment of heart wall motion Coronary arteriography for bypass patency
Time interval	1. Image acquisition occurs at a rate of 30 frames per second. 2. Preinjection mask image is recorded. 3. Contrast is injected. 4. Subtraction is performed at specified time interval. 5. Subtracted image becomes new mask. 6. New mask is subtracted from subsequent images at the predetermined interval. 7. Each new subtracted image becomes the new mask for the next interval subtraction. 8. Images are stored.	Cardiac angiography Imaging of moving structures
Postprocedure	1. Stored images are retrieved. 2. Images are manipulated or reviewed.	Stored image manipulation

Energy subtraction is based on the attenuation differences of the various types of tissue and the iodine in the contrast agent and on their relationship to the energy—peak kilovoltage (kVp)—of the x-ray beam. This method of subtraction requires equipment that differs from that used for temporal subtraction. The generator must be capable of switching kilovoltage during the exposures; there must also be a changing filtration system because this type of subtraction requires that images be recorded at two different energy levels (a low energy level and a high energy level). The two images can then be subtracted, and either bone or soft tissue can be removed from the subsequent images. One advantage to this type of subtraction is that motion artifacts can be reduced.[2]

Hybrid subtraction combines the best characteristics of temporal and energy subtraction methods. Images can be produced with the motion artifacts eliminated or reduced by subtracting the soft tissue via energy subtraction while the bone is eliminated via temporal subtraction.[3]

Temporal subtraction is by far the most common method of digital subtraction.

Once the digital subtraction images are produced, they can be either stored or manipulated. A useful component is the array processor, which can perform a series of image manipulations very rapidly. One such manipulation is **image reregistration (remasking)**. As discussed earlier, motion of any sort between the production of the images can interfere with the subtraction process by causing misregistration. The array processor shifts the contrast agent image up or down in relation to the precontrast agent mask image to compensate for any motion between the two images, a process known as image reregistration. This can be an extremely important option when performing digital subtraction in areas in which motion cannot be avoided, such as during cardiac imaging.

SUMMARY

Certain special procedures require that the image be recorded rapidly to capture the pathologic or physiologic processes being studied. To accomplish this, special image recording devices are necessary. There are two major categories of imaging devices: those that record the image directly and those that record the image indirectly.

The large-film rapid sequence changers can be categorized as direct image recording systems. Despite the different forms of recording media (e.g., cut film, spot film, roll film) transported in this category, all of the changers had similar operational periods: the transport period (when the film is in motion) and the stationary period (when the film is stopped and exposed).

The indirect image recording systems include the videotape recorder, videodisc systems, recordable CD M–DICOM 3 CD-ROM systems, serial spot filming devices, and cinefluorographic systems. All of these devices record the image indirectly; that is, they capture the images from the output phosphor of an image intensification system. These devices can be further subdivided into those systems that record the images from the electrical signal generated by the television camera (videotape and recordable CD-ROM systems) and those systems that record the images directly from the output phosphor of the II tube (serial spot filming and cinefluorographic cameras).

These recording systems can be used alone or in combination, depending on the configuration of the equipment.

REFERENCES

1. Digital Imaging and Communications in Medicine (DICOM) – PS 3.1 – 2003. Rosslyn, Virginia, National Electrical Manufacturers Association, 2003, p. 5.
2. Brody WR, Macovski A: Dual energy digital radiography, *Diagn Imag* 3:18, 1981.
3. Guthaner D, Brody WR, Lewis BD, Keyes GS, Belanger BF: Clinical application of hybrid subtraction digital angiography: Preliminary resutls, *Cardiovasc Intervent Radiol* 6:290, 1983.

SUGGESTED READINGS

Intensifying Screens, Grids, and Film

Bushberg JT, Seibert JA, Leidholdt E, Boone J: *The Essential Physics of Medical Imaging*, 2nd ed. Philadelphia, 2002, Lippincott Williams & Wilkins.
Holdsworth DW, Pollmann SI, Nikolov HN, Fahrig R: Correction of XRII geometric distortion using a liquid-filled grid and image subtraction. *Med Phys* 32(1):55–64, 2005.
National Electrical Manufacturers Association, 1300 N. 17th Street, Rosslayn, Virginia, 22209; accessed at http://medical.nema.org/.
Shephard CT: *Radiographic Image Production and Manipulation*. New York, 2003, McGraw-Hill.

Digital Radiography

Abella H: CTA matches DSA's safety for renal artery stenosis—Both techniques produce similar rates of side effects from contrast media, 2002, http://www.dimag.com/
Kaiser CP: Multidetector CT nudges MRA, DSA in neuroimaging—Convergence of hardware and software advances allows comprehensive head and neck evaluations in minutes, 2003, http://www.dimag.com/

Merjering EHW, Zuiderveld M, Viergever MA: Image registration for digital subtraction angiography. *Int J Computer Vision* 31(2/3):227–246, 1999.

Matsuda T, Yasuhara Y, Kano A, Mochizuki A, Ikezoe J: Effect of temporal subtraction technique on the diagnosis of primary lung cancer with chest radiography. *Radiat Med* 21(3):112–119, 2003.

Xiujiang R, Shaw CC, Xinming L, Lemacks MR, Thompson SK: Comparison of an amorphous silicon/cesium iodide flat-panel digital chest radiography system with screen/film and computed radiography systems—a contrast–detail phantom study. *Med Phys* 28(Issue 11):xx, 2001.

STUDY QUESTIONS

1. Simultaneous radiography in two planes is referred to as:
   - **a.** cineradiography
   - **b.** biplane radiography
   - **c.** indirect digital conversion
   - **d.** temporal subtraction

2. The standard for file formats for the archiving and communications of medical images that could be understood by equipment and systems manufactured by different companies is called the _____ standard.
   - **a.** NEMA
   - **b.** DACOM 3
   - **c.** DICOM
   - **d.** ACR

3. When rapid serial changers are used, there is a period of time during which the exposure contact was closed in relation to the cycle of the line voltage. This is referred to as the _____ time.
   - **a.** phase in
   - **b.** transport
   - **c.** zero delay
   - **d.** stationary

4. Which of the following terms is *not* associated with the term "analog"?
   - **a.** ambiguity
   - **b.** continuity
   - **c.** imprecision
   - **d.** discrete

5. The computer software program that converts the digital signal into a usable image is called a(n) _____.
   - **a.** algorithm
   - **b.** array
   - **c.** matrix
   - **d.** pixel

6. The process by which an image of the *differences* between two similar images is produced is referred to as:
   - **a.** quantization
   - **b.** digitization
   - **c.** subtraction
   - **d.** transformation.

7. In most digital systems in use today the maximum number of gray levels that can be produced for each pixel is:
   - **a.** 256
   - **b.** 512
   - **c.** 1024
   - **d.** 4096

8. Displaying a group of 16 shades of grays at a time is termed:
   - **a.** subtraction
   - **b.** masking
   - **c.** windowing
   - **d.** conversion

9. The radiographic system that uses cassettes equipped with a photostimulable phosphor plate is referred to as:
   - **a.** computed radiography
   - **b.** direct digital radiography
   - **c.** flat panel detection
   - **d.** fluoroscopy

10. The image intensifier input screen uses a(n) _____ scintillator to produce light when stimulated by x-ray photons.
    - **a.** amorphous selenium
    - **b.** barium platinocide
    - **c.** cesium iodide
    - **d.** calcium tungstate

3 *Automatic Injection Devices*

CHAPTER OBJECTIVES

After completing this chapter, the reader will be able to perform the following:

- Identify the need for automatic injection devices
- List the basic components of an automatic injector
- List and describe the advantages of a detachable injector head
- List and describe the advantages of dual syringe capacity
- Define the concept of flow rate
- Identify the factors that affect the flow rate
- Explain the injectors that are used for computed tomography (CT) and magnetic resonance imaging (MRI)

CHAPTER OUTLINE

AUTOMATIC INJECTORS

    Basic Components

    Optional Components

    Injector Operation

CT INJECTORS

MRI INJECTORS

SUMMARY

M any special radiographic procedures require an injection of contrast medium under specific controlled conditions. Performing these injections by hand would make it difficult to maintain a consistent flow rate. Maintenance of a sufficient dilution of contrast agent in the blood is also difficult to achieve with an injection made by hand.

Angiography requires the delivery of a specific amount and concentration of contrast agent to the target area. As the contrast agent enters the bloodstream, it is diluted. This dilution effect is dependent on several factors, such as the injection site, size of the vessel, and type and iodine concentration of the contrast agent. The target site determines the speed (rate of flow) of the injection. Vessel size also affects the concentration of the contrast agent. The larger the vessel, the greater the flow rate must be to maintain the proper concentration of contrast medium so that the desired anatomic features can be visualized radiographically. In some procedures, flow rates of 30 to 40 ml of contrast material per second are not uncommon.★ These injections must be performed with a mechanical device in order to achieve consistency in the flow rates. The flow rate is controlled by many factors, such as the viscosity of the contrast medium, catheter length, catheter diameter, and injection pressure. The flow rate or injection speed can be increased or decreased by varying any of these parameters.

Most current injectors are designed for operation as either high- or low-pressure injectors, thereby broadening their usefulness in many types of angiographic procedures. The Medrad Avanta injector (Fig. 3-1, *A*) is a multimodality system that can be utilized in the cardiac and angiography arena as well

---

★Milliliters will be used throughout this text as the unit of measure for liquid and gas volumes.

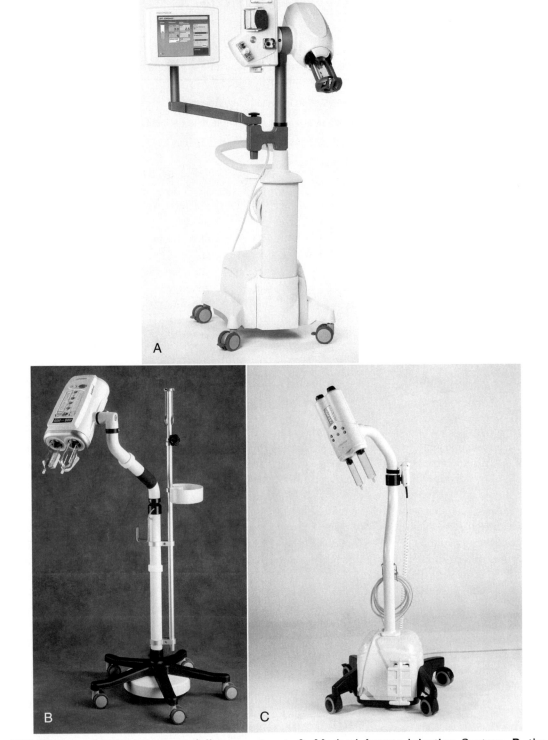

FIGURE 3-1. Medrad contrast delivery systems. **A**, Medrad Avanta Injection System, **B**, the Medrad Stellant CT Injector, and **C**, the Medrad Spectris Solaris EP MRI Injector System.

as for larger vessels and peripherals. The Medrad Avanta is capable of injecting contrast material in variable mode at low flow rates and low pressures, fixed mode at high flow rates and high-pressure injections, and fixed mode for saline flushing. Dedicated automatic injection systems such as the Medrad Stellant CT injection system and Spectris Solaris EP MRI injector are also available (see Fig. 3-1, *B* and *C*). These systems can be configured with options specific to each of their respective modalities.

AUTOMATIC INJECTORS

Basic Components

All automatic injectors have certain components in common; each is equipped with a control panel, syringe, heating device, and high-pressure mechanism.

Control Panel

Each of the automatic injection devices has a control panel that is used to set the parameters of the injection sequence (Fig. 3-2). Depending on the unit and the optional equipment purchased, the control panel will appear more or less intricate. The injector systems are equipped with a touch screen display for ease of programming. Almost all of the units available are digitally controlled and ergonomically designed for ease of use. Some of the systems allow the control panel to be removed from the unit and taken to the control area during the procedure.

The controls and indicators present on the control panel vary with the type of options available with the system. These controls are clearly marked for ease of operation. In the Medrad ProVis Mark V injector the control panel is segmented and sequenced to guide the setup procedure. The system's rotating and tilting console is easily read in a variety of lighting situations and throughout a range of distances. The Angiomat Illumena injector is also equipped with a tilting and rotating console that allows for viewing from a wide variety of angles.

Many of the systems come equipped with optional electroluminescent displays. This type of display can be easily read from a variety of angles and under a wide range of lighting conditions. Some of the systems also have graphical user displays for easy setup and system monitoring. The EmpowerCT provides a number of voice prompts (spoken cues) that can quickly alert the operator to potential problems.

Each of the systems is supplied with an instruction manual that should be referred to if questions concerning operation or troubleshooting arise. The manufacturers also make available product manuals and technical assistance on their websites.

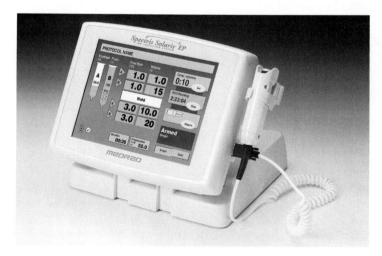

FIGURE 3-2. Medrad Spectris Solaris EP injector control panel illustrating a sample injection protocol.

Syringe

In all automatic injectors, the syringe is removable. Disposable syringes are available for use with all automatic injectors; these are presterilized and can be installed easily. The manufacturers also offer prefilled syringes for use with their systems. The syringes are completely disposable, thereby eliminating the possibility of cross-contamination from reusable parts. Syringe capacity varies with brand. The syringes come in a variety of sizes depending on the company and the automatic injector. These range from 60 ml to 200 ml with sizes of 125 ml, 130 ml, and 150 ml also available. The smaller syringes (60 ml) find wide usage in pediatric, neurologic, and coronary studies. The 130-ml and 150-ml syringes are mainly used in aortic, peripheral, hepatic, and left ventricular studies. The 200-ml syringe can be used when multiple studies are anticipated.

The syringe must be handled with care when preparing for a procedure because any abnormality can cause failure under operating conditions. It is wise to have extra syringes available in the special procedures suite so that if syringe failure or contamination occurs, a prolonged delay can be avoided. Figure 3-3 shows some syringes in use today. Latex-free syringes are also offered by the manufacturers to reduce the possibility of allergic reactions.

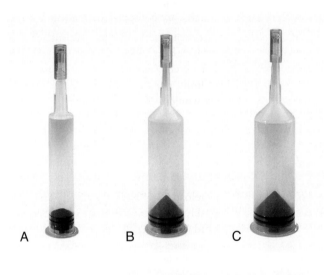

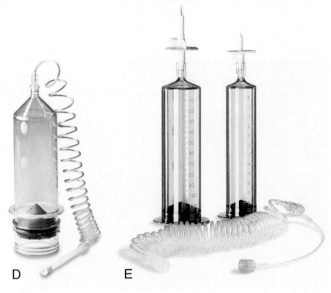

FIGURE 3-3. Automatic injection syringes. Medrad polypropylene disposable syringes: **A**, 60 ml, **B**, 150 ml, **C**, 200 ml, **D**, Medrad Stellant CT syringe, and **E**, the Medrad Solaris syringe kit.

Heating Device

The heating system is an electronic device that heats and maintains the contrast medium at or near body temperature and reduces the viscosity of certain contrast agents, thereby facilitating the setting of certain flow rates from the injector. It is usually located on the injector head close to the syringe. The syringe temperature is thermostatically controlled and is usually preset at the factory to a nominal 37° C (approximately 98° F). Heating time varies with the injector being used. Most injection device heaters can only maintain the temperature of the contrast agent. Therefore, the contrast agent should be prewarmed when using injection devices equipped with this type of heater.

Injector Power Heads and High-Pressure Mechanism

The injector power head is generally attached to an articulating arm that allows for a wide variety of positions during the injection. Digital displays are available on the power head indicating the protocol used and the amount of contrast available. Various configurations are available from free standing, attached to the injector module, and table or ceiling mounted power heads. Figure 3-4 illustrates some of the configurations available.

   The main type of high-pressure mechanism used on automatic injectors is the electromechanical system. This is simply an electric drive motor connected to a jackscrew that drives the piston into or out of the syringe. Figure 3-5 depicts a simplified version of an electromechanical high-pressure device. The high-pressure mechanisms of modern automatic injectors have several safety features built into them. The Medrad ProVis injector can prevent injections from exceeding their preset volume, flow rate, and pressure. There is also a mechanical stop that physically limits the injection volume to a preset amount. In the case of an electrical malfunction, the injection would still be limited by the device, which is not dependent upon electricity to function.

Optional Components
Double-Syringe Assembly

Also of interest is the double-syringe assembly, which allows preloading of two syringes. When one syringe has been emptied, the plunger is retracted and the assembly is turned 180 degrees to position the second syringe with minimum resulting time loss. The Medrad Mark V ProVis provides for varying configurations of the double syringe turret assembly. The syringe assembly can be configured as 60 ml/150 ml, 150 ml/150 ml, or 200 ml/200 ml on the same turret. Table 3-1 lists the syringe sizes and their applications. The E-Z-EM CT injector also is equipped with an injector head and display that swivels independently to allow for positioning the unit on either side of the CT gantry (see Fig. 3-6).

Safety Devices

Acceleration regulators and pressure-limiting devices can add optional safety features to the automatic injection device. The acceleration regulator allows the drive motor to be accelerated over a specific period of time, which reduces the possibility of catheter whip.

   Both simple devices, such as the rate rise control on the Angiomat Illumena, and sophisticated systems by which the flow rate may be selected according to various parameters, such as the Medrad universal flow module, are available. The latter not only can increase the flow rate to a specific level and maintain this level for the duration of the injection but also can achieve a final acceleration or deceleration of the flow rate after an initial level has been reached. With the Medrad Mark V ProVis injector, multiple-level injections can be programmed to allow for a wide variety of unusual flow patterns during the study. This is accomplished by having the flow rate change during the injection. The Medrad Mark V ProVis injector has the capability for four levels (flow rate and volume changes) per injection. Multiphasic and biphasic injection patterns as well as backflow studies and positive and negative accelerations are possible with this system. The rate rise is controlled in the Angiomat Illumena injector by digitally setting the transition time on the control panel.

Fundamentals of Special Radiographic Procedures

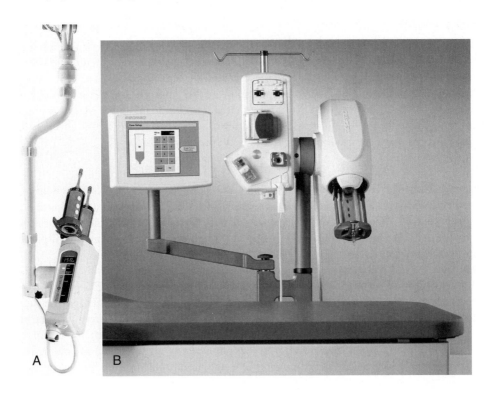

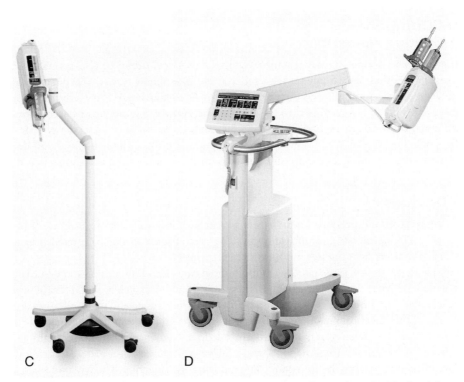

FIGURE 3-4. **A**, Medrad ProVis Counterpoise mounted configuration, **B**, Medrad Avanta table mounted configuration, **C**, Medrad ProVis free standing pedestal configuration, **D**, ProVis integrated pedestal mounted configuration.

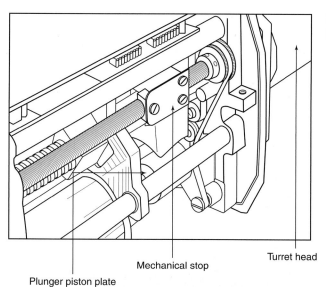

FIGURE 3-5. Typical electromechanical drive mechanism of automatic injectors.

Plunger piston plate

Mechanical stop

Turret head

TABLE 3-1   *Syringe Sizes and Their Associated Applications*

Syringe Size	Application
60 ml	Carotid arteriography
	Coronary arteriography
	Neuroangiography
	Pediatric angiography
	Renal angiography
150 ml	Aortography
	Hepatic angiography
	Peripheral angiography
200 ml	Multiple aortic studies

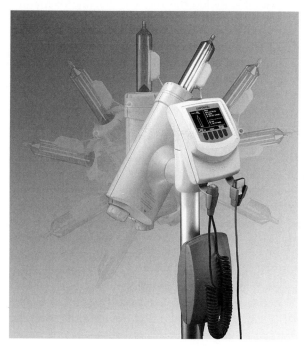

FIGURE 3-6. The E-Z-EM Empower CT injector rotating head for ease of positioning on either side of the patient couch.

Pressure-limiting devices set a maximum on the pressure permitted to be generated, thereby ensuring safe use of even low-pressure catheters. The pressure-limiting parameters for the Medrad Mark V ProVis will depend upon the syringe size and the flow scale (ml/s, ml/min, or ml/hr).

Volume-limiting devices are designed to set a maximum limit on the volume of contrast agent injected into the patient. The automatic safety stop device on the Medrad Mark V Plus will reposition itself automatically for each injection, providing for a recurring volume-limiting action and preventing the plunger from moving past a certain point.

Function-monitoring devices are available on all types of units. These devices may be simple, such as a ready light, or sophisticated, such as in the Medrad Mark V ProVis, which monitors the key functions and operation sequences of the injector. This device will alert the operator to an arming procedure or control setting that was overlooked as well as indicate both primary and secondary circuit features.

Most automatic injectors are designed to be triggered with the head pointed toward the floor to allow air bubbles that may be present to collect at the far end of the syringe and not be injected into the patient. Modern injectors also have some sort of air detection device to prevent the accidental injection of a large bolus of air into the patient. Although these units are equipped with such a device, it is not a substitute for visual inspection and careful attention to all aspects of the injection procedure.

The EmpowerCT injector system also provides an Extravasation Detection Accessory safety device on the system that will alert the technologist and abort the injection if variations indicate extravasation. The injector has a "help" feature included that will provide immediate assistance if there is a problem. It is similar to the help button in windows programs and can provide assistance in troubleshooting the unit in case of an operational difficulty. The CTA system also has an easy-to-read graphical readout screen showing status and volume of syringe filling in auto mode (Fig. 3-7).

Injector Operation

When programming the automatic injector, the radiographer must be concerned with one primary factor—the *flow rate*. Flow rate can be defined simply as the delivery rate (amount delivered per unit of time). It is dependent on the viscosity of the contrast agent, the length and diameter of the catheter, and

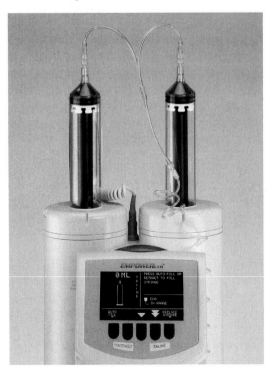

FIGURE 3-7. Closeup of the E-Z-EM injector head showing the readout display for manual and auto filling.

the injection pressure. The flow rate chosen for a specific procedure is governed by the procedure itself, the vessel entered, the patient, and the nature of the disease. Flow rates can vary from as low as 4 ml/s to as high as 30 to 40 ml/s, depending on these factors.

Constant Flow Rate

When constant flow injectors are used, the desired flow rate and injection time are set, and the selected volume in milliliters per second will be delivered regardless of the variables involved. For example, if a flow rate of 50 ml/s and a volume of 100 ml are required, they are programmed on the injector as 50 ml/s injection rate for 2 s. This setting will deliver the specific volume at the desired flow rate regardless of the viscosity of the contrast medium or any other parameters involved. Care must be exercised when flow rates are set because too high a flow rate may injure the patient or damage the catheter.

Constant flow rate injectors provide adjustable pressure during the injection. The unit changes the pressure to adapt to the parameters involved in the study. These types of injection systems are usually equipped with pressure-limiting devices that prevent the injector from producing pressures beyond the safety limits of the catheter being used. The radiographer is responsible for setting this factor on the injector before the study. It is important that the pressure limitations of the catheters being used are known. Some low-flow catheters have a maximum bursting pressure of 500 psi, while higher flow, reinforced-wall catheters have maximum pressures that may exceed 1000 to 1200 psi. If the pressure-limiting device for a low-flow catheter were set for a maximum of 800 psi, this would exceed the safe operating range and be potentially harmful to the patient.

Another consideration involves setting the pressure-limiting device too low for the parameters involved. Each combination of parameters used (catheter length, diameter, number of side holes, type and viscosity of the contrast agent, etc.) requires a minimum amount of pressure to maintain the selected flow rate. (This pressure should be below the maximum rating for the catheter involved.) If the pressure-limiting device was set below this minimum level, the injection would be made with a decreased flow rate. For example, assume that a particular set of parameters requires 450 psi to maintain a flow rate of 6 ml/s and the catheter is rated at 800 psi. If the radiographer sets the pressure-limiting device at 150 psi, the injector would not be able to produce the minimum pressure required for the desired flow rate; in this case, the flow rate would be reduced to 3 ml/s.

Varying the parameters used for a particular study can change the pressure required. If the maximum safe operating pressure is exceeded and the desired flow rate cannot be achieved with the selected parameters, other combinations should be considered. The types of changes that can be considered are summarized as follows:

1. Catheter diameter. The catheter with the **larger overall internal diameter** (ID) (lumen) will provide less resistance against the flow of contrast media and require less pressure to maintain a selected flow rate.
2. Catheter length. The catheter with the **overall greater length** will provide more resistance to flow than one that is shorter because the resistance is applied over a longer length of catheter tubing.

If the major parameters cannot be varied, the removal of nonessential components in the system can decrease the resistance to flow and drastically reduce the pressure needed to maintain the flow rate; this refers to any tubes or fittings that would be in the path of the syringe and the catheter.

If the components of the system cannot be varied, a reduction in the resistance can be accomplished by warming the contrast agent or using a contrast medium with a lower iodine concentration which would naturally have less viscosity, thereby reducing the resistance to flow. The contrast agent must not be heated above the nominal 37° C (approximately 98° F) or damage to the blood vessel could occur.

Injection Pressure

Electromechanically powered injectors usually indicate the actual pressures used during the injection procedure. The pressure range available is from 100 to 1000 psi, which allows a wide range of flow rates when combined with the variable parameters discussed previously.

Table 3-2 illustrates some basic parameters used for various procedures. It should be noted that these are only guidelines and that actual parameters may differ with the institution, physician, and patient. The guidelines are also recommended for unsubtracted imaging. If digital subtraction is used, the volumes can be reduced by 50% or diluted with normal saline to a 50% concentration.

CT INJECTORS

CT procedures require a high degree of control over the injection and its parameters to maximize the accuracy of the study. Injection systems used for CT have the same basic components as those used for angiography. The injector head can be either floor mounted or track mounted on an overhead system. In many cases, the console is mounted inside the control booth for maximum operator safety. The Liebel-Flarsheim CT 9000 ADV (Fig. 3-8) allows a variable flow rate, from 10 ml/hr to 10 ml/s. This

TABLE 3-2 *Basic Guidelines for Contrast Agent Rates and Volumes*

Anatomic Area	Volume/Second	Total Volume
Abdominal aorta	25 ml	50 ml
Thoracic aorta	35 ml	70 ml
Aortic bifurcation	15 ml	30 ml
Major vessels directly off aorta	10 ml	20 ml
Selective vessels	5 ml	10 ml

Adapted from data supplied to Medrad, Inc., by Jorge A. Lopez, MD, Assistant Professor, University of Texas, Southwestern Medical Center, Dallas.

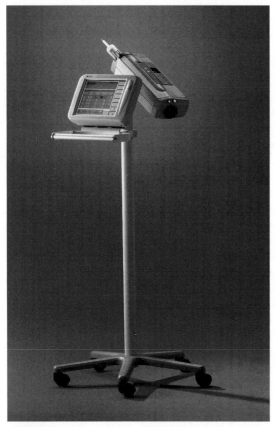

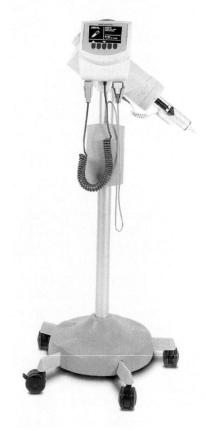

FIGURE 3-8. The Mallinckrodt Liebel-Flarsheim CT 9000 ADV injector system.

FIGURE 3-9. The E-Z-EM Empower CT injector system.

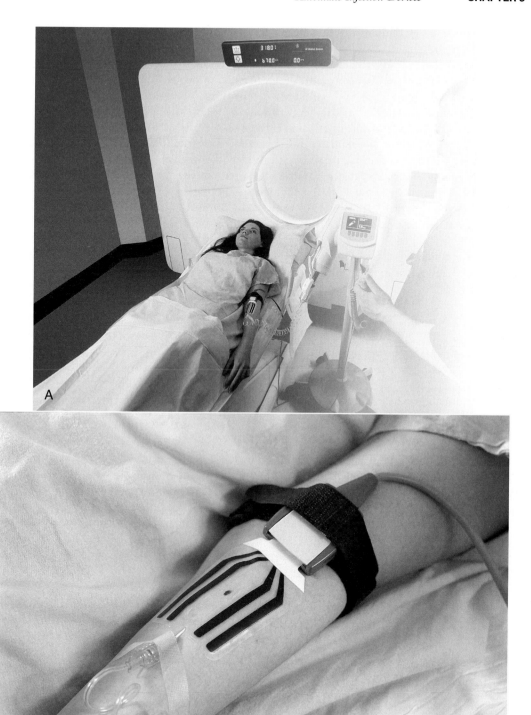

FIGURE 3-10. **A**, Extravasation device attached to a patient ready for the CT procedure. **B**, Closeup of the extravasation device.

unit also allows programming injection delays from 0 to 255 s in 0.01-s intervals for use during multiphasic studies.

The Empower CT injector (Fig. 3-9) has the same safety systems as the previously discussed injectors, including pressure limitation, tilt sensor lockout to prevent air embolism, voice prompts to alert operators to potential problems, and an extravasation detection accessory. The extravasation detector monitors the patient's skin impedance and alerts the technologist to the potential extravasation and also pauses the injection to further protect the patient (Fig. 3-10). The unit is also equipped with a feature that permits a pause in the injection; the injection can then be resumed on command. The parameters of the pause, such as the phase number, pause mode, elapsed time, and volume remaining, are displayed on the console. The display is a high-contrast electroluminescent display that is easily seen under ambient lighting conditions from a variety of different angles (Fig. 3-11). The Empower CT is also capable of storing more than 50 anatomically referenced preprogrammed procedures that can be recalled when needed. It also has a touch screen display allowing rapid system control by the technologist (Fig. 3-12).

With the Medrad Envision CT injection system, 1 to 8 phases per protocol can be programmed, allowing for a variety of different flow patterns during the study. The flow rate can be programmed from 0.1 to 9.9 ml/s, in 0.1-ml increments. A manual flow control dial allows for the adjustment of existing flow rates during the injection without having to abort the procedure. It is also capable of dual programming with the choice of flow rate/volume or flow rate/duration. The Envision CT also has a keep vein open (KVO) feature that minimizes the potential for clotting during pauses in the injection.

The E-Z-EM Empower injector system is manufactured with a dual-barrel injector head specifically designed for saline chase injections (Fig. 3-13). The routine use of a saline bolus "chaser" for certain CT studies may yield cost savings in terms of the contrast agent and present a decreased risk of contrast nephropathy. The chaser is administered immediately following the injection of the contrast agent. The purpose of the chaser is to provide better vessel enhancement while utilizing a lower dose of contrast medium.

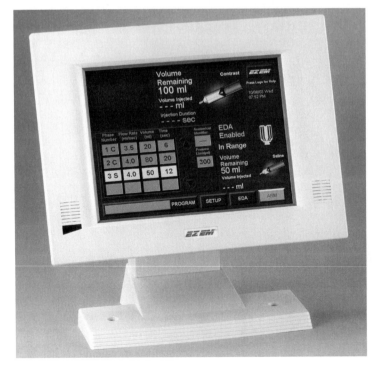

FIGURE 3-11. A closeup of the E-Z-EM Empower CT electroluminescent display.

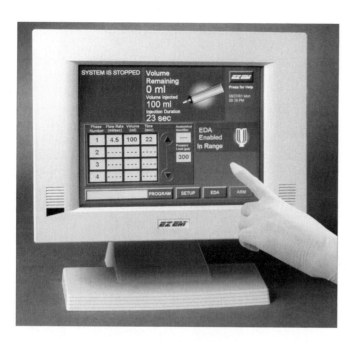

FIGURE 3-12. Closeup of the E-Z-EM Empower CT touch screen display.

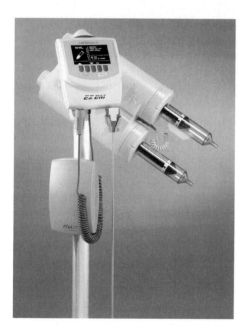

FIGURE 3-13. The E-Z-EM CTA injector system.

MRI INJECTORS

These injector systems must be manufactured of nonferrous materials in order to be safely used in the MRI suite. Injector systems used for these procedures are also equipped with similar safety features as the other injection systems. It is important that the capability to start and stop the injection be available from outside the magnet room. The Medrad Spectris Solaris EP (Enhanced Performance) and the Liebel-Flarsheim Optistar injector systems (Fig. 3–14) are equipped with a dual-syringe power head, which can provide for saline flush injections as well as single- and dual–phase contrast injections. The Solaris injector is designed to operate with magnets up to 3T. It also has an enhanced battery for more

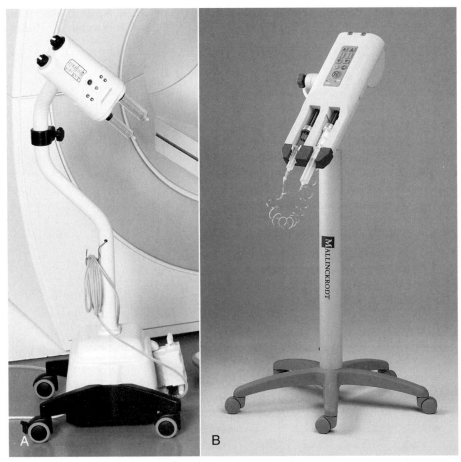

FIGURE 3-14. **A,** The Medrad Solaris injector system placed next to the magnet in the MRI suite. **B,** The Tyco-Mallinckrodt-Liebel Flarsheim Optistar MRI injector system.

injections between charges. The Spectris Solaris EP also has an integrated continuous battery charger (ICBC) that allows for conversion from battery to AC power within seconds and continuously charges the battery through an AC connection.

SUMMARY

Certain special procedures require the use of automatic injection devices. These devices vary by design but have certain features in common, including a syringe, a heating device, and a pressure mechanism. Automatic injection devices manufactured and in use today use an electromechanical high-pressure device. The constant flow rate delivery of contrast medium has become the standard. This implies that there will be a known amount of contrast agent delivered per unit of time regardless of the parameters of the system.

The delivery (flow rate) of the contrast agent to the patient is affected by any part of the system between the syringe and the patient that affects the resistance of the contrast medium to flow. Variables such as catheter ID, length, and side holes; contrast agent viscosity; and accessory items contribute to the resistance to flow. These factors should be considered when planning the study, and equipment choices should be made to optimize the delivery of the contrast agent.

SUGGESTED READINGS

Brown DB, Papadouris DC, Davis RV Jr, Vedantham S, Pilgram TK: Power injection of microcatheters: an in vitro comparison. *J Vasc Interv Radiol* 16(1):101–106, 2005.

Cohan RH, Ellis JH, Gardner WL: Extravasation of radiographic contrast material: recognition, prevention and treatment. *Radiology* 200:593–604, 1996.

Dorio PJ, Lee FT Jr, Hemseler M, et al: Using saline chaser to decrease contrast media in abdominal CT. *AJR Am J Roentgenol* 180:929–934, 2003.

Federle MP, Chang PJ, Scharmen C, Ozgun B:. Frequency and effects of extravasation of ionic and nonionic CT contrast media during rapid bolus injection. *Radiology* 206:637–640, 1998.

Funaki B: Central venous access: a primer for the diagnostic radiologist. *AJR Am J Roentgenol* 179(2):309–318, 2002.

Haage P, Schmitz-Rode T, Hubner D, et al: Reduction of contrast material dose and artifacts by saline flush using a double power injector in helical CT of the thorax. *AJR Am J Roentgenol* 164:1049–1053, 2000.

Herts BR, O'Malley CM, Wirth SL, Lieber ML, Pohlman B: Power injection of contrast media using central venous catheters feasibility, safety, and efficacy. *AJR Am J Roentgenol* 176:447–453, 2001.

Prince MR, Zhang Hong-Lei, Dong Q, Ersoy H: A Primer for dynamic MR injection. *Appl Radiol* 33:28–36, 2003.

Ruess L, Bulas DI, Rivera O, Markle BM: In-line pressures generated in small-bore central venous catheters during power injection of CT contrast media. *Radiology* 203:625–629, 1997.

Sanelli PC, Deshmukh M, Ougorets I, Caiati R, Heier LA: Safety and feasibility of using a central venous catheter for rapid contrast injection rates. *AJR Am J Roentgenol* 183(6):1829–1834, 2004.

STUDY QUESTIONS

1. Which of the following is not a part of the automatic injection device?
   a. acceleration regulator
   b. heating device
   c. rate/rise control
   d. receiving chamber

2. Which of the following factors affect the flow rate?
   i. catheter length
   ii. catheter diameter
   iii. miscibility of the contrast agent
   a. i only
   b. i and ii only
   c. i and iii only
   d. i, ii, and iii

3. The syringe temperature is regulated to a factory preset temperature of:
   a. 25° C
   b. 27° C
   c. 35° C
   d. 37° C

4. Which of the following statements is not true for constant flow rate injectors?
   a. The desired flow rate and injection time are set, and the selected volume in milliliters per second will be delivered.
   b. Too high a flow rate could possibly damage the catheter.
   c. Too low a flow rate could possibly injure the patient.
   d. These injectors provide a constant pressure during the injection.

5. Automatic injector safety devices include all but which of the following:
   a. detachable injector head
   b. volume-limiting device
   c. pressure-limiting device
   d. function monitoring device

Fundamentals of Special Radiographic Procedures

STUDY QUESTIONS (*cont'd*)

6. An acceleration regulator is a safety device that is used to prevent:
   a. catheter whip
   b. extravasation
   c. air embolus
   d. changing flow rates

7. When using an automatic injection device for digital subtraction angiography, the contrast agent should be:
   a. increased by 25%
   b. increased by 50%
   c. decreased by 25%
   d. decreased by 50%

8. The basic guideline for performing a contrast study of the abdominal aorta over a 2-s interval would be:
   a. 20 ml
   b. 35 ml
   c. 50 ml
   d. 70 ml

9. Which syringe volume would be used on an automatic injector for pediatric and neurologic angiography?
   a. 60 ml
   b. 100 ml
   c. 150 ml
   d. 200 ml

10. The safety feature found on the CT injection device that minimizes the potential for clotting during pauses in the injection is referred to as a(n):
    a. extravasation monitor
    b. air detection monitor
    c. KVO device
    d. catheter pressure fitting

4 *Instrumentation and Accessories*

Catheters used during diagnostic radiography act as pipelines for transporting the contrast agent from an external source to a location within the body. In special procedures, the instillation of contrast material by catheters allows the radiologist to selectively demonstrate specific anatomic areas. The most common use of catheterization is during vascular and cardiac interventional radiography (angiography), although catheters can also be used in many other nonvascular special radiographic procedures.

CATHETERS

Catheterization offers some definite benefits in radiography. When selective angiographic procedures are performed, the amount of contrast agent delivered to the patient is reduced. In these cases, a smaller amount of contrast agent delivered to a specific area through a catheter will maintain the proper concentration for good radiographic visualization. Direct injection into a remote vessel with the bolus traveling through the circulatory system to a specific location requires that a large amount of contrast material be injected to offset the dilution that occurs. If less contrast medium is used, the procedure is easier for the patient to tolerate; fewer subjective and objective symptoms are produced, and the patient is more relaxed and cooperative during the procedure. Other advantages of catheterization include the possibility of biopsy and the ability to measure pressures within the lumen of vessels or directly from the chambers of the heart.

Catheters are simply tubes of varying lengths and inside diameters with holes in each end that allow the contrast agent to flow through. Originally, catheters were adaptations of ureteral catheters that were constructed of rubber, but this soon gave way to the various thermoplastic catheters manufactured today. Catheters are manufactured out of Teflon, polypropylene, polyurethane, and polyethylene. Each of these materials possesses different characteristics that make them suitable for different procedures (Box 4-1). One major advance in catheter manufacturing was the development of the radiopaque polyethylene catheter, which allowed the radiologist to follow the path of the catheter through the body to its destination. Radiopaque catheters usually have different characteristics than the nonopaque varieties.

A wide variety of catheters and catheter systems are available for use during special procedure radiography. These range from the simple straight catheter with one end hole to complex catheter systems designed to perform more than one function. A discussion of every type of catheter and catheter system is beyond the scope of this textbook. However, the companies that manufacture catheters and accessories will provide catalogs illustrating their product lines. In most cases, the catalogs include data sheets that usually illustrate and reference each product and provide a short description of each catheter or accessory. These companies are also represented on the Internet and provide online catalogs with descriptions of their product lines. They also provide easy-to-use search engines to aid in finding a particular product.

All catheters manufactured today are disposable; that is, they are designed to be used once and then discarded. Some accessory items are still manufactured as "reusable." These items are designed to be cleaned, repackaged, and sterilized after the procedure. These must be inspected carefully during the cleaning process for any visible flaws. If any are noted, the item should be discarded.

The choice of the catheter or catheter system is made by the physician performing the procedure and is usually designated in the advanced procedure or catheterization laboratory procedure protocols. An understanding of the various standard catheters that are available is necessary. The interventional radiographer often is responsible for the ordering and maintenance of materials including the catheters used in the various procedures.

In some research institutions catheters are custom made by the physician to meet the specifics of the procedure being studied. Catheter tubing is available from certain manufacturers and can be custom formed. Appendix 1 illustrates the method of specialized catheter formation from standard catheter tubing.

BOX 4-1   *Advantages of Various Catheter Materials*

Teflon	Polyurethane	Polyethylene
Good memory—retains shape	High tissue compatibility	High tissue compatibility
High material strength	Increased lumen diameters	Contains no additives
Stiffer than other materials	Increased flow rate	Soft and flexible
Larger inner diameters	Low thrombogenicity	Better torque than polyurethane
Higher potential to kink	Ease of insertion and placement	
	Gas sterilized only	
	Low incidence of tissue trauma	

Size

Catheter sizes are expressed in inches or millimeters or by French number.

The gauge scale known as the French scale was developed by Charrière, a French instrument maker (1803–1876). On Charrière's gauge scale, 1 Charrière (or 1 French [1F][1]) is equal to a diameter of $^1/_3$ mm, with each consecutive Charrière differing from the previous one by $^1/_3$ mm. Table 4-1 lists the millimeter conversions for French numbers from 1 to 30.

If the diameter is expressed in inches, it is necessary to know that 1 in = 25.4 mm. To convert from inches to millimeters, simply multiply the number of inches by 25.4. For example, if the catheter diameter is 0.056 in, the conversion to millimeters is accomplished by multiplying 0.056 by 25.4 to give 1.42 mm as the catheter diameter.

Figure 4-1 illustrates a gauge scale that was used which listed size specifications for cardiovascular catheters, facilitating the conversion from inches to millimeters or to French size. The gauge scale also shows the relative sizes of various catheters from 3 French to 34 French. Table 4-2 lists the size specifications for a selection of both standard and thin-walled cardiovascular catheters.

Some companies imprint sizing information on the hub, the proximal portion of the catheter that provides an attachment for the injector or syringes. Diagnostic catheters have the French size, length, and guide wire size imprinted on the hub. Interventional catheters show the same information on the injectate hub, whereas the inflation hub shows the inflated balloon size in millimeters and the usable balloon length in centimeters.

Shape and Utility

The distal end of the catheter can be either straight or shaped. The shape of the catheter depends on the type of procedure being done and the anatomic part being imaged. Specialized shapes are used for a variety of studies including entry into smaller vessels during selective angiography (Fig. 4-2), cardiac electrophysiology studies, and ablation procedures. There are a wide variety of catheter shapes available; some possible configurations of the distal ends of catheters are illustrated in Figure 4-3.

Interventional radiology and cardiac catheterization have spawned the development of catheters that serve a variety of purposes. Catheters are available that contain attachments allowing various tests and measurements to be performed during the procedures. Other catheters are equipped with small balloons that mechanically occlude vessels and allow hemodynamic studies to be performed as well as providing hemorrhage control, segmental isolation, and selective distribution of contrast media or therapeutic drugs. Catheters are also manufactured and equipped with baskets or forceps that allow the

TABLE 4-1　*French Gauge Scale Conversions*

Charrière	OD (mm)	Charrière	OD (mm)	Charrière	OD (mm)
1	$^1/_3$	11	$3^2/_3$	21	7
2	$^2/_3$	12	4	22	$7^1/_3$
3	1	13	$4^1/_3$	23	$7^2/_3$
4	$1^1/_3$	14	$4^2/_3$	24	8
5	$1^2/_3$	15	5	25	$8^1/_3$
6	2	16	$5^1/_3$	26	$8^2/_3$
7	$2^1/_3$	17	$5^2/_3$	27	9
8	$2^2/_3$	18	6	28	$9^1/_3$
9	3	19	$6^1/_3$	29	$9^2/_3$
10	$3^1/_3$	20	$6^2/_3$	30	10

From *Instruments and Catheters for Radiography*. Solna, Sweden, Firma AB Kifa, 1970.
OD, outside diameter.

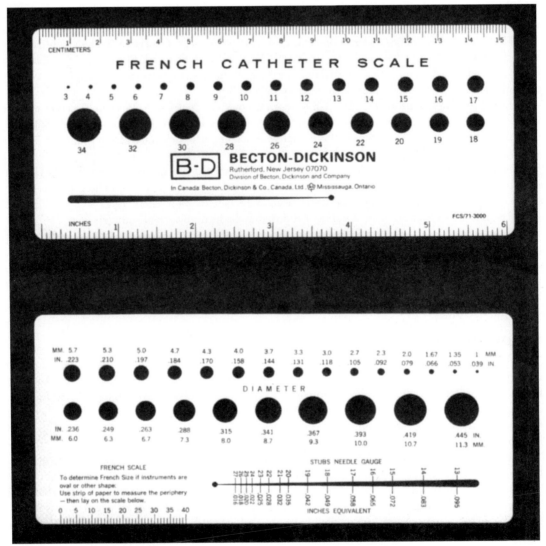

FIGURE 4-1. The Becton-Dickinson French catheter scale.

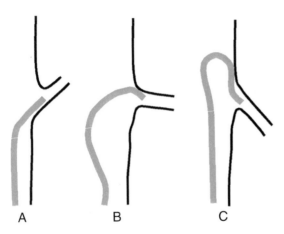

FIGURE 4-2. Catheter shapes used for different selective vessel access. **A,** Angled catheter for use when there is a low branch angle from aortic axis. **B,** Curved catheter shape when angle of selected vessel is between 60 and 120 degrees from the aortic axis. **C,** Recurved catheter used when the angle of the selected vessel is great.

A   B   C

TABLE 4-2 *Size Specifications for Cardiovascular Catheters*

| | Standard Wall | | | | | | | Thin Wall | | | | | |
| | Inside Diameter | | Outside Diameter | | Needle Equivalent | | | Inside Diameter | | Outside Diameter | | Needle Equivalent | |
French Size	in	mm	in	mm	ID	OD	French Size	in	mm	in	mm	ID	OD
3	0.014	0.36	0.039	1.00	23+	20+							
4	0.018	0.46	0.052	1.33	22+	18+	4	0.023	0.58	0.052	1.33	20	18+
5	0.026	0.66	0.065	1.67	19	16	5	0.034	0.86	0.065	1.67	19+	16
6	0.036	0.91	0.078	2.00	18+	15+	6	0.046	1.17	0.078	2.00	17+	15+
7	0.046	1.17	0.091	2.33	17+	13-	7	0.058	1.47	0.091	2.33	15+	13-
8	0.056	1.42	0.104	2.67	15+	12-	8	0.068	1.73	0.104	2.67	14+	12-
9	0.064	1.63	0.118	3.00	14+		9	0.078	1.98	0.118	3.00	13+	
10	0.072	1.83	0.131	3.33	13+		10	0.088	2.24	0.131	3.33	12+	
11	0.083	2.11	0.144	3.67	12-		11	0.098	2.49	0.144	3.67		
12	0.094	2.39	0.157	4.00			12	0.108	2.74	0.157	4.00		
14	0.144	2.90	0.183	4.67			14	0.128	3.25	0.183	4.67		

From *Cardiovascular Catheters and Accessories*. Glens Falls, NY, United States Catheter and Instruments Corporation.

ID, inside diameter; OD, outside diameter.

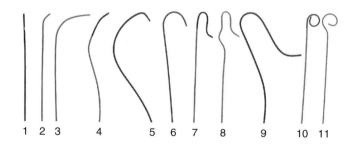

FIGURE 4-3. The distal ends of vascular catheters have different shapes for use in special procedures. 1, Straight. 2, Davis. 3, Multipurpose. 4, Headhunter. 5, Cobra. 6, Celiac. 7, Visceral. 8, Mickaelson. 9, Simmons. 10, Pigtail. 11, Tennis racket.

physician to remove foreign bodies or to perform biopsies. A variety of balloon catheters are also available. Figure 4-4 illustrates some of the types of interventional balloon catheters. Catheters that have permanently attached balloons have the capabilities of injecting contrast agents or therapeutic drugs either proximal or distal to the balloon, depending on the design. In some catheters, the design permits the balloon to be detached in situ and left in place to provide a permanent occlusion.

Guide Wires

Catheters inserted by the percutaneous catheterization method are threaded over a stainless-steel guide wire. The guide wire is basically composed of an outer case of tightly wound stainless-steel wire enclosing a wire core that may be either fixed or movable (Fig. 4-5). The inner core is a straight piece of stainless-steel wire. If the inner core is fixed, it is usually secured a short distance from the distal tip of the guide. This provides a flexible spring-wire tip that facilitates passage of the guide through sclerotic or tortuous vessels. The length of the standard flexible guide tip is 3 cm, but 7.5-cm flexible distal-tipped guides are also available.

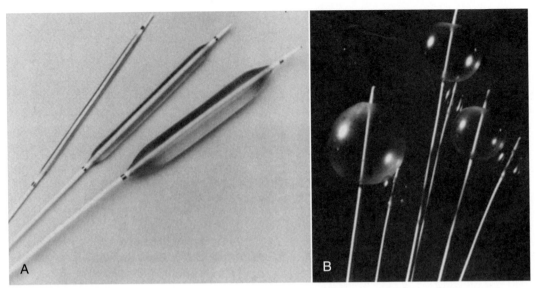

FIGURE 4-4. **A,** Balloon dilation catheters. **B,** Balloon occlusion catheters.

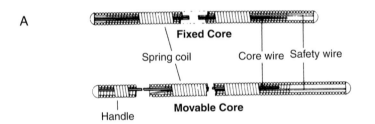

FIGURE 4-5. Basic construction of guide wires used during advanced procedures. **A** and **B** illustrate the straight and curved safety guide wire; **C** illustrates the movable core guide wire.

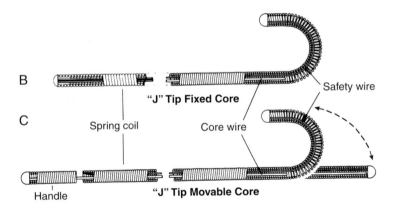

The movable-core spring guide has a movable inner core that can be used to vary the length of the flexible tip. When fully inserted, the inner core is used to straighten guides that have a precurved distal tip. When the inner core is withdrawn, the curve returns.

The length of spring guide wires ranges from 45 to 260 cm; guide wires used for exchanging catheters are usually more than twice the normal catheter length to prevent the loss of the guide while the catheter is being removed. Other lengths of guide wires can be made to order. The size of the guide chosen should be a minimum of 10 cm longer than the catheter.

Spring guide wires are very delicate instruments and should be handled with care. Spring guide holders serve as protective devices for the guide during sterilization and storage (Fig. 4-6). These holders can also be used as dispensers during the procedure, facilitating the handling of the guide wire and aiding in maintaining the distal end of the guide wire within the sterile field. It is generally recommended that spring guides be used only once and then discarded. If the guide is used more than once, a thorough inspection of the guide both before sterilization and during the procedure is recommended to prevent complications resulting from the use of a damaged guide.

NEEDLES AND ACCESSORIES

Needles are used extensively during procedures. The most frequently used are venipuncture needles. This type of needle is used for percutaneous vein punctures. They are disposable and are available in a wide range of gauges. Venipuncture needles are relatively inexpensive, and a generous supply in various gauges should be kept in the special procedure suite. These needles are measured according to the Stubbs needle gauge, which, like the French system for catheters, relates needle size to a whole number. The Stubbs number represents the outside diameter (OD) of the needle— the larger the Stubbs number, the smaller the OD of the needle. Box 4-2 illustrates some common needle sizes. The sizes of needle gauges in the Stubbs format range from 7, which is the largest, to 33, which represents the smallest. The 21-gauge needle is commonly employed in the practice of venipuncture.

Vessel access needles are necessary for all angiographic procedures. These are manufactured under a wide variety of eponyms by a variety of companies. Their main purpose is to provide access to the

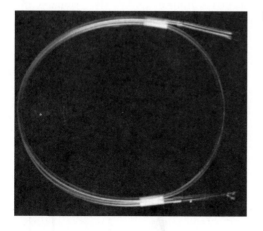

FIGURE 4-6.   A spring guide wire holder.

BOX 4-2	*Examples of Needle Sizing Using the Stubbs Needle Gauge System*		
Needle Gauge	**OD (in)**	**Needle Gauge**	**OD (in)**
27	0.016	21	0.032
26	0.018	20	0.0355
25	0.020	18	0.050
22	0.028	16	0.065

OD, outside diameter.

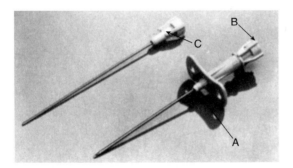

FIGURE 4-7. A typical sterile disposable arterial needle. The three-part set consists of an outer cannula (*A*), a sharp metal obturator (*B*), and a matching blunt tip obturator (*C*).

lumen of a vessel in order to introduce a guide wire and catheter. Most access needles are basically two- or three-piece sets (Fig. 4-7). Each set consists of an outer cannula with either a short bevel or a blunt tip, a sharp metal obturator, and a matching blunt-tip metal obturator These puncture needles are equipped with a specialized flange that facilitates holding the needle during the puncture. The sharp inner obturator has either a regular bevel or a trocar point. Figure 4-8 illustrates some common types of access needles that are available. Table 4-3 summarizes some common needle types used during angiography.

It is common during vessel access to require dilatation of the vessel wall and surrounding tissues in order to accommodate the catheter diameter that has been chosen for the procedure. Specialized vessel dilators are used for this purpose (Fig. 4-9). These are much stiffer than the catheters used during the procedure and are designed to be slipped over the guide wire in order to accomplish the dilatation. Successful dilatation is effected by using progressively larger dilators in small increments until the appropriate diameter has been reached.

The National Alliance for the Primary Prevention of Sharps Injuries (NAPPSI)[1] maintains the NAPPSI Primary and Secondary Prevention Needlestick Safety Device List. The list identifies

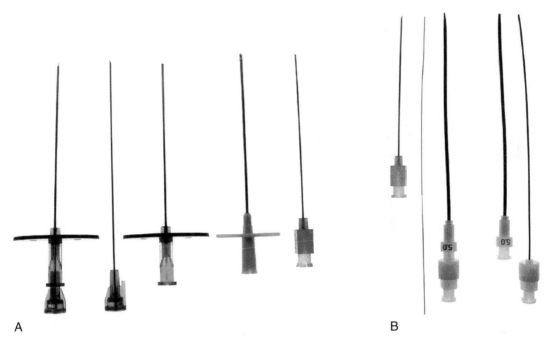

A   B

FIGURE 4-8. Illustration of specialized access needles used in angiography. **A,** Seldinger needle. **B,** Microaccess needle system.

TABLE 4-3　*Some Common Needles and Their Applications*

Needle Type	Description	Application
Angiocath	Needle with a beveled metal cannula and a Teflon sheath; the Angiocath comes in various sizes.	Used for cubital vein puncture for DSA, peripheral venography, and pediatric angiography.
Amplatz	A three-part needle with a beveled cannula, stylet, and fitted radiopaque Teflon outer sheath. The Amplatz needle comes in 16-, 18-, and 20-gauge sizes.	Used for femoral, brachial, and axillary artery puncture; for the femoral vein; and for vascular grafts.
PTCA needle (Chiba needles)	These are long, thin needles that usually are available in two sizes (22- and 23-gauge).	Used for percutaneous transhepatic cholangiography and splenoportography and as a percutaneous biopsy needle and fine needle aspiration procedures.
Potts-Cournand needle	A three-part needle with a beveled outer cannula and a hollow, beveled stylet and a blunt obturator. It is available in an 18-gauge size.	Used for arterial and venous puncture.
Seldinger needle	A two-part needle that has a thin-walled outer cannula with an inner stylet that can be beveled, diamond-shaped, or pointed. It is available in 16-, 18-, and 20-gauge sizes.	Used for arterial or venous puncture.
Butterfly needles	These are available in various gauges. They have small "ears" (wings) attached to the hub portion of the needle to facilitate entering the vessel.	These needles are generally used to enter smaller veins. They can be used during a wide variety of procedures.

DSA, digital subtraction angiography; PTCA, percutaneous transfemoral coronary angiography.

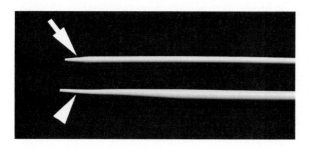

FIGURE 4-9. Specialized vessel dilators used to increase the diameter of the vessel wall and surrounding tissue. The arrow denotes a standard taper, and the arrowhead illustrates a longer taper for gradual dilation.

which devices provide primary prevention (eliminating the need for a needle or other "sharps" device) and which devices provide secondary prevention (devices that make the use of "sharps" safer). The list is adapted from the Exposure Prevention Information Network, International Health-Care-Worker Safety Center at the University of Virginia.

PROCEDURE TRAYS AND SETS

Prepackaged, sterile procedure trays are available for many special procedures. These contain all of the accessory items necessary to prepare the patient and perform the percutaneous puncture. Becton Dickinson and Company manufactures general procedure trays for those performing direct puncture and for those using the Seldinger technique for arterial catheter insertion. These sets are divided into two sections; the top section contains the materials necessary for patient preparation, and the bottom section contains the components for the particular procedural technique being performed.

Two commonly available prepackaged sets are the arthrography and myelography sets (Fig. 4-10).

Contents of a Prepackaged Arthrography Set
    One 5-ml Luer-Lok syringe
    One 10-ml Luer-Lok syringe
    One 30-ml Luer-Lok syringe
    One 18-g $\times$ 1$^1/_2$-in BD transfer needle
    One 20-g $\times$ 1$^1/_2$-in BD short bevel needle
    One 25-g $\times$ $^5/_8$-in BD needle
    One 3-in $\times$ 3-in gauze pad
    One absorbent fenestrated drape
    Two small basins
    Two absorbent towels
    One 2-oz medicine cup
    One 10-in connecting tube
    One adhesive bandage
    Two prep sponges

Contents of a Prepackaged Myelography Set
    One fenestrated drape
    Three prep applicators
    Two towels
    Five 3-in $\times$ 3-in gauze pads
    One removable antiseptic sponge
    One 5-ml BD syringe
    One 25-gauge $\times$ $^5/_8$-in BD Yale needle
    One mpule 5 ml Xylocaine
    One 21-gauge $\times$ 1$^1/_2$-in BD Yale needle
    One 18-gauge $\times$ 1$^1/_2$-in BD TW fill needle
    One 19-gauge $\times$ 1$^1/_2$-in BD TW filter needle
    One 10-in extension tubing set
    One 20-in extension tubing set
    One 3-in $\times$ $^3/_4$-in adhesive bandage
    Three specimen tubes

BD, Becton-Dickinson.
TW, Twinpack.

The myelography tray comes supplied with different accessories. Each tray contains a variety of items from each of three basic groups of equipment: (1) **prep group** (fenestrated absorbent drape, prep applicators, absorbent towels, 3- $\times$ 3-in gauze sponges, and removable antiseptic basin), (2) **anesthetic group** (5 ml Xylocaine, 5-ml syringe, 25-g $\times$ 5/8-in needle, 21-g $\times$ 1 to 1 $^1/_2$-in needle and 18-g $\times$ 1$^1/_2$-in transfer needle, and (3) **insertion and contrast removal group** (10-ml syringe, 20-ml syringe, 20-ml syringe, 10-in extension tubing, 20-in extension tubing, 3 in- $\times$ 3/4-in adhesive

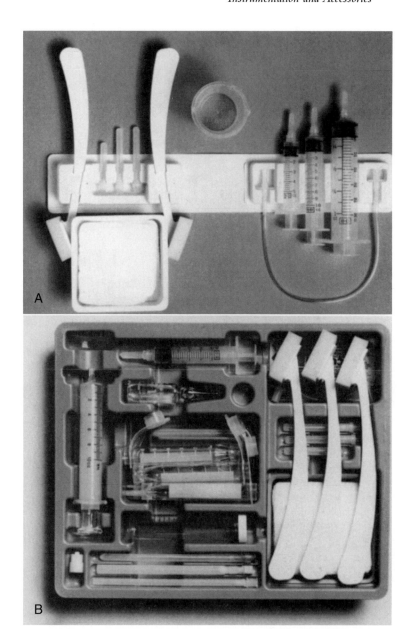

FIGURE 4-10. **A,** Sample prepackaged arthrography tray. **B,** Sample myelography tray for aspiration procedures.

bandage, male Luer-Lok cap, and specimen tubes). The trays can also be supplied with different myelography needles that match a variety of different clinical requirements.

ACCESSORIES

Accessory items that should be kept in the special procedure suite include adapters, connectors, manifolds (Fig. 4–11) and stopcocks.

Connectors are usually supplied as sets containing vinyl tubing with male and female Luer-Lok adapters. They are available in various lengths ranging from 10 in (25 cm) to 6 ft (180 cm) (Fig. 4–12). Connectors are also sterilized by autoclaving and should be thoroughly cleaned and rinsed after each use.

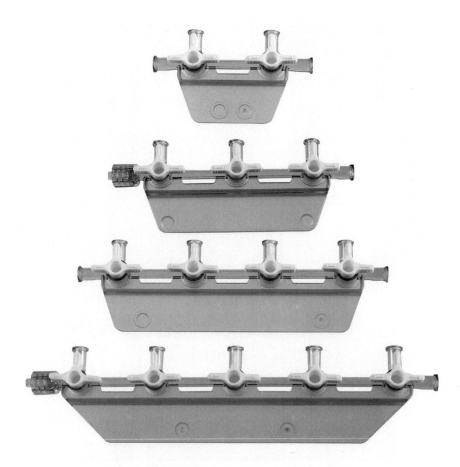

FIGURE 4-11. An accessory manifold device.

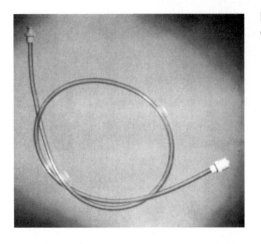

FIGURE 4-12. The sterile, disposable, flexible connector set with Luer-Lok fittings.

SUMMARY

Catheters are needed to direct the contrast medium to the desired location in the body. These simple tubes come in a variety of shapes and sizes. Catheters are made from Teflon, polyurethane, and polyethylene. Each material has advantages and disadvantages. Catheter sizes can be expressed as millimeters, inches, or in terms of the French gauge scale. The usual method of referring to catheter size is by its corresponding French number.

The distal end of a catheter can be equipped with devices that are used for a variety of different therapies. Balloon catheters are common devices used for reopening stenosed vessels. They can be equipped with or without stents that can act as supports inside the lumen of the blood vessel. Specialized catheters are available for use in the removal of foreign bodies from the vascular system, and some are outfitted with small lasers to effectively burn away plaque that blocks the vessels.

Needles are always found in the advanced procedure suite. They also come in a variety of shapes and sizes. Needles are sized by the Stubbs gauge scale. The higher the Stubbs number, the smaller the needle size. Combination needles are manufactured for specific methods of vessel entry. Prepackaged sterile trays are made for several different procedures, including myelography and arthrography. These kits contain all the needles and accessory items required for the procedure.

REFERENCE

1. The National Alliance for the Primary Prevention of Sharps Injuries. Accessed at http://www.nappsi.org.

SUGGESTED READINGS

Ahn WS, Bahk JH, Lim YJ, et al: The effect of introducer gauge, design and bevel direction on the deflection of spinal needles. *Anaesthesia* 57(10):1007–1011, 2002.

Baert SA, van Walsum T, Niessen WJ: Endpoint localization in guide wire tracking during endovascular interventions. *Acad Radiol* 10(12):1424–1432, 2003.

Baron, TH: Expandable metal stents for the treatment of cancerous obstruction of the gastrointestinal tract. *N Engl J Med* 344:1681–1686, 2001.

Fisher KL, Leung AN: Radiographic appearance of central venous catheters. *AJR Am J Roentgenol* 166:329–337, 1996.

Kessel D, Robertson I: *Interventional Radiology: A Survival Guide*. London, 2000, Churchill Livingstone.

Lin PH, Chronos NA, Marijianowski MM, Chen C, Bush RL, Conklin B, Lumsden AB, Hanson SR: Heparin-coated balloon-expandable stent reduces intimal hyperplasia in the iliac artery in baboons. *J Vasc Interv Radiol* 14:603–611, 2003.

Long AL, Sapoval MR, Beyssen BM, et al: Strecker stent implantation in iliac arteries: patency and predictive factors for long term success. *Radiology* 194:739–744, 1995.

Murphy M, Healey AE, Harper J, et al: Percutaneous removal of a right atrial catheter fragment: the value of the En Snare. *Nephrol Dial Transplant (England)* 19(10):2686–2687, 2004.

Todd DM, Hubner PJ, Hudson N, Sarma J, McCance AJ, Caplin J: Multicentre, prospective, randomized trial of 4 vs. 6 French catheters in 410 patients undergoing coronary angiography. *Catheter Cardiovasc Interv* 54:269–275, 2001.

Weintraub WS: Safety of 4 French catheters for diagnostic catheterization: smaller is better. *J Invasive Cardiol* 13(2):79–80, 2001.

Wunsche P, Werner C, Bloss P: Bending stiffness of catheters and guide wires. *Biomed Tech* 47(Suppl 1)Pt 1:150–153, 2002.

STUDY QUESTIONS

1. When selective angiography is performed, the amount of contrast agent administered to the patient is:
a. usually increased
b. usually decreased
c. increased by 2
d. not measured

STUDY QUESTIONS (*cont'd*)

2. A 2 French catheter inside diameter is equivalent to:
   a. $1/3$ mm
   b. $2/3$ mm
   c. 1 mm
   d. 3 mm

3. Catheters used for percutaneous insertion usually require that:
   a. the vessel be exposed for the insertion
   b. they be heated before insertion
   c. they be threaded over a guide wire during insertion
   d. they be manufactured out of a latex material

4. Which of the following is true for needles measured using the Stubbs needle gauge?
   i. The outside diameter of the needle is given.
   ii. The larger the Stubbs number, the smaller the outside diameter.
   iii. An 18-gauge needle measures 0.050 in inside diameter.
   a. i only
   b. i and ii only
   c. i and iii only
   d. i, ii, and iii

5. The device that is slipped over the guide wire to prepare the path for the catheter is called a:
   a. guide wire stiffener
   b. flexible tip catheter gauge
   c. vessel dilator
   d. introduction enhancer

6. In a prepackaged sterile tray, which of the following does not belong to the "prep" group of items?
   a. 3 in × 3 in gauze pads
   b. 20 in extension tubing
   c. fenestrated absorbent drape
   d. antiseptic basin

7. In a two-piece access needle, the portion of the needle that is inserted into the outer cannula portion is termed a(n):
   a. trocar
   b. dilator
   c. flange
   d. obturator

8. Catheter sizing information such as French size, length, and guide wire size may be found imprinted on the:
   a. catheter tip
   b. catheter hub
   c. body of the catheter
   d. catheter trocar

9. Catheters used to obstruct the flow of blood in a vessel are equipped with _____ devices.
   a. balloon
   b. obturator insert
   c. no side hole
   d. metal sheath

10. Which of the following is not an advantage of polyurethane catheters?
    i. low thrombogenicity
    ii. better torque
    iii. increased flow rates
    a. i only
    b. ii only
    c. iii only
    d. i and iii

5 *Introduction to Pharmacology*

CHAPTER OBJECTIVES

After completing this chapter, the reader will be able to perform the following:

- Define common terms used in pharmacology

- List the routes of administration of pharmacologic agents

- Identify the general guidelines for drug administration

- Identify the principles of intravenous (IV) therapy as well as the complications and equipment associated with it

- Differentiate between osmolality and osmolarity

- Define the principle of venipuncture

- Describe the calculations for intravenous flow rates

- Define conscious sedation

- Identify the various types of pharmacologic agents used in conjunction with the advanced radiographic and interventional procedures

- List the medications that could be used in cases of cardiac or respiratory emergencies

- List the principles of medication dose calculation

CHAPTER OUTLINE

TERMINOLOGY

    Agonists and Antagonists
    Drug Classification

ROUTES OF ADMINISTRATION

    General Guidelines for Parenteral Medication Administration

CONSCIOUS SEDATION

PHARMACOLOGIC AGENTS USED DURING ADVANCED PROCEDURES

    Preprocedure Pharmacologic Agents
    Emergency Medications
    Dose Calculations

SUMMARY

Throughout the 1990s it was sufficient for the special procedure radiographer to have a solid knowledge of the types of contrast agents as well as their action, purpose, and effects with regard to the patient. Beyond this, the broader realm of pharmacology was left to the physician and special procedure nurse. More recently, the practice of diagnostic and interventional radiography requires that the technologists be aware of the types and effects of various medications that are used in the procedures. These include drugs that are prescribed as preexamination medications, those used through the procedure, and the drugs that are available for the treatment of patient reactions. It is beyond the scope of this text to present an in-depth discussion of pharmacology; however, the basic principles of this science will be presented.

The American Registry of Radiologic Technologists (ARRT) requires the candidate for the advanced level examinations to have some understanding regarding the types and administration routes, indications, contraindications, and complications of various drugs used in cardiac and vascular interventional radiography.[1] Contrast agents represent a special category of materials; they will be discussed separately in Chapter 6.

TERMINOLOGY

Agonists and Antagonists

When a drug is introduced into the body its action usually begins when it attaches or binds itself to a specific target cell. Four common protein targets are considered binding sites for drugs. These are considered to be regulatory proteins such as enzymes, carrier molecules, ion channels, and receptors. This is a gross simplification of the mechanism of drug action; however, the interaction of the drug and **receptor** is an important beginning step in understanding the mechanism of drug action and cellular response.

When a drug binds itself to the receptors on specific cells or tissues and produces an effect, it is termed an **agonist.** On the other hand, the classifications of drugs that bind with certain receptor sites and prevent an action from happening are called **antagonists.** Antagonists are considered "blocking" drugs that bind to the receptor and prevent other drugs from producing an effect. They are also used at times to counteract the action of an agonist. This use or mechanism is called **competitive antagonism** because each class of drugs is competing for the receptor sites. The overall result will depend upon which class binds to the most receptor sites.

Drug Classification

This refers to the system used to identify drugs. Medications can be classified by their name(s), by their mode of action, or as prescription or nonprescription medications. Each drug that is developed begins its life with a **chemical name,** the nomenclature used to describe its chemical makeup. Once the chemical has been approved for availability on the commercial market, it is given its **generic name**. The generic name is derived from the chemical formula in some way and is considered to be nonproprietary. This name indicates that the basic chemical composition of the drug can be provided by several manufacturers. When a pharmaceutical house trademarks a name for its specific brand of the drug, it can then be classified by its **trade** or **brand name**.

Pharmacology is the study of drugs and their origins, chemical composition, preparations, and use. **Pharmacokinetics** refers to the mechanisms of bodily absorption, distribution, metabolism, and excretion of drugs. **Pharmacodynamics** is the action that various drugs have with body tissues.

ROUTES OF ADMINISTRATION

The route of administration will vary not only with the drug used but also the purpose that it has been designed for. The drugs used in vascular and cardiac diagnostic and interventional radiography fall into two major classifications: local and systemic.

The **local medications** are usually administered at a specific site and are injected into the tissues only in that particular area. The route is by direct injection, and the purpose of the drug is the reduction of sensation (pain) in the tissues of the surrounding area. These drugs are used at the beginning of the procedure, and they have an anesthetic and analgesic effect at the puncture site. The anesthetic effect of the "local" medication is almost immediate and is well tolerated by most adult patients. Box 5-1 lists some local anesthetics. Occasionally, one of the amides will be added to the contrast agent to reduce the discomfort and pain associated with the injection.

Local medications can also be administered by inhalation and topical application to the skin and other mucous membranes. Inhaled medication is used to produce a rapid response to local respiratory

BOX 5-1	*Local Anesthetics*
Classification	**Medication**
Amides	Lidocaine (Xylocaine)
	Bupivacaine (Marcaine, Sensorcaine)
	Mepivacaine (Carbocaine)
Esters	Chloroprocaine (Nesacaine)
	Procaine (Novocain)

conditions. The glucocorticoids and bronchodilators are administered by inhalation. Despite the fact that these drugs are given for local conditions, some of the medication will enter the systemic circulation and can be the cause of various side effects. Topical administration is a painless way of administering some medications with the probability of limited consequence.

Systemic medications produce a wide variety of effects to the patient. These drugs are usually used before the procedure begins, at times during the procedure, and often in emergency situations to alleviate a problem. The four major routes of administration for the systemic agents are oral, rectal, sublingual, and parenteral. The first three routes are self-explanatory, and their use will appear obvious. Inhalation can also be considered as a means of administering systemic medications as in the case of general anesthesia.

Oral medications are taken by mouth. The rectal route of administration is used if the patients are unable to take oral medication. This could be due to the inability to retain the drug in the stomach or because the drug would be adversely affected by the gastric contents. Sublingual administration of certain medications is used when quick action of the drug is required. These drugs are manufactured to dissolve quickly when placed under the tongue to provide a rapid effect. It can be seen that these three routes of administration of medication all utilize the digestive system to introduce the medication into the body. The **parenteral route** pertains to the administration of a medication other than the gastrointestinal tract. This is usually accomplished by injection.

There are five subdivisions of parenteral administration of medication: intravenous, intramuscular, intrathecal, intradermal, and subcutaneous. Each of these methods requires the use of a needle and usually a syringe. Intravenous (IV) fluid therapy is the exception to the use of a syringe as a part of the process. Refer to Chapter 4 for the discussion regarding needles and syringes.

Each of the parenteral routes of administration is similar in that the object of the procedure is to place a needle into a specific part of the body. Table 5-1 summarizes the locations for the injections as well as any specifics about the process.

General Guidelines for Parenteral Medication Administration

In this section we will discuss the general guidelines for the administration of parenteral medication. Table 5-1 illustrates the major differences in the various parenteral routes of medication administration. As mentioned earlier, medications can be administered to the patient in a variety of different ways: oral, rectal, topical, inhalation, and parenteral. The parenteral route of drug administration is subdivided into five separate areas: intravenous, intradermal, intrathecal, subcutaneous, and intramuscular.

The guidelines will be essentially the same for all routes of administration with the exception that the parenteral administration of medications is considered an invasive procedure and all standard precautions should be observed during the process. Strict aseptic techniques should be employed. The specifics of administration for each of the routes should be meticulously followed. The radiographer not only must be aware of the specifics of each parenteral route but must guard against inadvertent personal needle stick injury.

TABLE 5-1 *Summary of Parenteral Routes of Injection*

Parenteral Route	Description	Specific Criteria
Intravenous	Insertion of a needle into a vein	Needle held at 15–30-degree angle to patient's arm with needle bevel up. Use the smallest needle size for the product to minimize tissue damage. Most common sizes are 16–18 gauge.
Intramuscular	Insertion of a needle into a muscle	Use a 21–23 gauge needle (1$\frac{1}{2}$ inches) to ensure passage into deep muscle tissue. Needle is held at a 90-degree angle.
Intrathecal (intraspinal)	Insertion of a needle into the subdural, arachnoid, or lumbar areas.	Use a 16–25-gauge, 3$\frac{1}{2}$ inch long spinal needle.
Intradermal	Insertion of a needle into the dermis	A small syringe or needle combination is used, 26–27 gauge , $\frac{1}{4}$ to $\frac{1}{2}$ inch needle. The angle of insertion is 5–15 degrees.
Subcutaneous	Insertion of a needle into the loose connective tissue directly under the dermis	Use a 25-gauge, $\frac{5}{8}$ inch needle. An angle of 45–90 degrees can be used depending upon the body habitus of the patient. Larger, obese patients will require a 90-degree angle for insertion.

When any medication is administered it is important to follow some basic principles, known as the "Six Rights."[2] These basic rules should be followed whenever any medication is dispensed to a patient.

1. Administer the drug to the **RIGHT PATIENT**
2. Administer the **RIGHT DRUG**
3. Administer the **RIGHT DOSAGE**
4. Use the **RIGHT ROUTE** to administer the drug
5. Provide the drug at the **RIGHT TIME**
6. Complete the **RIGHT DOCUMENTATION**

As a part of the advanced procedure team, it is imperative to have a working knowledge of all of the medications commonly used for the specific procedure. This also includes any emergency drugs. In other words the radiographer must be knowledgeable about the medications given to the patient before, during, and after the procedure. This practice will help ensure that the patient will have the greatest possibility for a successful and uneventful procedure.

Many of the guidelines listed here are the same for routine patient care and communication. The difference is that all of the vascular and cardiac interventional procedures are invasive and have the potential to produce a number of different reactions. Extreme care should be exercised in adhering to these rules and guides. In almost every case some type of medication is administered to

---

BOX 5-2   *ISMP List of High Alert Medications*

Class/Category of Medications
- Adrenergic agonists, IV (e.g., epinephrine)
- Adrenergic antagonists, IV (e.g., propranolol)
- Anesthetic agents, general, inhaled, and IV (e.g., propofol)
- Cardioplegic solutions
- Chemotherapeutic agents, parenteral and oral
- Dextrose, hypertonic, 20% or greater
- Dialysis solutions, peritoneal and hemodialysis
- Epidural or intrathecal medications
- Glycoprotein IIb/IIIa inhibitors (e.g., eptifibatide)
- Hypoglycemics, oral
- Inotropic medications, IV (e.g., digoxin, milrinone)
- Liposomal forms of drugs (e.g., liposomal amphotericin B)
- Moderate sedation agents, IV (e.g., midazolam)
- Moderate sedation agents, oral, for children (e.g., chloral hydrate)
- Narcotics/opiates, IV and oral (including liquid concentrates, immediate and sustained release)
- Neuromuscular blocking agents (e.g., succinylcholine)
- Radiocontrast agents, IV
- Thrombolytics/fibrinolytics, IV (e.g., tenecteplase)
- Total parenteral nutrition solutions

Specific Medications
- IV amiodarone, antiarrhythmic drug (Pacerone)
- Alkaloid (colchicine injection)
- Heparin, low molecular weight, injection
- Heparin, unfractionated, IV
- Insulin, subcutaneous and IV
- IV lidocaine
- Magnesium sulfate injection
- Methotrexate, oral, nononcologic use
- Human B-type natriuretic peptide (nesiritide, Natrecor)
- Nitroprusside, sodium, for injection
- Potassium chloride for injection concentrate
- Potassium phosphates injection
- Sodium chloride injection, hypertonic, more than 0.9% concentration
- Warfarin

Institute for Safe Medication Practices: ISMP's List of High Alert Medications, 2003, http://www.ismp.org/MSArticles/highalert.htm.

---

the patient before, during, or after a procedure. It is the responsibility of everyone on the team to practice a heightened level of care in order to ensure patient safety from medication reactions due to human error. The Institute for Safe Medication Practices (ISMP) has identified some common medications that have been known to cause an increased risk for patient injury when errors are made. The organization recommends that when any of these drugs are administered safety strategies are in place to prevent any errors. Box 5-2 summarizes the ISMP List of High Alert Medications.[3]

Parenteral administration (by injection and not via the gastrointestinal tract) requires additional guidelines depending upon the subclassification of the injection route. The first 10 steps in any procedure for the administration of medication would be the same and are as follows:

1. Throughout the procedure follow standard precautions.
2. Wash hands thoroughly.
3. Be sure it is the **RIGHT PERSON**. Check the patient's identification and ask the patient's name.
4. Even if an informed consent has been negotiated, explain the procedure to the patient in terms the patient will understand.
5. Assemble the necessary equipment. Organize for use.
6. Be sure you have the **RIGHT DRUG**. Read the label several times.
7. Be sure you have the **RIGHT DOSAGE**. Check the order and any calculations that have been made.
8. Be sure you are administering the medication at the **RIGHT TIME** (preprocedure, during the procedure, or postprocedure).
9. Put on protective gloves.
10. Locate and cleanse the appropriate site. Be sure you are using the **RIGHT ROUTE**.
11. Complete the **RIGHT DOCUMENTATION**.

Table 5-2 lists the procedures for each of the parenteral routes of administration with the exception of the intrathecal route, which is discussed in detail in Chapter 21.

Intravenous Therapy

Intravenous therapy involves the introduction of a fluid through a vein. This is accomplished using an intravenous cannula such as a needle or one of the special angiocatheters. The location or insertion site can be either in a central or a peripheral vein. In most cases the peripheral sites are used. These include the veins of the hand; the veins of the arm (antecubital, radial, ulnar, cephalic), and the external jugular vein.

The main purpose of this type of therapy is the management of the fluids in the body. The body is composed of over 65% water, and fluid management is vitally important for the balance of electrolytes, blood volume, and other nutritional materials required for intra- and extracellular equilibrium. In the normal, healthy patient this is accomplished automatically even under situations in which there is a minor fluid loss. Extracellular fluids are the body fluids consisting of the interstitial fluid and blood plasma. Approximately one quarter of the body's water is located outside the cells. Most of this water is found in the **interstitial space**. Interstitial fluid fills the spaces between most of the cells of the body. Less than 8% of the body's fluid is located in the intravascular space. Three quarters of all the water is found within the cells of the body. These intracellular fluids are within cell membranes throughout the body and contain dissolved solutes essential to fluid and electrolyte balance and metabolism. Electrolytes are substances that ionize when dissolved in water and as such are able to conduct a current. Calcium is an electrolyte that is necessary for the conduction of nerve impulses responsible for the contraction of skeletal muscle. All of these substances are necessary for normal body metabolism. Table 5-3 lists the various electrolytes present in the body's fluids.

The therapeutic introduction of fluid materials becomes necessary under certain conditions, such as trauma, surgical procedures, illness, and factors contributing to an increased level of stress. Ernest H. Starling, a British physiologist, proposed that a balance exists at the level of the capillary membranes when the fluid entering the circulation and that leaving the circulation are the same. His theory described the capillary wall as a semipermeable membrane that allowed salt solutions to pass through it (by osmosis). In order to balance the concentration on both sides of the membrane, the osmotic pressure forced movement of fluids from the tissue into the circulation. In other words, the fluids will move toward the side of the semipermeable membrane that contains the largest proportion of these solutes.

TABLE 5-2 *Generalized Guidelines for Parenteral Administration of Medication*

Intravenous*	Intradermal	Intramuscular	Subcutaneous
Set up equipment. Open sterile packages using aseptic technique.	Select appropriate injection site usually 3–4 fingerwidths below the antecubital space.	Select appropriate injection site in a large, deep muscle. Assess the size and integrity of the muscle. Some sites are the ventrogluteal muscle, dorsogluteal muscle, deltoid muscle, and the vastus lateralis muscle.	Select appropriate injection site. Best sites are located in vascular areas such as outer areas of upper arms, abdomen (iliac crests to rib margins), scapular areas, upper ventral and dorsal gluteal areas.
Prepare IV tubing. Check solution for expiration date. Open infusion set while maintaining sterility. Place roller cap below drip chamber and set to off position.	Elbow and forearm should be extended. Cleanse site outward in circular motion. Remove cap from needle. Stretch skin over site with opposite hand.	Ensure that the patient is in a comfortable position depending on the injection site.	Choice of needle is determined for each patient by grasping skinfold between thumb and forefinger. Needle should not be more that half the depth.
Remove the protective sheath from the IV bag and insertion spike, then insert proper end of infusion set into the port in the bag. Prime the tubing by squeezing the drip chamber several times until the chamber is $^1/_3$–$^1/_2$ full. Remove protective cap from other end of tubing and slowly open the compression valve until fluid is seen at the needle adapter. Reset the compression valve to the off position. Be sure air bubbles are out of the tubing and replace the protective cap on the tubing.	Needle bevel should be up; insert needle at a 5- to 15-degree angle until resistance is felt. Advance needle another $^1/_8$ inch (needle tip should be seen through the skin). Inject medication slowly against resistance.	Cleanse the area using a circular motion from in to out to a diameter of approximately 2 inches. Remove cap from needle. Stretch the skin over the injection site prior to needle insertion. This provides a "Z-track" injection path that forms a self-seal after the skin is released.	Cleanse area using a circular motion from in to out to a diameter of approximately 2 inches. Remove cap from needle. Hold syringe between thumb and forefinger as if holding a dart.
Select the injection site (usually distal to the vein that is chosen). Place a tourniquet about 5–6 inches above the injection site. It should only restrict the flow of blood in the vein, not the arteries. Look for a well-dilated vein.	A small skin wheal should appear. Withdraw needle while applying alcohol swab. Do not massage site. Cap and discard needle according to regulations Remove gloves and wash hands. Observe patient for signs of allergic reactions.	Hold syringe as if holding a dart between thumb and forefinger. Insert needle into the muscle quickly at an angle of 90 degrees. Slowly pull back on plunger; if blood appears, withdraw needle and begin procedure again. If not, inject medication slowly. The slow injection rate (10 ml/s) reduces the patient's pain. Withdraw needle after injection and apply gentle pressure. Do not massage the site.	Squeeze skin to make a fold at injection site; insert needle quickly at a 45–90-degree angle, then release skinfold. Slowly pull back on plunger; if blood appears, withdraw needle and begin procedure again. If not, inject medication slowly.

Continued

TABLE 5-2 *Generalized Guidelines for Parenteral Administration of Medication (cont'd)*

Intravenous*	Intradermal	Intramuscular	Subcutaneous
If none immediately are visible, try one of the following methods to achieve the desired result; stroke the area from the distal to proximal position, have the patient open and close the hand, slightly tap over the vein or apply a warm compress for a short period of time over the area.		Discard needle and syringe. Dispose of additional supplies. Remove gloves, wash hands. Observe patient for any changes such as localized pain, numbness, tingling, allergic symptomatology, disorientation.	After injection, withdraw needle and place a swab over the area. Discard needle and syringe. Dispose of additional supplies. Remove gloves, wash hands. Observe patient for any changes such as localized pain, urticaria, eczema, wheezing or dyspnea, and disorientation.
Cleanse the site using circular motion from inward to outward with appropriate cleansing agent.			
Perform venipuncture. Look for blood return to indicate that the vein has been entered. If intracatheter is used, advance $1/4$ inch, remove stylet, and advance catheter into vein. If using butterfly needle, insert until hub rests against skin at puncture site.			
Stabilize catheter release tourniquet and connect needle adapter, administration set, or heparin lock to the hub of the needle.			
Release the compression clamp to begin IV drip.			
Secure the IV catheter or needle using institutional guidelines including a loop of infusion			

TABLE 5-2 *Generalized Guidelines for Parenteral Administration of Medication (cont'd)*

Intravenous*	Intradermal	Intramuscular	Subcutaneous
tubing. If using a butterfly needle, it can be secured by using the "U" or "H" method of taping.			
Adjust the flow rate, or if using a heparin or saline lock flush with 1–3 ml heparin or saline, respectively.			
Discard needle and syringe. Dispose of additional supplies.			
Remove gloves, wash hands.			
Observe patient for any changes such as inflammation at site, extravasation, and bleeding at puncture site. Check vital signs every hour.			

*A discussion of venipuncture and the use of heparin or normal saline locks is presented in the section, "Intravenous Therapy."

TABLE 5-3 *Major Electrolytes and Their Function in the Body*

Electrolyte	Chemical Symbol	Function
Bicarbonate	HCO_3^-	Neutralizes acidosis when blood pH has dropped to hazardous levels
Calcium	Ca^{2+}	Has a major role in muscle contraction Involved in the transmission of nervous impulses
Chloride	Cl^-	Involved in fluid balance and renal function
Magnesium	Mg^{2+}	Essential for many enzyme processes in the body Important for neurochemical transmissions Affects the central nervous, neuromuscular, and cardiovascular systems
Phosphate	HPO_4^-	Essential as a buffer Regulates storage and use of energy received from metabolism
Potassium	K^+	Important for the transmission of electrical impulse
Sodium	Na^+	The main electrolyte in interstitial fluid Regulates water allocation Needed for the transmission of nervous impulses.

Osmolarity and Osmolality

Certain concepts must be understood prior to a discussion of intravenous therapy. Starling's principle is not only applicable to intravenous therapy; it is thought that many of the reactions caused by the administration of contrast media are the result of this osmotic action. The terms **osmolarity** and **osmolality** are used quite extensively in describing different solutions, including the various classes of positive contrast media, and must be understood in order to understand their actions within the body. A review of osmosis is necessary in order to understand the concepts of osmolarity and osmolality.

Osmosis is defined as the passage of a solvent (water) through a semipermeable membrane into a solution of higher solute (a salt or a substance dissolved in a solution) concentration that tends to equalize the concentrations of solute on the two sides of the membrane. In the body, human plasma is considered to be isotonic. In order to maintain this isotonic state, everything administered into the body must be equated to the sodium chloride equivalent of the human plasma, because sodium chloride is a major determinate of blood osmolarity.

Any substance dissolved in a solution can be considered a solute. Although osmosis is not limited to the actions resulting from the administration of IV therapy solutions or contrast media, the discussion of this concept will relate to the action of water as the solvent and contrast medium as the solute. Osmosis is the tendency for a solvent, such as water, to move through a permeable or semipermeable membrane so as to become mixed with a solute, such as contrast medium, to create a solution that is equal in osmotic pressure on both sides of the membrane. This movement of the solvent (water) is from a solution that is lower in solute (contrast medium) concentration to the side of the membrane that is higher in solute (contrast medium) concentration. Osmotic activity will continue until the concentration of the solutions on both sides of the membrane is equalized. In essence, osmosis is the movement of water through the membranes separating the body's compartments.

Osmolarity and osmolality refer to the **osmotic pressure** of a solution. This pressure is the mechanism that controls the movement of the water across the membrane. Osmolarity refers to the concentration per volume of solution (milliosmols per kilogram of solution), while osmolality refers to weight or milliosmols per kilogram of water. These two terms are often used interchangeably, and although they both relate to osmotic pressure it can be seen that they are actually different measurements. In most cases, there is little difference in these measurements; however, in certain cases the discrepancy can be considerable. Osmolality is the term that should be applied when discussing the intravenous therapy solutions and radiopaque contrast media.

An important fact is that the **solute** does not usually pass through the membrane and only the **solvent** moves to equalize the solution's concentration. Under certain circumstances, however, the solute can filter into the interstitial fluid via endothelial cell clefts. This can occur because of the high osmolality of the mixture of the solute and blood.

In the central nervous system the endothelium has a continuous basement membrane, and the cells are connected by tight junctions. This is referred to as the **blood-brain barrier**. The blood-brain barrier will normally hold back the passage of a number of solutes serving as a protective guard to the body. The blood-brain barrier is the anatomic/physiologic aspect of the brain that separates the parenchyma (organ tissue) of the central nervous system from the blood. Current theory is that the blood-brain barrier prevents or slows the passage of various chemical compounds and other potentially harmful substances from the blood into the tissue of the central nervous system.

The ultimate goal of intravenous therapy is to prevent or correct fluid and electrolyte (solute) disturbances. Depending upon the purpose, intravenous fluids can be hypotonic, hypertonic, or isotonic. Solutions that are similar in content to physiologic fluids are said to be **isotonic**. Depending upon the source of information, an isotonic solution ranges between 240 and 375 mOsm. Isotonic solutions are also considered to be equivalent to a 0.9% weight/volume NaCl solution, which is equivalent to that of blood plasma. This type of solution does not exert any osmotic action in either direction at the capillary level.

Hypertonic solutions generally are greater than 375 mOsm. In the attempt to achieve balance, these solutions will move fluid across the semipermeable membrane at the capillary level and into the intravascular spaces, causing the cells to shrink and get smaller. These solutions have a greater solute concentration than blood plasma, and fluid is needed to achieve balance.

When a solution is less than 240 mOsm it has lower concentration of solutes than blood plasma and is considered **hypotonic**. In order to achieve balance, the fluid from the vascular space moves across the semipermeable membrane and into the cells. This influx has a tendency to cause the cells to expand and get larger.

The importance of the definitions listed here is that the technologist should be aware of the osmolality of the solution that is being introduced into the patient. The IV solution packs, referred to as "bags," are labeled with the osmolality. This can be easily compared with the range for isotonic solutions, and the radiographer can quickly determine which of the three types of solutions is being administered.

Intravenous therapy when used during advanced radiologic procedures serves several functions. Among these functions, the intravenous port provides a ready access to the vein for the rapid introduction of emergency medication; however, fluid management is the primary purpose, especially when contrast agents are administered. The patient should be well hydrated during contrast examinations to reduce the probability of an adverse reaction. The patient's condition and the type and amount of contrast agent will govern the type and flow rate of the intravenous fluid. Box 5-3 summarizes the reasons that IV therapy is employed.

| **BOX 5-3** | *Summary of Indications for IV Therapy* |

Maintenance of fluid and electrolyte balance
- Age related
- Illness related
- Surgical reasons
- Dehydration

Maintenance of IV access for medication administration
- During a surgical procedure
- During interventional or diagnostic angiography
- Extended use via a normal saline or heparin lock
- Trauma

Parenteral nutritional supplementation

Venipuncture. The general guidelines for initiating an IV line have already been discussed for intravenous fluid replacement utilizing a metal needle and extension tubing for connection to a bag or bottle of IV fluid. Depending upon the nature or purpose for entering the vein the difference between the collection of a specimen or the introduction of a bolus of medication via a vein, and placing a long-term access port is minimal.

Venipuncture is generally accomplished utilizing a metal needle attached to a syringe or a device called a Vacutainer tube. In either case the process is the same. The steps are as follows:

Venipuncture Procedure for Injection or Collection
- Collect necessary equipment.
  - Disposable gloves
  - Needle (gauge is dependent upon several factors)
    The vein used for the procedure
    The viscosity of the medication
    The method of injection
  - Vacutainer set if collection is the purpose of the procedure (consists of a double-ended needle attached to a plastic tube)
  - Angiocatheter (intracatheter) if long-term access is the purpose of the procedure
  - Medication if injection is the purpose of the procedure
  - Alcohol swabs or povidone iodine solution
  - Dressing, tape, or adhesive bandages (Band-Aids)
- Check patient's identity and the physician's order.
- Discuss the process with the patient.
- Wash hands thoroughly.
- Put on disposable gloves.
- Cleanse area to be punctured using the appropriate solution.
- Apply a tourniquet above the puncture site—opening and closing the hand facilitates the identification of the vein.
- Stabilize the vein by pulling back on the skin toward the patient's hand.
- Hold the syringe or Vacutainer so the needle bevel is up.
- Smoothly insert the needle at an angle of 15 to 30 degrees and advance it into the vein.
- Blood will flow back into the syringe or Vacutainer when a successful puncture has been accomplished. Remove the tourniquet before injection of medication.
- Ensure that there is no air trapped in the needle before injecting any medication if injection was the purpose of the procedure. (Check for extravasation during injection.)
- Gently slide the Vacutainer tube over the inside needle without disturbing the placement of the needle in the vein. Blood will collect in the tube. Tubes may be switched during the collection of the specimen.
- When the injection or collection is completed, remove the needle and apply gentle pressure over the puncture site using a small gauze square.
- Dispose of syringes and other equipment as per institution policy.

Long-term IV access is accomplished in the same manner as that described for venipuncture. However, instead of a syringe/needle combination or Vacutainer set, a special venipuncture set called an Angiocath is used. The angio- or intracatheter uses a special needle that is equipped with a short Teflon or polyethylene catheter. There are two types of Angiocath sets available: the "over the needle" or "through the needle" cannula. The catheters are designed to remain in place for longer periods than metal needles and will normally cause fewer reactions. They are manufactured in various gauges to suit the different types of therapies and patients. Indwelling plastic catheters inserted over a guide wire are also used for long-term medication administration. Peripherally inserted central catheters, or PICC lines, are one example of this type of system.

The method of heparin or normal saline lock placement is similar to the procedure using a metal needle or butterfly assembly, which is discussed later in Table 5-6. The insertion is made with the bevel up at a 15- to 25-degree angle a little distal to the intended site of puncture. The needle is a bit different, having a catheter over the needle. In this case the needle is used to puncture the vein, and the catheter ultimately remains in the vein to provide access. Once the vein has been punctured and blood is seen at the hub (a sign that the vein has been successfully accessed) the stylet can be loosened and the catheter advanced into the vein over the stylet until the hub is close to the entry site. Once the stylet (needle) has been loosened it should not be reinserted into the catheter. This can cause damage to the catheter, creating a foreign body embolus. When the stylet is removed, a needle adapter or heparin lock should be attached to the hub. Once this is completed the intracatheter must be secured so that it cannot be easily dislodged from the vein. There are two methods of securing the intracatheter to the skin: standard dressing and transparent dressing. The following steps should be taken to secure the intracatheter using the standard method referred to as the **chevron method**:

- Using an approximately 3-inch piece of $\frac{1}{2}$-inch tape, place it under the catheter (adhesive side up) and cross it over the catheter, taping it to the skin.
- Using a second piece of $\frac{1}{2}$-inch tape, place it over the catheter hub and attach it to the skin.
- Place a 2- × 2-in piece of gauze over the puncture site and secure with tape.

If a transparent dressing is used, the following steps apply:

- Using the aseptic technique, carefully clean and dry the insertion site.
- Remove the dressing from its packaging and place it directly over the puncture site. The hub of the needle should be covered but not the extension tubing.

Equipment Necessary for Intravenous Therapy. In most cases it will be highly unlikely that the radiographer will have to initiate intravenous therapy without specialized training and competency testing. Familiarity with the procedure will enable the radiographer to assist the nurse or physician performing the procedure. The collection of the equipment is the first step in the process. Table 5-4 summarizes the necessary equipment for intravenous therapy initiation.[4]

Intravenous therapy is used for four primary reasons: fluid and electrolyte therapy, medication therapy, total nutritional supplementation therapy, and blood therapy. It is important to understand what the IV therapy is being used for in order to have the proper solutions and equipment available.

TABLE 5-4   *Equipment Used in Establishing Intravenous Therapy*

IV Fluid Infusion	Heparin or Normal Saline Lock	Items Required for Either Setup
Administration set—adult or pediatric	IV plug (injection cap)	Correct IV solution pack
0.22 micro mm filter if required by institution protocol	Short piece of extension tubing for loop	IV catheters sized to patient and reason for therapy
Extension tubing	1–3 ml normal saline or heparin flush (as ordered)	Alcohol or povidone iodine swabs
IV pole or means of suspending the bag	Syringes and 25-gauge needles	Disposable gloves Tourniquet Arm board (if necessary) Nonallergenic tape Towel or sterile drape for use during cleansing area Gauze or transparent dressing as per institution

The choice of solutions is based on their osmolality: isotonic, hypotonic, and hypertonic. Table 5-5 lists some IV solutions and their usage. These are grouped by their respective classifications. This list is not a complete listing of the solutions that are available for treatment. In many cases other medications are added to the solution as they are being infused into the patient. A discussion of the various medications that can be administered by means of the infusion or through the heparin lock is beyond the scope of this text.

TABLE 5-5 *Intravenous Solutions and Their Usage*

Solution/Osmolality	Usage
Isotonic solutions (240–375 mOsm)	
Normal saline—0.9% NaCl Osmolality 308 Osm/L	Restoration or expansion of extracellular fluidvolume
	Used as a replacement for Na^+ and Cl^- electrolytes
	Will not cause hemolysis of red blood cells
	Can be administered with blood and blood products
Ringer's solution Osmolality 309 mOsm/L	Does not provide free water
	Replaces the following solutes; K^+, Na^+, Cl^-, Ca^{2+}
	Does not contain lactate
Ringer's lactate solution Osmolality 273 mOsm/L	Similar to the electrolyte composition of blood serum and plasma
	Used to treat fluid losses from burns and lower GI tract
	Corrects electrolyte depletion
10% Dextran 40 in 0.9% normal saline	Plasma volume extenders in cases of hypovolemia
	Available in several concentrations
10% intralipids Osmolality 290 mOsm/L	Provides fatty acids and calories
20% intralipids Osmolality 330 mOsm/L	Provides fatty acids and calories
D_5W—5% dextrose in water Osmolality 250 mOsm/L	Provides free water to both extra- and intracellular spaces
	Promotes renal elimination of solutes
	Does not provide electrolytes
D_5 1/4 normal saline—5% dextrose and 0.45 NaCl Osmolality 320 mOsm/L	Maintenance of body fluids when Na^+ and Cl^- are also required
Hypotonic Solutions (<240 mOsm)	
Solution / Osmolality	Usage
1/2 normal saline—0.45% NaCl Osmolality 154 mOsm/L	Provides free water
	Assists renal function
	Replaces normal daily fluid losses
	No calories or electrolyte replacement except for Na^+ and Cl^-
Hypertonic Solutions (>375 mOsm)	
$D_{10}W$—10% dextrose in water Osmolality 500 mOsm/L	Acts as an osmotic diuretic
	Supplies calories
	Does not contain electrolytes
	Supplies free water
$D_{10}NS$—10 % dextrose and 0.9% NaCl Osmolality 810 mOsm/L	Fluid replacement
	Electrolyte replacement (Na^+) and (Cl^-)
	Supplies calories
D_5LR—dextrose in lactated Ringer's solution Osmolality 524 mOsm/L	Similar to electrolyte composition of blood serum and plasma
	Used to treat fluid losses
	Corrects electrolyte depletion
	Adds calories for nutrition

Calculation of IV Flow Rates. Physician's orders will normally specify the amount of fluid and medication that is to be administered over a specific time. In some cases the intravenous tubing will be connected to an infusion pump (Fig. 5-1). The Baxter Healthcare Clear Link activated valve provides for connection to IV tubing without the need for a needle insertion offering protection for both the patient and health care personnel (Fig. 5-2). These devices will normally perform the flow

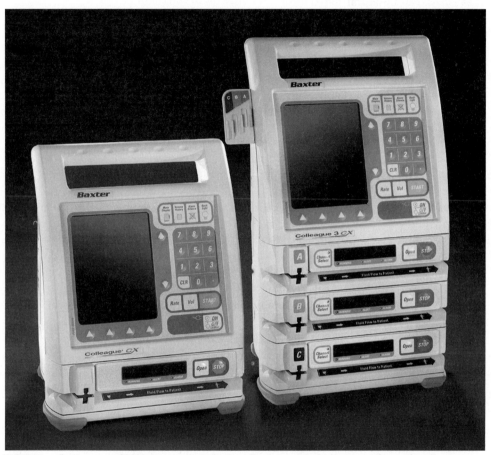

FIGURE 5-1.   Colleague CX Volumetric Infusion Pump with Colleague Guardian Feature.

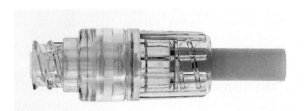

FIGURE 5-2.   Clear Link activated valve for use with intravenous therapy systems.

rate calculation automatically after inputting the parameters. It is important to check the accuracy of the flow rates and the medication type when these devices are used to avoid unnecessary complications. Merely programming in the figures does not automatically ensure that everything will go as planned. All team members must remember to follow the "Six Rights" of medication administration.

At times the dose or flow rate must be calculated manually. Two factors are usually calculated; the dose (volume) administered per hour and the number of drops per minute. The formulae are as follows:

$$\text{Total volume (ml)/time (hours)} = \text{ml/hr}$$

$$\frac{\text{(ml/hr)(gtt/ml)}}{60 \text{ min}} = \text{gtt/min}$$

The first formula calculates the amount (total dose) that the patient is to receive over a total period of time (usually hours). The formula breaks the total amount of medication into an amount to be given over a 1-hour time span. Let's look at an example of this calculation.

Assume that the physician's order was to administer 2000 cc of fluid over 4 hours. Using formula 1 the calculation per hour is:

$$\frac{2000 \text{ ml}}{4 \text{ hr}} = 500 \text{ ml/hr}$$

The next part of the calculation, to arrive at the number of drops (gtt) per minute (expressed as gtt/minute), requires a knowledge of the drop factor, gtt\ml, the drops per ml provided by the particular infusion set or pump. Generally speaking there are microdrip and macrodrip infusion sets. The drops per milliliter (gtt/ml) varies with each type.

Microdrip infusion sets = 50–60 gtt/ml

Macrodrip infusion sets = 10–20 gtt/ml

The formula used to calculate the number of drops per **minute (gtt/min)** is:

$$\frac{\text{(ml/hr) (gtt/ml)}}{60 \text{ min}} = \text{gtt/min}$$

In the preceding example of 2000 ml per 4 hours, initially the amount to be dispensed in 1 hour (500 ml) was calculated. Assuming an infusion set that is calibrated to a microdrip factor of 50 gtt/ml, formula 2 can be used to arrive at the gtt/min or the number of drops per minute required to administer the ordered dose. The factors are 500 ml/hour (calculated with formula 1), 50 gtt/ml (infusion set drip factor), and 60 minutes in each hour (time conversion).

$$\frac{\text{(500 ml/hr) (50 gtt/ml)}}{60 \text{ min/hr}} = 416.6 \text{ gtt/min}$$

The number of drops per minute for these parameters calculates out to be 416.6 drops/min. This number represents the flow rate of the medication that is being administered to the patient. Once the proper drip factor (gtt/min) is known, the IV flow can be easily regulated by counting the drops for 15 s and multiplying the result by 4. The tube clamp can be adjusted to maintain this flow rate.

Complications of IV Therapy. Intravenous therapy involves some risk to the patient. It is an invasive procedure and as such can result in both local and systemic problems. Table 5-6 summarizes some of the local and systemic reactions that can result from IV therapy.

TABLE 5-6   *Summary of Complications during IV Therapy*

Problem	Causes	Signs/Symptoms
Local Reactions/Problems		
Dislodged catheter	Improper taping of catheter or loosened tape.	Check to see if catheter has backed out and if there is any fluid infiltration in the surrounding tissue
Thrombosis	Injury to the vein wall causing thrombus formation	IV flow stopped Pain at the site, reddened vein
Phlebitis	Access unit left in too long Thrombophlebitis at catheter tip Incompatible IV solution	Area over vein swollen or puffy Increased temperature Vein feels hard on palpation Redness along vein
Catheter occlusion	Lock not flushed Line clamped too long Solution flow interrupted	Backflow of blood in the line Pain or discomfort at puncture site No visible increase in flow rate when bag is raised
Extravasation	Catheter dislodged Vein punctured	No backflow of blood Swelling at or above puncture site resulting in tightening of skin Decreased skin temperature at puncture site
Vasovagal reaction	Anxiety causing vasospasm Can result from pain	Vein collapse (during insertion) Reduced blood pressure Sweating, faintness, or dizziness accompanied by nausea
Damage to nerves or tendons	Improper technique Catheter or needle secured too tight	Numbness Extreme pain Feeling of electric shock (nerve injury)
Systemic Reactions/Complications		
Allergic reaction	Reaction to medication	Anaphylactic symptoms: Urticaria Wheezing Bronchospasm Itching Cardiac arrest
Infection Septicemia Bacteremia	Poorly secured catheter Poor aseptic technique Catheter left in place too long Phlebitis	Fever Chills Malaise
Air embolism	Empty bag or bottle Line not purged before bag or bottle replaced	Reduced blood pressure Unconsciousness Weakened pulse Respiratory distress
Circulatory overload	Flow rate too rapid Improper calculation of flow rate	Respiratory distress Increased blood pressure Discomfort and neck veins distended

CONSCIOUS SEDATION

During short-term surgical, diagnostic, and therapeutic procedures the patient can be administered a pharmacologic agent that produces a form of **conscious sedation** in which he or she has a depressed level of consciousness but will respond to verbal commands and physical stimulation. The pharmacologic agents that are commonly administered are the benzodiazepines (e.g., midazolam) and narcotic analgesics (e.g., fentanyl). These drugs are given usually in small doses that produce a light sedation in which the patient can maintain airway reflexes and respond to stimuli.

It is important that all patients under conscious sedation be monitored continuously both throughout the procedure and during the recovery phase. The monitoring parameters should include blood pressure, respirations, oxygen saturation via pulse oximeter, heart rate and rhythm, as well as the level of consciousness. Oxygen should be available to the patient in all medical treatment rooms.

Adverse patient reactions are possible, and the imaging suite and recovery space should have an emergency crash cart equipped with a defibrillator, suction device, positive pressure breathing machine, and a variety of airways. The personnel responsible for the patients should be adequately trained in the recognition of cardiac arrhythmias, oxygen administration, and advanced cardiopulmonary resuscitation. Reactions are generally specific to the type of medications administered, and knowledge of their actions and adverse complications should be understood.

PHARMACOLOGIC AGENTS USED DURING ADVANCED PROCEDURES

The ARRT certification handbook for both cardiac and vascular interventional radiography content specifications lists a number of drug types and administration routes that may be utilized in the diagnostic/interventional suite or prescribed for the patient. Table 5-7 lists the general categories of drugs, their uses, and their routes of administration. Dose information is not included as this is particular to the patient and condition. The choices of dose and drug are made by the physician.

Preprocedure Pharmacologic Agents

Two classes of pharmacologic agents are used to medicate patients before angiography—sedatives and analgesics. Some of the agents span both classes and produce effects that are considered both sedative and analgesic. In addition, certain agents have a concomitant effect when used in conjunction with other pharmacologic agents. Dosages should be individualized to the patient's age, weight, and overall health status. The characteristics and recommended rate and routes of administration should be known and understood before administration of any pharmacologic agent.

Sedatives

Sedatives are administered to decrease the activity of the central nervous system (CNS). Excessive stimulation of the CNS can cause an individual to become more alert, anxious, and irritable. In the extreme, excessive stimulation can even cause convulsions. Sedatives reduce the desire for physical activity and have a calming or tranquilizing effect on the patient. The net effect is that the patient experiences a reduction in anxiety level relating to the procedure. Some frequently used sedatives are diphenhydramine, promethazine hydrochloride, hydroxyzine hydrochloride, and phenobarbital.

Phenobarbital (Nembutal). This agent is classified as a barbiturate and a nonspecific CNS depressant. Barbiturates produce what is considered to be dose-dependent depression of the CNS. The action of this agent is short in duration (4 to 6 hours). An intramuscular dose of 150 to 200 mg can produce a hypnotic effect. The average intramuscular dose for angiography premedication ranges from 75 to 100 mg. Phenobarbital is contraindicated in patients with hepatic disease, emphysema or other breathing disorders, or porphyria.

TABLE 5-7   *Summary of Drug Types*

Category	Description/Use	Route of Administration	Examples
Analgesics	Reduce pain without loss of consciousness; however, in some individuals a loss of consciousness can occur. Classed as opioids, nonopioids, and other.	Opioid: Parenteral Oral/parenteral Oral Oral/parenteral Oral Nonopioid Oral Oral	Fentanyl Morphine Codeine Meperidine Oxycodone Naproxen Ibuprofen
Antiarrhythmics	Treat alterations in the rhythm of the heart	Oral Oral Oral Oral/parenteral Oral/parenteral Oral/parenteral Oral/parenteral Parenteral Parenteral	Beta-blockers Metoprolol Propranolol Nadolol Calcium channel blockers Verapamil Diltiazem Amlodipine Digoxin Adenosine Lidocaine
Antibiotics	Treat bacterial or fungal infections	Parenteral Oral/parenteral Oral/parenteral Oral/parenteral Oral/parenteral Oral/parenteral Oral/parenteral	Aminoglycosides, Cephalosporins Macrolides Lincosamides Penicillins Sulfonamides Tetracyclines
Anticoagulants	Aid in hindering the coagulation of the blood	Oral/injection	Warfarin Heparin Lepirudin
Antiemetics	Prevent vomiting	Oral/rectal/injection	Metoclopramide hydroxyzine Prochlorperazine
Antihypertensives	Used in the treatment of high blood pressure (hypertension); usually accompanied by treatment with diuretic.	Oral Oral/parenteral	Metoprolol Vasotec
Antiplatelets	Used to destroy blood platelets	Oral Oral/parenteral Parenteral	Aspirin Tirofiban Epoprostenol
Anxiolytics	Helps to reduce anxiety such as generalized anxiety, phobias, panic disorders, post-traumatic stress disorder	Parenteral Oral Oral Oral/parenteral Oral/parenteral Parenteral Oral/parenteral	Benzodiazepines Midazolam Diazepam (Valium) Clonazepam Oxazepam Barbiturates Lorazepam Thiopental Phenobarbital

TABLE 5-7   *Summary of Drug Types (cont'd)*

Category	Description/Use	Route of Administration	Examples
Beta-blockers	Combine with and block beta-receptors—used to decrease the heart rate and force of contractions and lower high blood pressure; can be used to treat arrhythmias	See Antiarrhythmics and Antihypertensives	See Antiarrhythmics
Calcium channel blockers	Used to treat some forms of angina pectoris and some cardiac arrhythmias	See Antiarrhythmics	See Antiarrhythmics
Diuretics	Increase the excretion of urine; also used to treat congestive heart failure	Angiotensin-converting enzyme (ACE) inhibitors Oral Oral Loop diuretics Oral/parenteral Oral/parenteral Thiazides Oral Oral	Enalapril Perindopril Furosemide Torasemide Bendroflumethiazide Hydrochlorothiazide
Narcotics	Dull the senses, relieve pain, induce sleep; controlled substances that have a wide range of potential for abuse	See Analgesics	See Analgesics
Sedatives	Reduce excitement or nervousness, produce a calming effect; also produce sleep or loss of consciousness	See Anxiolytics	See Anxiolytics
Thrombolytics	Used to eliminate or break up a thrombus—blood clots remaining attached to the wall of vessels	Oral Parenteral Parenteral Parenteral Parenteral Parenteral	Warfarin Streptokinase Alteplase Duteplase Heparin Low molecular weight heparins (LMWHs)
Vasoconstrictors	Cause narrowing of blood vessels	Parenteral	Levophed
Vasodilators	Cause widening or dilation of blood vessels	Parenteral Oral/parenteral Oral/parenteral/transdermal	Nitroprusside Ethanol Nitroglycerine

Hydroxyzine Hydrochloride (Vistaril). Hydroxyzine is indicated for the relief of the anxiety, tension, and psychomotor agitation experienced by the patient before a diagnostic or interventional angiographic procedure. It also controls the nausea and vomiting that can be attendant with the administration of the contrast agent. The only contraindication is previous sensitivity to the agent. It should be noted that hydroxyzine has a concomitant effect when used in conjunction with other CNS depressants. The usual dose is 25 to 100 mg administered intramuscularly.

Promethazine Hydrochloride (Phenergan). This drug belongs to the family of drugs generically called the phenothiazines and functions primarily as an antihistaminic agent. It also has an antiemetic, anticholinergic (drying) effect. One of the major side effects of this drug is its ability to produce sedation. The duration of its action is short (4 to 6 hours). It is usually contraindicated when large amounts of other types of CNS depressants have been administered; it can be given in combination with other CNS depressants, but concomitant effects usually occur. Promethazine can intensify the action of the other drugs, and dosages should be adjusted to counter its influence. The usual dose ranges from 25 to 50 mg administered orally or intramuscularly.

Diphenhydramine (Benadryl). This drug is also primarily an antihistaminic agent. Diphenhydramine's sedative side effect makes it useful as premedication for angiographic procedures. It exhibits a marked anticholinergic effect that may be undesirable. The usual dose ranges from 25 to 50 mg administered intramuscularly or orally.

Analgesics

Analgesics are agents administered to reduce pain and are classified as narcotics (strong) and nonnarcotics (mild).

Narcotic analgesics are either derived from opium or synthetically produced to create the same pharmacologic effect. These agents can relieve pain without producing a loss of consciousness, and their use can lead to a physical dependence. Morphine, codeine, and hydromorphone (Dilaudid) are some naturally occurring opioids. Meperidine (Demerol), fentanyl (Sublimaze), and propoxyphene (Darvon) are representative of synthetic narcotic analgesic agents.

The narcotic analgesics primarily affect the CNS and the gastrointestinal system. They can alter the patient's mental alertness, are usually antitussive, and have the potential to cause physical dependence if used for chronic treatment. The narcotic analgesics usually produce nausea and vomiting as well as a depression of the respiratory system. The effects of the narcotic analgesics can be reversed with naloxone (Narcan). Among the contraindications to the use of this class of analgesics are a hypersensitivity to morphine and conditions such as severe CNS depression, bronchial asthma, head injury, acute alcoholism, cardiac arrhythmias, biliary obstruction, convulsive disorders, and increased intracranial pressure.

The agents most often used as premedication analgesics are morphine, meperidine, and fentanyl.

Morphine Sulfate. This analgesic is a naturally occurring opioid. The amount of agent used in the normal adult ranges from 2 to 20 mg administered intramuscularly. The onset of the analgesic effect usually occurs within 15 to 20 minutes, and its duration is from 3 to 6 hours. The effect on the patient's respiratory and gastrointestinal systems is moderate.

Meperidine (Demerol). This agent is also administered intramuscularly and has a dose range of 75 to 150 mg. It acts within 10 to 15 minutes and lasts 2 to 4 hours. Meperidine has a moderate probability of causing respiratory depression and gastrointestinal distress. This agent is usually administered with diazepam (Valium) to offset its negative effects.

Fentanyl (Sublimaze). Fentanyl is a reasonably fast-acting analgesic, with effects occurring within 5 to 15 minutes. It is also administered intramuscularly in the dose range of 0.05 to 0.1 mg. This drug has a high risk of causing respiratory depression, and the patient should be carefully monitored throughout the procedure.

Other Pharmacologic Agents

Each institution has its own armamentarium of drugs that are used before, during, and after the procedure. The list may differ from the group of agents discussed in this text; however, the radiographer or cardiovascular and interventional technologist should become familiar with each of the agents and their action, dose, and adverse reactions. If the biliary tree is undergoing study, the patient may also be given antibiotic treatment before the procedure begins as a prophylactic measure to prevent infection. The initial dose is administered as a preventive measure, and treatment is usually continued for 24 hours after an uncomplicated procedure.

Several other pharmacologic agents can have significant use in the special procedure suite—diazepam (Valium), naloxone (Narcan), and atropine.

Diazepam (Valium). This drug is used to relieve the anxiety the patient experiences before the procedure. Diazepam can reduce the requirement for opioid analgesics and is an adjunct for the relief of painful acute musculoskeletal conditions. It can be administered in conjunction with some of the narcotic analgesics, such as meperidine.

Naloxone (Narcan). Narcan is a narcotic antagonist that prevents or reverses the effects of the opioid narcotic analgesic agents. Its action can be demonstrated within 2 minutes. Its usual dose range for an adult is from 0.4 to 2 mg, administered intravenously.

Atropine. This drug can reduce the effect of laryngospasm. Although it has not found a place as a premedication for special procedures, it is a bronchodilator and is sometimes given as a preoperative agent to reduce salivation and excessive secretions in the respiratory tract. Atropine can prevent the cholinergic effects of some of the pharmacologic agents, such as cardiac arrhythmias, hypotension, and bradycardia.

Emergency Medications

As stated earlier in the introduction, the special procedure radiographer must be familiar with the types of medications that are administered to the patient before, during, and after the procedure. The radiographer should also be knowledgeable about those medications that are administered in emergency situations. We have already seen some of the medications that could be used as preangiographic agents and during the examination. It is equally important for the radiographer to have a familiarity with some of the drugs that are commonly found on the emergency drug cart. When an emergency occurs, there is little time to search for the proper medication. The locations, containers, and general dosages of these medications should be known and readily at hand. A number of reactions that occur during and after the examination fall under the allergic reaction category. Table 5-8 lists several medications that are commonly found on the emergency cart at most institutions.

Dose Calculations

In most cases today, medications come from the manufacturer already prepared for administration to the patient. This preparation is usually referred to as dose packaging. This form of medication will almost always be found on the emergency cart because time plays an important part in the successful treatment of the patient. In some cases the amount of medication must be calculated. The reasons for this include calculation of dose by body weight, body surface area, as a portion of a vial, from a stock solution, or as a calculation during intravenous therapy. The mathematical formulae for dose calculations should already be known from basic mathematics and general radiography. The ratio and proportion are frequently used to calculate dosage, and these basic formulae should be familiar to all who work in such situations.

Dose calculations are based on amounts expressed as weight, volume, and equivalents, depending upon the medication. Drug measurements are categorized using one of three systems. In the early days of pharmacology medication, measurement was made using the **apothecary system**. This oldest form of measurement has been primarily phased out by the **metric system**. Calculations of medications in the health care field are primarily accomplished using the metric system of measurement. The **household system** of measurement is the third system of measurement. Dose calculations using this system are used by patients and relatives in home care situations. Although this system is somewhat inaccurate, it is the one that is the most familiar to the population in general.

Although the apothecary system is infrequently used, the radiographer should be familiar with the symbols associated with the weight and volume units of measure. These units are summarized in Table 5-9. In this system the dosage quantities are usually written as lower case Roman numerals (e.g., i, ii, iii, iv). Amounts greater than 10 are expressed as the Arabic numbers (e.g., 11, 12) with the

TABLE 5-8 *Emergency Medications*

Medication	Route of Administration	Dosage	Indication
Alpha-adrenergic drug class			
Norepinephrine			
Levophed	Intravenous	1–10 g/min	Causes contraction of
Epinephrine			smooth muscle resulting
Adrenaline	Intravenous	0.5–1.0 ml of 1:1000 solution	in vasoconstriction; used to treat hypotension, increase blood pressure, and maintain circulation
Aminophylline	Intravenous	6–10 mg/kg	Bronchial dilator, used to treat bronchospasm
Atropine	Intramuscular Intravenous, oral	0.4–1 mg	Increases heart rate Preoperative medication Antagonist to cholinergic drugs
Benadryl (diphenhydramine)	Intravenous Intramuscular	10–50 mg 400 mg/day (max)	Acute allergic reactions Urticaria Dermatitis
Dopamine	Continuous intravenous infusion	800 mg in 500 ml D_5W	Shock Cardiac stimulant increasing cardiac output and renal blood flow High doses can cause vasoconstriction
Diazepam (Valium)	Intramuscular Intravenous	5–10 mg 10 mg	Convulsions Antianxiety medication
Glucocorticoids			
Solu-Cortef	Intravenous Intramuscular	100–500 mg 100–500 mg	Anti-inflammatory
Solu-Medrol	Intravenous	10–40 mg	
Hyoscyamine	Intravenous, oral	0.25–1.0 mg	Same as atropine
Lidocaine	Intravenous	50–100 mg	Ventricular tachycardia Ventricular fibrillation
Organic acid diuretics			
Lasix (furosemide)	Intravenous, oral	40 mg/2 ml	Used to relieve edema;
Demadex (torsemide)	Intravenous	10–20 mg	also referred to as "loop" diuretics
Morphine	Intravenous Intramuscular Subcutaneous	5–10 mg 2–20 mg 2–20 mg	Analgesic, relieves pain and produces sedation
Nitrites and nitrates			
Nitroglycerine	Sublingual	0.15–0.6 mg	Antianginal class of drugs used
Transderm-Nitro	Intravenous Patch (cutaneous)	2.5–15 mg	to reduce pain when blood flow to the heart is reduced
Promethazine	Intravenous Intramuscular	25 mg	Adjuncts to pre- and postoperative medications to minimize anesthetic irritability; reduces nausea and vomiting
Verapamil	Intravenous	5–10 mg	Produces vasodilation, used to treat angina and supraventricular tachycardia

TABLE 5-9 *Apothecary Units of Measurement*

Weight		Volume	
Unit	Symbol	Unit	Symbol
grain	gr	minim	min
dram	dr	fluidram	fl dr
ounce	oz	fluidounce	fl oz
		pint	pt
		quart	qt

The following symbols should not be used: ʒ, ℥ . These are considered to be error-prone abbreviations and appear on the ISMP "List of Error Prone Abbreviations, Symbols and Dose Designations," 2004, accessed at http://www.ISMP.org.

exception of 20 and 30, which are expressed as **xx** and **xxx,** respectively. Any amount less than one is expressed as a fraction (e.g., $^5/_8$, $^7/_8$) with the exception of one half which is written as **ss**. Equivalents between weight and volume are as follows:

- 1 minim = 1 grain (1 minim of fluid weighs the same as 1 grain)
- 1 grain = 0.065 gram
- 60 grains or 60 minims = 1 dram or 1 fluidram
- 8 drams or 8 fluid drams = 1 ounce or 1 fluidounce

The **metric** system is the preferred method of measurement of medication. The common units of drug measurement in the metric system are the liter (volume) and the gram (weight). Specifically, the milliliter (1/1000 of a liter) represents the amount that can fit in a space measuring one centimeter (1/100 of a meter) on each side, commonly known as one cubic centimeter (cc). Unlike the apothecary system the doses are written in Arabic units, and fractions are generally decimal equivalents. The common symbols of measurements in the metric system are summarized in Table 5-10.

Conversions of weights and volume are commonplace in the calculation of doses using the metric system. It is essential for the radiographer to master these simple conversions in order to make calculation simple and accurate. Some common equivalents are as follows:

- 1 (milliliter) ml = 1 (cubic centimeter) cc
- 1000 ml = 1 liter (L)
- 1000 (micrograms) mcg = 1 (milligram) mg
- 100 milligrams = 0.1 (gram) g

The household system of measurement is not used in the health care setting. All of the units are written in Arabic numbers. Some examples of measurements in the household system are found in Table 5-11.

Occasionally it will be necessary to convert between systems. This can usually be learned with some practice. Certain basic equivalents can make these conversions a little simpler:

- 1/60 grain (gr) is equivalent to 1 milligram (mg)
- 1 grain (gr) is equivalent to 60 milligrams (mg)

TABLE 5-10 *Metric Units of Measurement*

Weight		Volume	
Unit	Symbol	Unit	Symbol
microgram	mcg*	milliliter	ml
milligram	mg or mgm	cubic centimeter	cm³*
gram	g, Gm, or gm	liter	L or l
kilogram	kg		

*The abbreviations "µg" and "cc" are no longer valid. (April 1, 2004—JCAHO "Do not use list.")

TABLE 5-11	*Some Symbols Used in the Household System of Measurement*		
Weight		**Volume**	
Unit	**Symbol**	**Unit**	**Symbol**
Ounce (dry)	oz	Drop (gutta), drops	gt , gtt
Pound	lb	Teaspoon	tsp
		Tablespoon	tbsp

- 15 grains (gr) is equivalent to 1 gram (gm)
- 60 drops (gtt) is equivalent to 1 teaspoon (tsp)
- 1 teaspoon (tsp) is equivalent to 5.0 milliliter (ml)
- 1 milliliter (ml) is equivalent to 15 drops (gtt)

Calculation of Solutions

Calculations of solutions are usually expressed as percentages and can be stated in three ways depending on how the solution was prepared. We already discussed the concept of solution and solutes when we addressed osmolality. The three categories of solutions are volume to volume (v/v), weight to volume (w/v), and weight to weight (w/w). Tables 5-9, 5-10, and 5-11 illustrate the common symbols for measurements in both weight and volume.

When checking dosages of solutions it is important to identify which of the three categories is being used. In all cases the final equivalent should equal 100 parts. When working in the **volume to volume** category the 100 parts are measured by volume; for example, a 20% volume to volume solution of NaCl (sodium chloride) in water would contain 20 ml of 100% sodium chloride solution plus a sufficient amount of solvent (usually water) to make 100 ml of the final solution.

A **weight to volume** measurement would relate a specific amount (weight) of a solute into enough solvent to make 100 parts by volume. Using the example of a 20% solution of NaCl in a weight to volume category, 20 g of sodium chloride would be added to a sufficient amount of solute to make 100 ml of the weight to volume solution.

Finally, in the **weight to weight** category, the final solution has a certain amount of solute (by weight) in a certain weight of solution to give 100 parts by weight. Again using a 20% NaCl solution, in this category 20 g of NaCl is added to 80 g of solute (water) to make 100 g of a 20% NaCl solution.

Calculation by Age or Weight

Radiographic studies are performed on the pediatric patient as well as the adult. It should make sense that there must be a difference in dosage between patients in each of these categories. The patient's weight also plays a factor in how much medication should be administered. Over the years there have been several different rules for calculating pediatric dosage (Young's rule, Cowling's rule, and rules by Dillings and Gabius). To aid in the process of adjusting pediatric dose, a benchmark by various ages and weights needs to be in place for each of the groups (Box 5-4).

No matter which formula we use it is always assumed that the adult weight is 150 lb and age is 150 months. The formula for adjustment by **age** is shown below:

$$\frac{\text{Patient's age (months)} \times \text{Adult dose}}{\text{Adult's age (150 months)}} = \text{Pediatric dose}$$

If the calculation was being based upon the weight of the individuals, the formula would look similar with the exception that the age would be replaced by the weight of the individuals.

$$\frac{\text{Patient's weight} \times \text{Adult dose}}{\text{Adult weight (150 lb)}} = \text{Pediatric dose}$$

The radiographer may not be called upon often to perform such calculations; however, being alert and knowing the difference between an adult dose and a pediatric dose could prevent a serious injury.

BOX 5-4	*Weight Benchmarks for Various Age Groups*	
Group	**Weight**	**Age**
Infant	<40 lb	0–24 months
Child	<150 lb	25–150 months
Adult	>150 lb	>150 months

SUMMARY

Pharmacology is a very complex area of study. The materials presented in this chapter were by no means covered in depth. The radiographer must be familiar with pharmacologic terminology, common medications used in diagnostic and interventional radiography, simple dose calculations, and the four major methods or routes of administration and their divisions.

The Six Rights of parenteral drug administration were presented: the right patient, right drug, right dosage, right route, right time, and right documentation.

A discussion about osmolality and osmolarity was covered. This segment has relevance in this chapter as well as in Chapter 6 in relation to contrast agents commonly used. The discussion included the different types of solutions that are commonly used: isotonic, hypotonic, and hypertonic.

The major types of medications were also discussed listing some common medications and their routes of administration. In performing angiographic and interventional studies the radiographer will be required to have at least a familiarity with the types of medications used as well as some of their common dosages, indications, and complications. Common emergency medications were listed, and their common doses discussed. This was not a complete listing of what might be found on the angiography suite's emergency cart, but it represents a catalogue of the more common drugs generally found in emergency carts. The radiographer should be familiar with the contents of the department's emergency cart.

The coverage on intravenous therapy included the method of inserting the Angiocath, some common solutions that are used, and the method of calculating the drop factor for proper dosage. Venipuncture was also discussed, and the equipment used for this and intravenous therapy was listed.

A segment on dose calculations was included, describing the three major categories of measurements: the apothecary, metric, and household. Calculations were described for adult and pediatric doses of drugs by volume, weight, and age. If additional information about the various medications is desired, the Suggested Readings should provide numerous detailed resources for the radiographer.

REFERENCES

1. Content Specifications for the ARRT Advanced Level Examination. Accessed at www.ARRT.org
2. Snyder K, Keegan C: *Pharmacology for the Surgical Technologist*, 2nd ed. St Louis, 2006, WB Saunders.
3. Institute for Safe Medication Practices: ISMP's List of High Alert Medications. Accessed at http://www.ismp.org/MSAarticles/highalert.htm, December 2003.
4. Perry AG, Potter PA: *Clinical Nursing Skills and Techniques*, 4th ed. St Louis, 1998, Mosby.

SUGGESTED READINGS

Bass A, Kinter L, Williams P: Origins, practices and future of safety pharmacology. *J Pharmacol Toxicol Methods* 49(3):145–151, 2004.

Centers for Disease Control and Prevention: Guideline for infection control in health care personnel. *Infect Control Hosp Epidemiol* 19(6):445, 1998.

Douglas SA, Ohlstein EH, Johns DG: Techniques: cardiovascular pharmacology and drug discovery in the 21st century. *Trends Pharmacol Sci* 25(4):225–233, 2004.

Godfraind T: TiPS, a venture in pharmacology. *Trends Pharmacol Sci* 25(4):167–169, 2004.

Pratt WB, Taylor P: *Principles of Drug Action: The Basis of Pharmacology*, 3rd ed. New York, 1990, Churchill Livingston.

Pugliese G, Salahuddin M: *Sharps Injury Prevention Program. A Step-By-Step Guide.* Chicago, 1999, American Hospital Association.

Rang HP, Dale MM, Ritter JM, Moore PK: *Pharmacology*, 5th ed. New York, 2003, Churchill Livingstone.

Roth S, Lyon M, Nakatsu K: Presentation and discussion of pharmacology. *Clin Invest Med* 23(1):90-92, 2000.

Thompson's PDR, 58th ed, Montvale, NJ, 2004, Thomson Publishing.

STUDY QUESTIONS

1. Which of the following routes of administration is not considered to be parenteral?
   a. intravenous
   c. sublingual
   b. subcutaneous
   d. intramuscular

2. An antagonist of a drug is usually one that:
   a. works in synergy with another drug
   b. blocks the action of another drug
   c. causes the patient to react
   d. should not be administered as a parenteral drug

3. Normal saline 0.9% NaCl is considered to be a(n):
   a. hypertonic solution
   b. hypotonic solution
   c. isotonic solution
   d. solution that has no value in IV therapy

4. Which of the following is not considered to be one of the six rights of medication administration:
   a. right place
   b. right dosage
   c. right patient
   d. right route

5. An analgesic drug is one that helps the patient:
   a. fight off allergic reactions
   b. come out of shock
   c. relieve pain
   d. fight off bacteria

6. Which of the following is a unit of volume in the metric system?
   a. microgram
   b. kilogram
   c. milligram
   d. cubic centimeter

7. Swelling at or above the puncture site during or after the injection is an indication of:
   a. urticaria
   b. dyspnea
   c. extravasation
   d. thrombus formation

STUDY QUESTIONS (*cont'd*)

8. When making calculations for pediatric patients the adult weight is always considered to be:
   a. >40 lb
   b. >60 lb
   c. >100 lb
   d. >150 lb

9. Diazepam is considered to be an _____ drug.
   a. antihistaminic
   b. antianxiolytic
   c. anti-inflammatory
   d. analgesic

10. Urticaria, wheezing, and bronchospasm are considered symptoms of a(n) _____ reaction.
    a. inflammatory
    b. bacteremic
    c. allergic
    d. air embolism

6 *Contrast Media*

CHAPTER OBJECTIVES

After completing this chapter, the reader will be able to perform the following:

- Identify the necessity for the use of contrast agents
- List the types of contrast agents that are currently available
- Describe the classes of contrast agents
- Describe the evolution of the organic iodine contrast media
- Define the characteristics of a good contrast agent
- Describe the excretory pathways of the various contrast agents
- Define informed consent as it applies to contrast media studies
- List and describe the general precautions that should be applied to every contrast medium study
- Identify the reactions and complications resulting from the use of contrast agents
- List the specialty contrast agents

CHAPTER OUTLINE

TYPES

    Negative Contrast Agents
    Positive Contrast Agents

CLASSES OF RADIOPAQUE CONTRAST MEDIA

    Evolution of the Organic Iodine Class of Contrast Media
    Characteristics of Radiopaque Contrast Media

EXCRETORY PATHWAYS

GENERAL PRECAUTIONS

REACTIONS

    Overdose Reactions
    Anaphylactic Reactions
    Cardiovascular Reactions
    Psychogenic Reactions
    Activation System—Triggering Reactions

COMPLICATIONS

    Extravasation

SPECIALTY CONTRAST AGENTS

SUMMARY

All of the examinations designated as special or advanced procedures require the introduction of some type of material into the area of interest to provide contrast. This is necessary because the differences in density among the various tissues in the body are too small to provide adequate contrast for visualization of anatomic details. To compensate for this, it is necessary to increase or decrease the density of the organ to provide the desired contrast. Most of the studies in this text depend on the use of intravascular contrast agents to yield diagnostic information. The use of contrast media has increased with the increase in the use of computed tomography (CT), magnetic resonance imaging (MRI), and digital subtraction angiography (DSA).

Some of the familiar, so-called routine special procedures (e.g., barium enemas, excretory urograms) as well as the advanced procedures increase the subject density by the addition of a radiopaque substance that renders the organ radiopaque. In some cases, however, it may be undesirable to increase the density of an organ. In these situations, the density of the organ can be decreased by the addition of a radiolucent substance.

Unlike the pharmaceuticals discussed in Chapter 5, the amounts used are much greater than those used for therapeutic drugs. They are designed to remain in the organ of interest for a very short period of time and are not designed to cause any changes either biologically or chemically in the body.

Contrast agents can be classified into two broad groups, depending on their interaction with x-radiation—positive contrast agents (radiopaque) and negative contrast agents (radiolucent).

TYPES

Negative Contrast Agents

The absorption of x-rays by a substance is dependent upon several factors, one of which is the atomic weight of the substance. Those materials that have lower atomic weights will attenuate less radiation. The resultant remnant radiation will produce a greater radiographic density (darker image) on the image receptor. This characteristic is useful when the objective is to demonstrate an anatomic structure against the dark background or to provide a silhouette image of the structure.

Examples of **radiolucent**, or **negative**, contrast agents are air, oxygen, carbon dioxide, and nitrous oxide. Most of the available gasses have been used as negative contrast agents with varying results; however, the four gases listed here are the most commonly used negative (radiolucent) contrast agents. The negative contrast agents can also be used in conjunction with a positive contrast agent. One common procedure that uses this combination of contrast agents is the double contrast barium enema.

Air and oxygen may be dangerous during certain procedures because they can cause gas emboli, but carbon dioxide and nitrogen do not pose the risk of gas emboli and can be used with relative safety. They are also able to be absorbed rapidly by the body. This factor can be advantageous when rapid absorption is desired, but in cases in which many radiographs are taken, it is a definite disadvantage.

Positive Contrast Agents

Because of their high atomic numbers, positive contrast agents cause an increase in the attenuation of x-rays and are considered to be **radiopaque**. They produce an area of decreased radiographic density on the image receptor. Contrast agents that are radiopaque contain elements with high atomic numbers such as iodine, bromine, and barium. When these substances are used to fill organs, they essentially make the organ radiopaque, and the image appears clear or white on the radiograph. They can take the form of tablets, powders, and liquids and can be introduced into the body through a variety of routes. They are relatively nontoxic in most cases, but certain patients may exhibit reactions of varying severity, especially to agents containing iodine. In some cases, small doses of these agents may cause death.

The positive contrast agents used during the advanced procedures discussed in this text will be organic iodine compounds.

CLASSES OF RADIOPAQUE CONTRAST MEDIA

Contrast agents used for intravenous injections fall into one of two major classes: ionic and nonionic. The **ionic compounds** are further subdivided into **high osmolality ionic compounds (HOCA)** and

low osmolality ionic compounds (LOCA). All of the positive contrast agents used for intravenous injection are organic iodine compounds that use iodine as the substance that provides the contrast.

Osmolarity and osmolality were discussed in Chapter 5. The **blood-brain barrier** separates the parenchyma (organ tissue) of the central nervous system from the blood, preventing or slowing the passage of potentially harmful substances from the blood into the tissue of the central nervous system. The hyperosmolality of the ionic organic iodine contrast agents is at the root of many of the major reactions that occur during radiographic procedures. One example of such a reaction is the degradation of the ionic contrast agents into electrically charged particles that can potentially disrupt the heart's electrical activity, thereby increasing the risks for arrhythmia.

It has been demonstrated that the nonionic contrast agents produce fewer adverse drug reactions. This has been attributed to the osmolality of the material. The ionic compounds have a greater tendency to pass the blood-brain barrier owing to their hyperosmolality. The following list provides the osmolalities of the various types of organic iodine contrast agents and both plasma and cerebrospinal fluid:

Agent	Osmolality
High osmolality ionic compounds	1800–2100 mOsm/kg water
Low osmolality ionic compounds	600–850 mOsm/kg water
Nonionic compounds	300–484 mOsm/kg water
Plasma	280–295 mOsm/kg water
Cerebrospinal fluid	301 mOsm/kg water

As evidenced from the list of osmolalities, the ionic compounds have two to seven times the osmolality of the cerebrospinal fluid and the blood, creating an increased potential for reactions to these agents.

The **nonionic compounds** have demonstrated clinically a marked reduction in adverse drug reactions relating to their use in special procedures. Another feature of this type of contrast agent is that patients are much more comfortable during the study. Also, there are fewer subjective side effects. This has the combined effect of producing less anxiety in the patient, and psychogenic responses are less likely to occur. Because the nonionic contrast media are less apt to damage the blood-brain barrier, they demonstrate a very low neurotoxicity. The nonionic agents also exhibit a high compatibility with other intravascular medications used during angiography and the treatment of allergic reactions.

This would lead one to think that it would be advantageous to use nonionic contrast agents exclusively in radiography. Adopting a policy of this nature would be easy from a medical standpoint, but there are economic considerations that make the decision difficult. The cost of the nonionic contrast agents is somewhat greater than that of ionic agents. At the present time, the ionic contrast agents are still used; however, the nonionic or low osmolality contrast media have become the primary type of agent used in the diagnostic and interventional arena. Most institutions screen their patients for a variety of risk factors, and based on this information the radiologist will select the dose and type of contrast media to be used. Depending upon the results of the screening process, it is possible to reduce the use of the low osmolality contrast media. In some institutions the use of nonionic contrast media is restricted to high-risk patients or individuals in which the history identifies a high potential for reaction. This type of protocol can result in a substantial economic saving without a corresponding increase in moderate or severe reactions. Almost all of the institutions performing angiographic studies are using the nonionic contrast agents exclusively despite the drawbacks of cost and lack of adequate reimbursement. The American College of Radiology has developed guidelines for the use of the low osmolality and nonionic contrast media.[1]

Evolution of the Organic Iodine Class of Contrast Media
Ionic Organic Iodine Compounds

The ionic contrast agents used for vascular studies are salts of organic iodine compounds such as benzene. The basic configuration can be drawn as a six-sided ring structure (Fig. 6-1, *A*). The locations

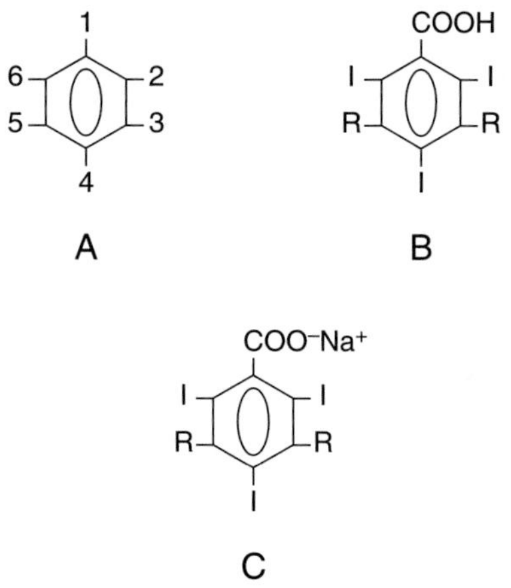

FIGURE 6-1. Basic foundation structure of the organic iodine compounds. **A**, Basic ring structure with the positions 1 through 6 marked. **B**, Basic structure with iodine atoms added to the 2, 4, and 6 positions. The COOH structure designates this as an acid. *R* indicates positions where side chain molecules are attached. **C**, Schematic illustration of the material as a salt, showing the cation and anion.

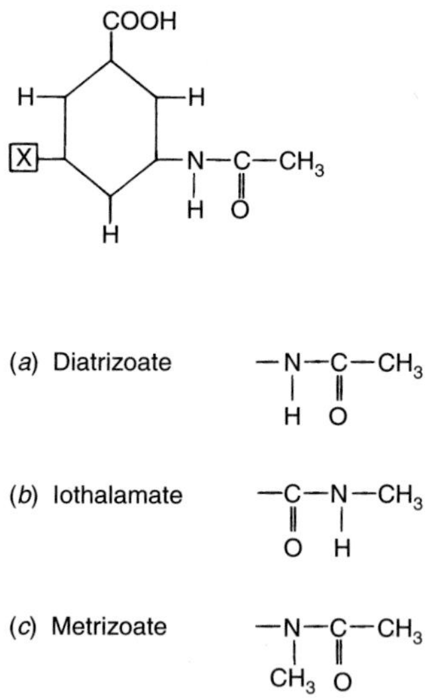

FIGURE 6-2. Basic structure of the anions of the organic iodine compounds used during angiography. The three side chains, diatrizoate (*a*), iothalamate (*b*), and metrizoate (*c*), can be substituted in the block marked *X* on the basic structure to form the different compounds.

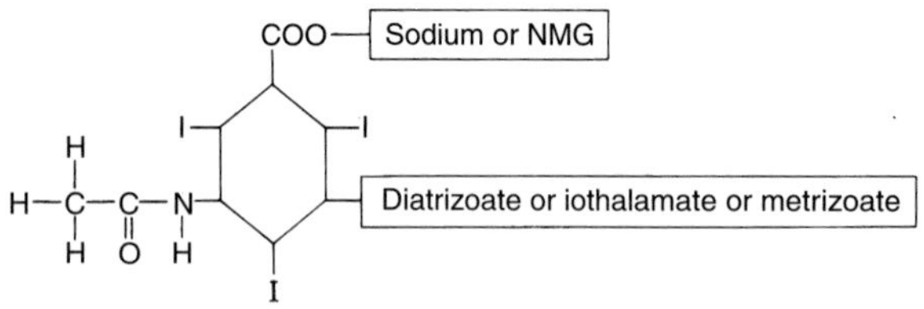

FIGURE 6-3. Basic structure combined with the anionic side chains and cations to form an organic iodine compound.

marked 1 through 6 on the illustration represent places where chemical structures can be attached. Figure 6-1, *B*, shows the placement of the iodine atoms on the molecule. The addition of iodine atoms in the 2, 4, and 6 positions and the conversion of the acid molecule (COOH) to a salt (Fig. 6-1, *C*) are the basis for the organic iodine compounds used today. The locations marked with the letter "R" are the sites used to place various side chains. The side chains initially were amino groups that helped to decrease the toxicity of the compound.

The anions of the common angiographic contrast media begin as organic benzoic acid compounds. The different angiographic contrast agents have the same basic ring structure but can differ in the side chains located at the 3 and 5 position (Fig. 6-2). Different side chains are used to improve solubility and tolerance to the material. The anions are combined with a cation to form a salt (Fig. 6-3). The major cations used to form the compound can be either sodium or meglumine (*n*-methylglucamine). Each of these salts has different characteristics and will affect the patient differently.

When injected into the patient, the ionic organic iodine compounds disassociate to form two particles: an **anion** (negatively charged) and a **cation** (positively charged). These conventional contrast agents are considered to be 3:2 compounds; that is, they deliver three atoms of iodine for contrast to two particles to provide osmolality.

Experimental results have shown that the meglumine salts are less toxic than the sodium salts of the organic iodine contrast agents. However, the sodium salts are less viscous than solutions of the meglumine salts with the same iodine content.

The ionic contrast agents currently available for angiographic use are either meglumine salts or combinations of meglumine and sodium salts. The toxicity of the low–viscosity, sodium salt contrast agents can be reduced somewhat by the addition of calcium and magnesium to the solution.

Nonionic Contrast Agents

These substances were developed because the high osmolality of the ionic contrast agents was thought to be responsible for the majority of the undesirable side effects. The basic structure of the nonionic compounds is the same as that of the conventional agents. However, the various side chains added to the basic building block create a substance that does *not* disassociate (i.e., separate into an anion and a cation) (Fig. 6-4). They are considered to be 3:1 compounds—they contribute three iodine particles in solution to provide contrast and only one particle to provide osmolality. The ionic compounds are 3:2 in that they also contribute three iodine particles for contrast and two particles for osmolality.

Osmolality depends on the number of particles in solution. The nonionic compounds exhibit less osmolality than conventional ionic contrast agents because they provide fewer osmotically active particles. This results in fewer patient reactions.

Although their chemical structure differs, nonionic contrast agents are as effective as ionic agents in providing the necessary contrast during special procedure radiography. Their main advantage is in the reduction of both subjective and objective side effects in the patient.

Low Osmolality Ionic Contrast Agents

This type of contrast agent overlaps characteristics of the two previously mentioned types of substances; the compound uses the same basic building block but forms what is called a monoacid dimer. This compound is an ionic contrast agent, but it has the same type of compound ratio as the nonionic substances. The contrast agent illustrated in Figure 6-5 is a 6:2 compound; that is, it provides six iodine particles for contrast and two particles for osmolality. This type of contrast agent lies between ionic and nonionic agents in the mediation of side effects. Its advantages are that it more closely mimics the nonionic compounds and is not as costly.

Characteristics of Radiopaque Contrast Media

In the selection of a radiopaque contrast agent, certain characteristics such as viscosity, toxicity, iodine content, miscibility, and persistence must be considered. The ultimate choice of the contrast agent is usually

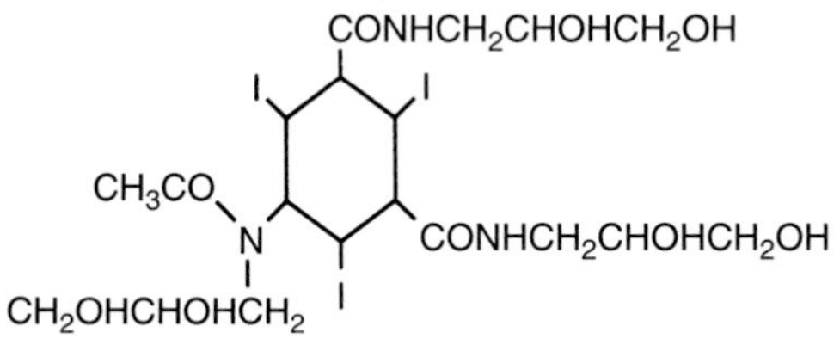

FIGURE 6-4. Chemical structure of iohexol (Omnipaque), an example of a nonionic contrast agent from Nycomed.

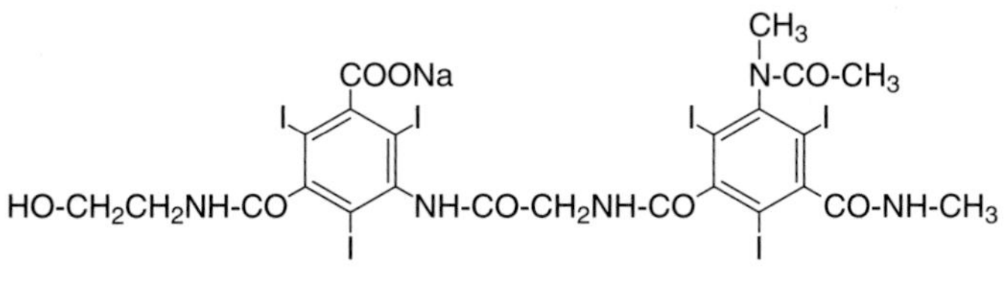

FIGURE 6-5. Sodium ioxaglate, a monoacid dimer, is a low osmolality compound with a 6:2 ratio of iodine atoms to particles in solution.

left to the physician performing the procedure, but the radiographer should understand the characteristics of contrast agents to be able to use them intelligently and efficiently during special procedures.

Iodine Concentration

The iodine atoms attached to the basic contrast agent structure are responsible for providing the radiopacity of the substance. As the iodine concentration of the contrast agent increases, the viscosity also increases. Compounds of the meglumine salts have a greater increase in viscosity than those of sodium salts. In considering the use of contrast agents during vascular procedures, viscosity becomes an important factor when long, small-bore catheters are used. More viscous contrast agents require greater injection pressures to deliver the same amount of material, increasing the possibility of patient trauma and catheter damage.

The iodine concentration itself is an important physical characteristic; it can be determined easily if the iodine content of the substance and the amount dissolved in its solvent are known. The iodine content is usually expressed in milligrams per milliliter or per cubic centimeter. Information relating to the physical characteristics of the contrast agents can be found in the product data sheet that is packaged with the contrast agent.

In comparing contrast agents, the amount of iodine delivered per second to the patient should be considered because contrast agents with a greater amount of meglumine salt usually have a lower iodine content as a result of the increased weight of the meglumine ion. Therefore, the amount of iodine delivered per second will be smaller. To illustrate this, if we compare the iodine content of Hypaque (sodium 50%) with that of both Conray (meglumine 60%) and Renografin 60% (meglumine 52%, sodium 8%) (Table 6-1), it can be seen that the Hypaque has a greater iodine content. It should be noted that Hypaque 50% contains 100% sodium salt, whereas Renografin 60% is a mixture of sodium and meglumine salts, and Conray 60% contains 100% meglumine salt. Table 6-2 illustrates the characteristics of some of the low osmolality and nonionic contrast agents.

Miscibility

The miscibility or immiscibility of a contrast agent is an important factor in vascular procedures. Angiographic contrast media must be completely miscible with the blood to prevent any possibility of contrast medium embolization.

Persistence

A final factor to consider regarding choice of contrast agent is the agent's persistence within the body. Because radiopaque agents instilled either directly or indirectly into body organs are foreign substances, it is important that they be excreted rapidly from the body. However, they should remain and

TABLE 6-1 *Characteristics of Some Ionic Intravascular Contrast Media*

Agent	Iodine Concentration %	Iodine Content mg/ml	Iodine Content %	Chemical Components Anion	Chemical Components Cation*	Viscosity (cP) 25° C	Viscosity (cP) 37.5° C	Sodium Content mEq/ml	Sodium Content mg/ml
Hypaque 60%	28 – 31%	282	28	Diatrizoate	Mg (60%)	6.22	4.18	0.001	0.02
Conray 60%		282	28	Iothalamate	Mg (60)%	6.10	4.0	0.0014	0.03
Renografin 60		288	29	Diatrizoate	Mg (52%)	6.0	3.9	0.16	3.76
Hypaque 50%		300	30	Diatrizoate	Na (8%) Na (50%)	3.25	2.5	0.8	18.1
Meglumine Diatrizoate 76%	36 – 40%	358	36	Diatrizoate	Mg (76%)	13.7	9.2	0.04	0.91
		370	37	Diatrizoate	Mg (66%)	13.94	9.1	0.19	4.48
Renografin 76		385	39	Diatrizoate	Na (10%)	13.4	8.35	0.39	9.0
Hypaque M75					Mg (50%) Na (25%)				

*Mg, Meglumine; Na, sodium; Ca, calcium.

TABLE 6-2 *Characteristics of Some Low Osmolality and Nonionic Contrast Media*

Agent	Iodine Content		Viscosity (cP)		Type
	mg/ml	%	25° C	37.5° C	
Visipaque	320	32	26.6	11.8.	Low osmolality
Visipaque	270	27	12.7	6.3	Low osmolality
Hexabrix	320	32	15.7	7.5	Low osmolality
Amipaque	170	17	2.9	1.8	Nonionic
Amipaque	300	30	12.7	6.2	Nonionic
Omnipaque	180	18	3.1	2.0	Nonionic
Omnipaque	240	24	5.8	3.4	Nonionic
Omnipaque	300	30	11.8	6.3	Nonionic
Omnipaque	350	35	20.4	10.4	Nonionic
Optiray	160	16	2.7	1.9	Nonionic
Optiray	240	24	4.6	3.0	Nonionic
Optiray	300	30	8.2	5.5	Nonionic
Optiray	320	32	9.9	5.8	Nonionic
Optiray	350	35	14.3	9.0	Nonionic

From Ansell G: *Notes on radiological emergencies*, London, 1996, Churchill Livingstone.

concentrate in the body organs long enough to provide an adequate radiographic study. This is an important criterion in the design of a suitable contrast agent.

Selective Localization

In most cases the contrast agent is delivered directly to the site of interest. There are times such as in excretory urography when the contrast agent is introduced at a distance from the site of interest. Most of the organic iodine compounds have a property referred to as selective localization. That is to say, they will collect at a site some distance away from their source of introduction. Selective localization is also the basis for the elimination of the organic iodide compounds. In most cases the compounds are eliminated through the urinary system because they have been designed to selectively locate at this location. In the case of the substances used during cholecystography, either by the oral route or through parenteral administration in the antecubital vein, their use of the body's physiology will enable them to collect in the gallbladder, essentially being excreted through the hepatic portal system.

This principle is used frequently during SPECT (single photon emission computed tomography) and PET (positron emission tomography) nuclear medicine examinations in order to have the radiopharmaceutical collect at a particular location utilizing the natural physiologic processes of the biochemical compound bound to the radionuclide. The results of most nuclear medicine procedures are the assessment of the metabolic processes occurring in the body at specific sites. These modalities will be discussed in Chapter 11.

Given the extensive use of selective catheterization during vascular diagnostic procedures, selective localization has become more a part of the **route of elimination** of the substance rather than a means to get it to a specific location. Most of the positive contrast agents are eliminated through the urinary system, and the results of the blood urea nitrogen (BUN) and creatinine tests become an important part of the preprocedural history. If the urinary system is already stressed, the additional load on the system caused by the introduction of a substance that selectively localizes in this area could be the cause of some major patient reaction.

EXCRETORY PATHWAYS

The **excretory pathway**, the route used to remove the positive contrast agent from the body, is an important characteristic of a good contrast agent. Two main routes are used for the elimination of the positive contrast agents used in the vascular and interventional studies: the urinary system and the hepatic portal system. Those agents that utilize the hepatic portal system are primarily used to study the organs associated with the system.

The primary route of elimination of most of the organic iodide compounds is through the urinary system. Therefore, it is important to know the status of the kidney's ability to perform this task before the examination. The results of both the BUN and creatinine tests should be checked to determine renal status. Renal insufficiency is indicated if the BUN exceeds 30 mg/dl and the creatinine is above 1.5 mg/dl. The physician should be notified regarding the results of these tests prior to the injection.

GENERAL PRECAUTIONS

The following is a summary of some general precautions to be taken before and after the administration of contrast media:

Before injection
    Discuss the procedure with the patient
    Obtain an informed consent from the patient
    Establish a set of baseline vital signs

Know the patient
    Check the chart for history of allergy or hypersensitivity
    Check the results of the patient's blood work:
        Blood urea nitrogen
        Creatinine
        Prothrombin time, in cases of arterial access
        Partial thromboplastin time
        Platelet count
    Check whether patient has other medical problems
        Hepatic or renal disease
        Pregnancy
        Multiple myeloma
        Congestive heart failure
        Graves' disease
        Homozygosity for sickle cell disease
        Known or suspected pheochromocytoma (solid tumors of neurogenic origin)
        Severe cardiovascular diseases
        Bronchial asthma
        Hyperthyroidism

Know the procedure
    Contraindications and limitations to the specific special procedure
    Know the possible reactions that can occur with the contrast agent used
    Check emergency equipment
    Know location and contents of crash cart

After injection
    Know where physician may be reached
    Evaluate patient's vital functions for abnormalities
        Respiration
        Pulse
        Blood pressure
        Presence of cyanosis
    Remain with and monitor the patient for at least 20 minutes after injection

REACTIONS

The onset of reactions is variable; approximately 70% of reactions occur within 5 minutes of the injection, whereas 16% occur more than 5 minutes after the injection and 14% occur 15 minutes after the injection. It is advisable that the radiographer remain with the patient for at least 15 minutes after the injection.

When a particular contrast agent is being used, the radiographer should read the supplied product data sheet. Information provided about the contrast agent includes description, indications and contraindications, administration and dosage, warnings or precautions, and adverse reactions or complications. The section on adverse reactions or complications can prepare the radiographer for the possible types of reactions that the agent can produce.

A vital part of the preprocedural protocol should include a detailed history of previous reactions to medications, the presence of chronic illnesses, pregnancy, lactation, and current medications.

The mechanism of patient reaction to contrast media is not fully understood. It is a complex issue, because there is no accurate way to predict a reactive event, and the causative factors vary greatly. Reactions can occur in patients receiving contrast agents for the first time, yet patients receiving subsequent doses after experiencing a reaction may have fewer symptoms or no additional reactions.

Contrast agent reactions are considered adverse drug reactions. Some of the problems experienced by patients can be classified as allergic reactions. Some can be attributed to the hyperosmolality of the contrast agent administered, and some are related to the chemotoxicity or specific, intrinsic chemical and pharmacologic characteristics of the substance.

The incidence of renal failure after the administration of a contrast medium can be decreased with proper hydration. If the patient is able to take fluids by mouth, a minimum of 500 ml of fluid should be administered prior to the procedure and an additional 2500 ml of fluid should be taken over the 24-hour period following the examination. If intravenous hydration is necessary, the infusion of a 0.45% or 0.9% saline solution should be administered at the rate of 100 ml per hour starting 4 hours before the procedure and continuing for the 24-hour period after the study.[2]

The reactions that occur during contrast examinations can be classified into one of five major groups: overdose, anaphylactic, cardiovascular, psychogenic, and activation system–triggering reactions.

Overdose Reactions

It should not be implied from this classification group that some patients are deliberately overdosed with the contrast agent. However, under certain conditions, some patients may be predisposed to inadvertent contrast agent overdose. Infants, adults with acute renal failure, adults with cardiac failure in the beginning stages, and adults with hepatic failure and ascites are particularly at risk of receiving an excessive osmotic load. A dose that is considered to be within normal limits for the general population may, in fact, be an overdose in patients with these conditions. Obtaining a thorough history from the patient can in most cases identify patients who might be at risk for this type of reaction.

Anaphylactic Reactions

These responses are considered to be allergic-type reactions caused by a hypersensitivity to the substance. They are usually of mild to medium severity and are easily recognized and treated. Once again, the patient's history can give the radiographer a hint as to the potential for this type of reaction. Questions relating to any previous allergic reactions should be included in the preprocedure protocol, including inquiries about food allergies, asthma, hay fever, or hives. The patient should also be questioned concerning any previously identified allergic reaction and whether or not it occurred during a medical procedure. If a previous reaction is identified, a detailed description of the reaction and any treatment given should be documented, and the information should be transmitted to the physician performing the procedure.

Cardiovascular Reactions

These reactions tend to cause peripheral vasodilation and a decrease in systemic blood pressure, which can result in reflex tachycardia. Because they are related to the effect of the vagus nerve on the cardiovascular system, they are referred to as vasovagal or vagal-type reactions. Vasovagal reactions can affect myocardial contractility and cardiac electrophysiology and can ultimately be serious. The most severe type of cardiovascular reaction is cardiac arrest. The patient's vital signs should be monitored before, during, and after the procedure.

Psychogenic Reactions

Psychogenic factors are important mediators of some major reactions. If patients are overanxious, they may respond to the subjective side effects produced as a result of the introduction of the contrast agent with an autonomic response. The response becomes the basis for the adverse reaction. Substances less likely to cross the blood-brain barrier and enter the central nervous system reduce the likelihood of reactions precipitated by this mechanism.

Activation System—Triggering Reactions

The activation of a variety of systems (complement, coagulation, fibrinolysis, and histamine) can be triggered as a response to damage to the vascular endothelium at the injection site. These systems do not cause the same type of reaction in every patient because of individual variations in the presence and action of inhibitors in the pathways. Histamine release, tissue damage, thrombus formation, and hemolysis are some manifestations of these types of reactions.

Because the reaction to the administration of a contrast agent is not predictable, all patients should be monitored closely during the procedure. The importance of assessing the patient before the procedure cannot be overemphasized. This will give the radiographer a baseline value from which to measure the patient's condition throughout the procedure. The radiographer should become familiar with the signs and symptoms of these types of reactions; a summary of some mild, moderate, and severe types of reactions and their signs and symptoms is given in Box 6-1. The radiographer should be familiar with these symptoms and note any changes in the patient during the procedure. If any of the symptoms appear, the physician should immediately be notified and the incident documented.

The possibility of a reaction should always be anticipated, and proper emergency medication should be available in the special procedure suite. The following is a list of typical emergency equipment:

> Oxygen wall system and oxygen tank and masks
> Airways (pediatric and adult)
> Suction apparatus
> Physiologic saline
> Emergency drugs (by physician preference)
>   Diphenylhydramine hydrochloride
>   Phenylephrine hydrochloride
>   Metaraminol
>   Hydrocortisone sodium succinate
>   Epinephrine
> Syringes and needles for drug injection
> Aromatic spirits of ammonia
> Blood pressure device (sphygmomanometer) and stethoscope

<table>
<tr><td colspan="2">

BOX 6-1   *Symptoms of Reactions to Contrast Agents Administered Intravenously*
</td></tr>
<tr><td>

Mild to Moderate Symptoms</td><td>

Severe Symptoms</td></tr>
<tr><td>

Nausea*
Flushing
Sneezing
Shivering
Chest pain
Facial swelling
Abdominal pain
Pain at injection site
Heat sensation*
Vascular pain
Vomiting*
Itching*
Hoarseness
Coughing
Urticaria*
Edema
Warm feeling</td><td>

Dyspnea
Sudden drop in blood pressure
Loss of consciousness
Paresthesias
Convulsions
Tissue necrosis
Cardiac arrest
Paralysis</td></tr>
</table>

*These symptoms were found to be the most frequent by Katayama H, et al: Adverse reactions to ionic and nonionic contrast media. *Radiology* 175:622, 1990.

COMPLICATIONS

Although they are infrequent, complications resulting from diagnostic angiography do occur. The use of newer techniques, equipment, and patient evaluation has reduced the frequency of complications. Singh and coworkers propose grouping the complications into three categories: those occurring at the puncture site, systemic complications, and complications induced by the catheter during the procedure.[3] The Society of Interventional Radiology (SIR) Standards of Practice Committee recognizes that the invasive arteriographic procedures is a proven safe, diagnostic procedure but that the potential for complication does exist. In their 2004 Quality Improvement Guidelines for Diagnostic Arteriography they have summarized the indications and relative contraindications for the various arteriographic procedures.[4]

In a previous review the Standards of Practice Committee of Cardiovascular and Interventional Radiology classified potential complications by outcome. They referred to the effect of the complication on the patient or the level of treatment required, if any. Table 6-3 represents the SIR outcomes classification of arteriographic complications.[4]

Attention should be given to the potential for drug interactions between the contrast medium and any medication that the patient is taking. One such instance is the administration of contrast medium when the patient is being treated for type 2 diabetes with Glucophage (metformin hydrochloride). The combination of contrast medium and metformin hydrochloride increases the risk for a buildup of lactic acid in the blood. This condition is referred to as **lactic acidosis**. The manufacture of lactic acid is a normal physiologic process of the mitochondria in the production of energy through the breakdown of sugars and fat. Lactic acid is a waste product resulting from the process. Under normal circumstances the lactic acid is broken down into simpler products and is eliminated from the body. Under certain circumstances the mitochondria are damaged, and lactic acid is not broken down but accumulates in the body, causing lactic acidosis. The symptoms of this condition include nausea, vomiting, weight loss, muscle weakness, dyspnea, abdominal pain, and cardiac rhythm abnormalities.

TABLE 6-3 *Outcomes Classification of Complications to Arteriographic Procedures*

Classification Level	Resultant Potential Outcomes
Minor Complications	No therapeutic intervention
	Minor therapeutic intervention
	Admission for observation—minimum 24 hours
	No permanent effect
Major Complications	Requires therapeutic intervention
	Observation for < 48 hours
	Major therapeutic intervention
	Hospitalization for > 48 hours
	Permanent effects
	Death

The radiographer should check the patient's serum creatinine level before the procedure. If it is within the normal level, which is under 1.5 mg/dL, the risks attendant to the use of a contrast medium are reduced. If the creatinine levels are greater than the normal limits, the use of metformin should be suspended or replaced with another medication at least 2 days before the procedure to reduce the risk of lactic acidosis. In any case the hydration of the patient is essential before and after the administration of the contrast medium. Prior to the procedure the physician should be alerted to the patient's creatinine levels and medication regimen.

Among the various complications occurring at the puncture site such as hematoma, occlusion, and pseudoaneurysm, extravasation of the contrast agent also has been seen with relative frequency.

Extravasation

Extravasation is a complication that can result from any injection and can be prevented through observation and careful needle or catheter insertion. **Accidental extravasation**, the escape of fluid into surrounding tissue, is a relatively common complication resulting from the injection of the contrast agent. In most cases in which a small amount of contrast agent is used, extravasation generally results in a minimal amount of damage. In examinations requiring large amounts of contrast agent, extravasation can cause severe damage to the skin and subcutaneous tissue. Extravasation seems to occur most often during computed tomography and lower limb venography, although this complication can occur as a result of any intravenous injection. Certain risk factors may predispose a patient to this type of complication, and Box 6-2 summarizes some of them.

In order to minimize the potential for extravasation, the injection of the contrast agent should be directly monitored. In cases in which the patient presents a high-risk profile, extra attention should be given to the injection. Intravenous injections should be carefully performed, preferably using plastic catheters for power injection.[5] Institutions have developed formal policies concerning injury caused by extravasation, and these should be followed as stipulated. It is also essential to document the incident, including patient symptoms, any immediate treatment, and notification of the physician in charge. The documentation should be done in accordance with the policy for treatment of this type of complication.

If extravasation occurs, the physician involved in the study should be immediately notified. If the departmental policy recommends elevation of the extremity above the level of the heart, it should be accomplished without compromising the arterial or venous flow. Additionally, the application of warm or cold compresses can help reduce the potential injury to the site. Each department should have its own protocol for immediate treatment and reporting.

SPECIALTY CONTRAST AGENTS

The organic iodine compounds have found widespread use in special procedure radiography and computed tomography (CT). However, they do not possess the characteristics necessary to function as

---

BOX 6-2   *Risk Factors for Extravasation*

- Tourniquets not released during injection
- Improper use of automatic injection devices
- Indwelling catheters in place for more than 24 hours
- Tapes and bandages over IV access site (prevents adequate monitoring of injection site)
- Injections into small peripheral veins, especially in the dorsum of the foot and hand
- Multiple attempts to gain vessel access
- The use of metal needles rather than plastic catheters
- The use of high osmolar contrast agents
- Examinations requiring large amounts of contrast agents
- Abnormal circulation caused by:
  - Atherosclerotic vessels
  - Diabetic vascular disease
  - Venous thrombosis
- Patients with a history of compromised lymphatic or venous drainage
- Increased risks in infants, children, the elderly, and chronically ill patients

---

contrast agents during magnetic resonance imaging (MRI) procedures. Iodinated contrast media function through absorption and subsequent attenuation of the x-ray beam. MRI does not use x-radiation to produce images; therefore, the usefulness of the iodinated compounds is limited. The substances used for contrast production in this specialty alter the microchemical environment to change the relaxation times (T1 and T2) and thereby increase the signal intensity.

The substance that has found favor as an intravenous contrast agent in MRI is gadolinium diethylenetriamine penta-acetic acid (Gd-DTPA). This substance is a metal chelate. Metal ions tend to bind with certain body tissues, such as in the kidneys, liver, heart, brain, bone, spleen, and lungs. As a result, they can remain in the system for a long period of time and can cause undesirable side effects. If the metal ion can be linked with a substance that prevents such binding, it can be used safely. The process of chelation makes the metal ion available for use while eliminating the negative effects of tissue binding within the body. DTPA is the chelating agent used in the production of Gd-DTPA.

The side effects of this agent are minimal and include a slight transient increase in serum bilirubin (up to 15 mg/dl above normal), mild headache, rash, gastrointestinal upset, nausea, vomiting, and hypotension. This substance has not demonstrated toxicity to organ systems such as the heart, brain, kidney, or liver, which would be primary target organs if decomplexation of the substance occurred.

The primary excretory pathway is via the kidneys; approximately 80% of the Gd-DTPA is eliminated within 3 hours. Approximately 98% is eliminated from the body through urination and defecation within 1 week of administration. It should be noted that because the primary method of excretion is via the urinary system, the use of the substance in patients who exhibit poor renal function or advanced renal disease is contraindicated.

The usual effective dose of Gd-DTPA compounds such as Magnevist is 0.2 ml/kg, not to exceed a total of 10 ml per 15 seconds.[6] This dose is sufficient for most MRI studies. Increases above this level have demonstrated decreased signal intensity. Other chelated forms of Gd are being researched that would provide better contrast with smaller doses, but these have not emerged in clinical use.

SUMMARY

Contrast agents can be divided into negative and positive varieties. Negative contrast agents silhouette the anatomy against a radiolucent background, whereas positive contrast agents produce areas of decreased density on the finished radiograph. Commonly used negative contrast agents are air, carbon dioxide, oxygen, and nitrous oxide. The positive contrast agents are primarily substituted benzoic acid compounds. They differ in the types of side chains and the extent of carbon atom substitution. They all use iodine to provide the contrast in the organ, but they vary in the number of particles that provide the osmolality of the substance. They are divided into agents that are ionic and those that are nonionic in nature. There is a category of iodinated compounds that are considered to have a lower osmolality than the purely ionic agents. Nonionic compounds have been proved to cause fewer reactions than other varieties, but the economic considerations have delayed these from gaining universal use. These compounds are usually used in high-risk cases.

Reactions to contrast agent injection cannot be predicted. These are grouped according to their severity: mild, moderate, and severe. An emergency drug cart should be present in the special procedures, CT, or MRI suite. The radiographer should know the departmental protocol for activities that should be carried out before, during, and after the study. A common complication during the injection of the contrast agent is extravasation; prevention is the best tool for reducing its occurrence. A department protocol should be established for patient evaluation and for monitoring and reporting any incidents that might occur.

The important physical characteristics of contrast agents—viscosity, toxicity, iodine content, miscibility, and persistence—are usually considered when a contrast agent is chosen for a specific special procedure. MRI has its own specific criteria for contrast agent selection. The iodinated contrast agents are not effective during these types of procedures. Gd-DTPA, a metal chelate, is the most widely used substance for MRI.

REFERENCES

1. American College of Radiology: *Manual on Contrast Media*, ed 4.1, Reston, Va, 2001, ACR.
2. Maddox TG: Adverse reactions to contrast material: recognition, prevention and treatment. *Am Fam Physician* 66(7):1229–1234, 2002.
3. Singh H, Cardella J, Cole P, Grassi CJ, McCowan T, Swan T, Sacks D, Lewis C: Quality Improvement Guidelines for Diagnostic Arteriography. *J Vasc Interv Radiol* 14:S283–S288, 2003.
4. Standards of Practice Committee of the Society of Cardiovascular and Interventional Radiology: Standards for interventional radiology. *J Vasc Interv Radiol* 2:59–65, 1991.
5. Bellin M-F, Jakobsen JÅ, Tomassin I, Thomsen HS, Morcos SK, members of the Contrast Media Safety Committee of the European Society of Urogenital Radiology (ESUR): Contrast medium extravasation injury: guidelines for prevention and management. *Eur Radiol* 12:2807–2812, 2002.
6. Product Data Sheet, Berlex Imaging, Montville, NJ, Sept 2005, http://www.berlex.com/html/products/pi/Magnevist_Pl.pdf.

SUGGESTED READINGS

Bettmann MA, Heeren T, Greenfield A, Goudey C: Adverse events with radiographic contrast agents: results of the SCVIR Contrast Agent Registry. *Radiology* 203:611-620, 1997.

Cohan RH, Ellis JH, Garner WL: Extravasation of radiographic contrast material: recognition, prevention and treatment. *Radiology* 200:593–604, 1996.

Hong SJ, Wong JT, Bloch K: Reactions to radiocontrast media. *Allergy Asthma Proc* 23(5):347–351, 2002.

Jackson R: Using metformin safely. X-ray with caution. *Diabetes Self Manag* 21(2):14, 17, 2004.

Martinelli G, Petrini F, Gamberini E: Adverse reactions to contrast media: treatment. *Radiol Med* 107(4 Suppl 1):42–52, 2004.

Morcos SK, Thomsen HS, European Society of Urogenital Radiology: European Society of Urogenital Radiology guidelines on administering contrast media. *Abdom Imaging* 28(2):187–190, 2003.

Morcos SK, Thomsen HS, Webb JA: Prevention of generalized reactions to contrast media: a consensus report and guidelines. *Eur Radiol* 11(9):1720–1728, 2001.

Murphy KP, Szopinski KT, Cohan RH, Mermillod B, Ellis JH: Occurrence of adverse reactions to gadolinium-based contrast material and management of patients at increased risk: a survey of the American Society of Neuroradiology Fellowship Directors. *Acad Radiol* 6(11):656–664, 1999.

Nakamura I, Hori S, Funabiki T, et al: Cardiopulmonary arrest induced by anaphylactoid reaction with contrast media. *Resuscitation* 53(2):223–226, 2002.

Parra D, Legreid AM, Beckey NP, et al: Metformin monitoring and change in serum creatinine levels in patients undergoing radiologic procedures involving administration of intravenous contrast media. *Pharmacotherapy* 24(8):987–993, 2004.

Sanchez-Perez JF, Villalta Maria Garcia, Ruiz Sara Alvarez, Garcia Diez Amaro: Delayed hypersensitivity reaction to the non–ionic contrast medium Visipaque (Iodixanol). *Contact Dermatitis* 48(3):167, 2003.

Thompson NW, Thompson TJ, Love MH, et al: Drugs and intravenous contrast media. *BJU Int* 85(3):219–221, 2000.

Thomsen HS, Morcos SK: Prevention of generalized reactions to CM. *Acad Radiol* 9(Suppl 2): S433–435, 2002.

Thomsen HS, Morcos SK, and members of the Contrast Media Safety Committee of the European Society of Urogenital Radiology (ESUR): Management of acute adverse reactions to contrast media. *Eur Radiol* 14:476–481, 2004.

STUDY QUESTIONS

1. Which of the following would not be a risk factor for extravasation?
   a. the use of metal needles in place of plastic catheters
   b. venous thrombosis
   c. abnormal circulation caused by atherosclerotic vessels
   d. tourniquets not being released during the injection

2. The anatomic/physiologic structure that prevents various chemicals and other harmful substances from passing to the central nervous system from the blood is called the:
   a. parenchyma
   b. dura mater
   c. blood-brain barrier
   d. intima

3. The basic structure that is used to create most of the organic iodide contrast agents is:
   a. gadolinium
   b. pyridine
   c. benzene
   d. metrizoate

4. Which of the following are considered to be an activation triggering type of reaction?
      i. nausea
      ii. thrombus formation
      iii. hemolysis
   a. i only
   b. i and iii only
   c. ii and iii only
   d. i, ii, and iii

5. The excretory pathway for the majority of the organic iodide compounds is through the:
   a. respiratory system
   b. process of defecation
   c. urinary system
   d. hepatic portal system

6. Which of the following is not a characteristic of informed consent?
   a. full disclosure to the patient of the risks involved
   b. competency of the patient
   c. authorization of the procedure by the patient
   d. usually done after the procedure is completed

STUDY QUESTIONS (*cont'd*)

7. The process of making a metal ion useful without the probability of it binding to the tissues in the body is called:
   a. concentration
   b. ionization
   c. chelating
   d. osmolarity

8. As the iodine concentration _____ the viscosity of the substance will _____ .
   a. increases, decrease
   b. increases, increase
   c. decreases, increase
   d. decreases, remain unchanged

9. Osmolarity of a solution refers to the _____ of the solution.
   a. volume
   b. weight
   c. viscosity
   d. miscibility

10. Renal insufficiency is indicated if the BUN exceeds _____ mg/dl and the creatinine is above _____ mg/dl.
    a. 10, 0.15
    b. 15, 0.30
    c. 20, 1.5
    d. 30, 1.5

7 *Principles of Patient Care*

CHAPTER OBJECTIVES

After completing this chapter, the reader will be able to perform the following:

- Identify the general principles for all special studies

- Identify the need for strict confidentiality

- List and describe the components of the patient preexamination and history

- Identify the need for pharmacologic awareness

- Identify the need and describe the process for obtaining an informed consent

- Identify the need for preprocedure equipment preparation

- Describe the need and process for proper documentation

- Describe the process of patient instruction

- Describe the patient's preprocedural, intraprocedural, and postprocedural care

- Define contrast material administration and filming

- Identify the risks associated with the catheterization procedure

- Identify the requirements for patient discharge

CHAPTER OUTLINE

The discussion of patient care in this chapter will be limited specifically to patient care throughout the procedure. Sterile techniques such as gloving, gowning, and sterile field maintenance will not be revisited. This material is presented in depth in several radiography reference texts and should already be well known and practiced by the advanced radiographer. These texts have been referenced in the bibliography at the end of the chapter. The intent of this chapter is to present the responsibilities of the radiographer to the patient before, during, and after the procedure.

Advanced level radiography is becoming increasingly complex. The radiographer is an integral member of the angiographic or interventional team having additional responsibility for the process and the patient. The additional responsibilities include some of the activities that were designated to the nursing staff assisting at the study. These additional responsibilities also make the individual more vulnerable to litigation. Attention to three major areas can provide protection for the advanced practitioner: knowledge, careful attention to details, and documentation.

The knowledge needed includes not only the equipment and the procedure but also pharmacology and some basic nursing procedures. Much of this knowledge will be learned during the training process; however, it is incumbent upon the radiographer to practice these skills and constantly strive to improve them.

The importance of careful attention to details cannot be stressed enough. Subtle changes in the patient throughout and after the procedure can be indicators that, if noticed promptly, could enable the radiographer to short circuit a major reaction or side effect. This attention to detail should also extend into the familiar realm of equipment preparation and care. Regular maintenance of a quality assurance program and consistently following a routine check-off procedure can eliminate most equipment failure problems. The check-off procedure is also a valuable tool for minimizing equipment-related patient injury.

Finally, documentation demonstrates that the individual has exhibited professionalism. Properly done, documentation provides an accurate record of the particulars of the procedure and the actions of the radiographer. It indicates a responsibility for performing at a high standard of patient care. Documentation also can provide the advanced level practitioner with an excellent defense during subsequent litigation.

GENERAL PRINCIPLES

All advanced radiographic studies, diagnostic and interventional, are performed following the same general procedure:

- Strict confidentiality
- Preexamination history, consultation
- Pharmacologic awareness
- Signed and witnessed informed consent
- Properly prepared equipment
- Proper documentation
- Patient instruction and preprocedural care
- Intraprocedural care
- Contrast administration, filming and performance of interventional treatment, if scheduled
- Postprocedural care and instructions
- Awareness of the risks associated with catheterization and contrast medium administration
- Patient discharge

In this chapter, we consider the basic principles of patient care common to all angiographic procedures. There may be some variations during the clinical performance of the examinations owing to differing hospital and departmental protocols; however, every angiographic examination should include all of the elements listed here.

Confidentiality

The passage of the Health Insurance Portability and Accountability Act of 1996 (HIPAA) and its subsequent revisions in 2001 and 2002 changed the way that health care providers treat patient information. The privacy and security aspects of the act were implemented in 2003 and regulated electronic transaction standards, privacy standards, security standards, and the use of unique identifiers to protect patient information. Most of the regulations do not affect the operations of advanced procedures and would not necessarily impact on daily practice. The privacy standards, however, should be understood so that inadvertent violations to the act will not occur. The protected information would include any information that includes the patient's name, birth date, medical record number, or any indicator that could identify the information as belonging to a particular individual.

Initially, the patient must be made aware of the institution's privacy policy. This is usually done in the admitting office, and patients generally are required to sign that they received and understood the policy.

Family members usually accompany the patient to the institution for the procedure. They are usually anxious to speak with the health care practitioner regarding the outcome of the procedure and the status of the patient's treatment. The patient must authorize any communication with family members regarding the patient's health status before any information is disclosed by the health professional. In any case the act states that the amount of information given should be limited to the minimum necessary for the situation.

The advanced procedure team must have safeguards in place to protect the patient's information. The safeguards should include the security of the patient's chart, which should be stored away from any public access area. Protection of the patient's rights also pertains to any public display of the patient's radiographs or digital images. Conversations among members of the advanced procedures team must always be carried out in a secure manner. These conversations should be made in a private location, and reasonable measures should be taken so as not to be heard.

Both intentional and unintentional violations of the HIPAA regulations can result in either criminal or civil penalties. The criminal penalties include a monetary fine up to $250,000 and a prison term of up to 10 years. Civil violations carry a monetary fine of $25,000 per violation.

Preexamination History and Consultation

Depending upon the situation, a consultation with the physician prior to the day of the procedure should provide the patient with the indications, aims, nature, and risks of the study. Angiography can be performed on an inpatient basis or on an outpatient basis through ambulatory surgery. At times the physician performing the study will meet with the patient on the day of the procedure.

During this meeting the procedure should be clearly explained, and any potential therapeutic interventions should be discussed as well. A short history of the patient is taken to determine what symptoms or signs warranted the procedure, and previous surgery should be discussed along with a review of the patient's organ systems, current medications, chronic illnesses, and allergies that could potentially provoke any reactions to the contrast agent. The physician should also perform a physical examination to assess the proposed puncture site to determine any contraindications for vessel access. Depending on the access site, the physician should physically check the following parameters. In the case of femoral access lower extremity pulses and the physical appearance of the limbs should be examined and noted. When the brachial artery approach is chosen, proximal and distal pulses should be taken.

The patient's chart should also be assessed to review any previous examinations as well as to review the patient's blood work. Although there are no hard and fast rules as to the type of blood work that is necessary, if any, this part of the preprocedure history may be moot. Depending upon the patient, the procedure, and hospital or physician protocol, possible blood work could include any combination of the following tests: hemoglobin and hematocrit, blood urea nitrogen (BUN), creatinine, prothrombin time (PT), platelet count, international normalized ratio (INR), and activated partial thromboplastin time (aPTT). The results should be reviewed and pertinent information should be noted on the patient's chart, such as the status of the patient's renal function, bleeding tendency, and whether there have been previous reactions to contrast agents. Box 7-1 lists the normal values for a variety of laboratory tests.

The physician is responsible for informing the patient of the preprocedural instructions and preparation for the procedure. These instructions will vary somewhat depending on institution and physician preference; however, it is important that the patient be well hydrated prior to the procedure.

BOX 7-1 *Normal Adult Laboratory Values*

LABORATORY TEST	NORMAL VALUES
Chemistry	
Bilirubin (total)	0.1–1.0 mg/dl
Bilirubin (direct)	0.3 mg/dl
Blood urea nitrogen (BUN)	10–22 mg/dl
Creatinine	
Female	0.6–1.3 mg/dl
Male	0.8–1.5 mg/dl
Potassium	3.6–5.0 mEq/L
Sodium	139–147 mEq/L
Alkaline phosphatase	16–95 IU/L
Hematology	
Hematocrit	
Female	37%–47%
Male	42%–52%
Hemoglobin	
Female	12–16 g/L
Male	14–18 g/L
Platelet count	150,000–400,000/mm³
White blood cell count (total WBC)	5000–10,000/mm³
Arterial Blood Gas (ABG)	
pH	7.35–7.45
Partial pressure for carbon dioxide (Pco_2)	35–45 mEq/L
Partial pressure for oxygen (Po_2)	80–100 mm Hg
Oxygen saturation	90%–100%
Coagulation	
Prothrombin time (PT)	10–13 s
Partial prothrombin time (PTT)	22–35 s
International normalization ratio (INR)	0.8–1.2
Activated clotting time (ACT)	150 s

Outpatients are instructed to consume clear liquids until about 2 hours before the procedure rather than fasting. On the other hand, if the patient is an inpatient, he or she may be required to fast for 6 to 8 hours prior to the study. In an effort to promote good hydration, continuation of a clear liquid diet is usually desired until 2 hours prior to the procedure. If the patient is admitted to the facility, there will probably be orders for overnight intravenous hydration, using half normal saline at 75 to 100 ml/hr. In these cases the patient will arrive in the department with the intravenous line in place. The physician determines if the patient should continue taking medication on the day of the procedure. It should be noted that certain exceptions may be required concerning the patient's medication. It is advisable to question the patient about any medications that were taken before arriving at the facility. Box 7-2 lists some of the medications and the reasons for their restriction. Premedication is usually administered in the angiography suite after the patient's peripheral pulses and vital signs are taken.

Pharmacologic Awareness

The basic principles of pharmacology for advanced level radiographers have already been discussed in Chapter 5. It is important for the radiographer to be aware of the type of medications administered to

BOX 7-2	*Restricted Medications*
Medication	**Reason for the Restriction**
Warfarin	Withheld for several days; substitute heparin treatment. Heparin should be stopped 2–6 hr before the procedure and 1–6 hr after the study.
Glucophage	Can result in lactic acidosis. Should be restricted 48 hr before and after the procedure.
Diuretics	May be suspended for angiography. Patient should be well hydrated for the procedure.
Insulin	Morning dose should be cut in half to reduce the risk of hypoglycemia.

the patient before, during, and after the study. This familiarity should include knowledge about the potential side effects and adverse reactions and possible concomitant effects of a variety of medications. Reference materials that would assist the radiographer in obtaining this knowledge are the *Physician's Desk Reference, Mosby's Drug Consult,* and the manufacturer's data product sheets that accompany the medications.

Informed Consent

Informed consent must be obtained from the patient prior to the procedure. This is usually accomplished on the day of the procedure or during the preexamination history and consultation. Informed consent is a legal condition which implies the following: **disclosure** of risks involved with the procedure, **understanding** by the patient, the **authorization** or **voluntary permission** to perform the procedure, and the **competence** of the patient to negotiate the document. Each institution has its own consent form that must be used. It is a violation of the patient's rights to perform a procedure without first obtaining informed consent. One benefit to the process is that a familiarity with the procedure can help to gain patient cooperation.

The process of obtaining the informed consent is primarily one of communication. The American Medical Association policy regarding informed consent is as follows:

H-140.989 Informed Consent and Decision-Making in Health Care
- Health care professionals should inform patients or their surrogates of their clinical impression or diagnosis; alternative treatments and consequences of treatments, including the consequence of no treatment; and recommendations for treatment. Full disclosure is appropriate in all cases, except in rare situations in which such information would, in the opinion of the health care professional, cause serious harm to the patient.
- Individuals should, at their own option, provide instructions regarding their wishes in the event of their incapacity. Individuals may also wish to designate a surrogate decision-maker. When a patient is incapable of making health care decisions, such decisions should be made by a surrogate acting pursuant to the previously expressed wishes of the patient, and when such wishes are not known or ascertainable, the surrogate should act in the best interests of the patient.

Continued

Continued

- A patient's health record should include sufficient information for another health care professional to assess previous treatment, to ensure continuity of care, and to avoid unnecessary or inappropriate tests or therapy.
- Conflicts between a patient's right to privacy and a third party's need to know should be resolved in favor of patient privacy, except where that would result in serious health hazard or harm to the patient or others.
- Holders of health record information should be held responsible for reasonable security measures through their respective licensing laws. Third parties that are granted access to patient health care information should be held responsible for reasonable security measures and should be subject to sanctions when confidentiality is breached.
- A patient should have access to the information in his or her health record, except for that information which, in the opinion of the health care professional, would cause harm to the patient or to other people.
- Disclosures of health information about a patient to a third party may only be made upon **consent** by the patient or the patient's lawfully authorized nominee, except in those cases in which the third party has a legal or predetermined right to gain access to such information.

From BOT Rep. NN, A-87; Reaffirmed: Sunset Report, I-97; Reaffirmed: Res. 408, A-02. American Medical Association – Copyright ©2004. Accessed at http:www.ama-assn.org.

The elements of the consent for angiographic procedures should include, at minimum, the following areas of the procedure; vessel access, catheter management, and pharmacologic aspects of the study including contrast agents, premedication, drugs used during the study, postprocedure medication, and complications. The patient must be aware of the intent of the consent document as well as the attendant risks of the procedure. The consent form is usually cosigned by witnesses to indicate that they witnessed the patient sign the form. It is not recommended that the witness be an individual who is involved with the procedure. The consent form may be negotiated on the day of the procedure, although this depends on individual hospital protocol.

Many factors can affect the patient's ability to make a decision about the procedure that they are about to have done. Some of these factors include stress, known mental illness, immature mental capacity, and the premedication that the patient has received.

Patients can also be influenced through persuasion, manipulation, or coercion to sign the consent form. Coercion or active deception is considered unethical when obtaining a valid informed consent. Deceitful misrepresentation and omission of some of the information can be considered unethical as well. It is acceptable, however, to offer the patient logical arguments for this choice, and in some cases patients might request this type of advice based upon the perceived expertise of the health care practitioner. As in any situation, the patient has the right not to hear the risks involved in the procedure but the request must come from the patient and not the individual seeking to obtain the consent.

Equipment Preparation

The specific equipment, contrast agents, and accessories needed for angiography have been discussed. The radiographer is responsible for the preparation of the angiographic suite before the patient arrives for the procedure. The equipment should be checked to ensure that it is functional, and the accessory items necessary to the procedure should be set out. There should be an adequate supply of these items in the angiographic suite to be used as replacements as needed. The radiographer should discuss the procedure with the physician to determine if there is a possibility of intervention. If so, the radiographer should ensure that the items required for the interventional procedure are also available.

Documentation

It is important to record accurate notes concerning the patient's condition and treatment before, during, and after the study. Any reactions or difficulties must also be charted. The hospital's risk management protocol should be followed for every special procedure performed. Each member of the angiographic team should know his or her responsibilities concerning the care of the patient as well as the type and amount of records charting required for the study.

It is of vital importance to report any abnormal or unusual occurrences, including contrast agent reactions, extravasation of contrast agents, and accidental injury. Each institution will have some type of incident report protocol that should be followed. Generic incident report forms require details about the type of incident, the time the incident occurred, who was involved, and what treatment, if any, was administered. This report will serve to document your observation of the situation, alert the risk management department of the incident, and allow them to review the situation and recommend an appropriate course of action.

A policy and procedure manual should be available and periodically reviewed with the angiographic team. It is essential that *all* members of the team be familiar with the protocols for the various procedures performed in the department. Review of policies and procedures should be carried out on a periodic basis and so documented, and any revisions to the manual should be clearly explained and discussed with the members of the team.

Each facility will have a specific protocol for documentation indicating the type of system used as well as the individual(s) responsible for maintaining the patient record. In some cases separate notations by the physician, nurse, or advanced level practitioner will be required. In some facilities one individual may be designated to document the procedure. In any case the record should be objective and accurately describe the patient's condition, progress, and any departure from the normal course of action.

Patient Instruction and Preprocedural Care

When the patient arrives in the department, he or she should be properly identified. The radiographer should consult the chart for information pertinent to the procedure. At this time, the order for the study should be confirmed. The procedure should be explained to the patient to establish a rapport and ensure the patient's cooperation during the procedure. The various members of the special procedure team should also be introduced.

If the study is being done through ambulatory surgery, the patient should be instructed to change into a hospital gown and subsequently transported to the angiographic suite.

The special procedure nurse or the radiographer will check the patient's peripheral pulses and secure a set of baseline vital signs. If any premedication has been ordered, the nurse will administer it at this time.

Intraprocedural Care

The most important aspect of intraprocedural care of the patient is continuous monitoring for abnormal changes. Benchmark measurements are taken of the patient's vital signs prior to the study. This includes the oxygen level in the blood as measured by the pulse oximeter. Besides continuous pulse oximetry during the procedure, continuous cardiac monitoring should be carried out. The patient will have an intravenous line to provide for additional hydration as well as an access point for any medication that may be necessary. Blood pressure should be monitored every 5 to 10 minutes, and the patient's status including respiratory rate, overall condition, and state of sedation should be recorded.

Oxygen should be available and supplied to the patient in the event that the O_2 saturation falls below the 90% level. It is important to monitor and protect the patient's airway in case of emergency. It is possible for a variety of reactions to occur during the study; however, careful observation of the patient and his or her vital signs can be an early alert of a possible adverse event. It should be remembered that reactions do not all happen immediately but can occur after some delay. Continuous and thorough observation of the patient is the best defense against having a minor incident escalate into a major catastrophe.

In many cases conscious sedation is provided to relieve the anxiety and discomfort of the procedure. It should be remembered that the patient is able to respond to commands under these conditions. This is usually administered as a cocktail of Versed (midazolam) and fentanyl (Sublimaze). The cocktail is administered intravenously at the onset of the procedure and is followed by smaller doses throughout the study.

Contrast Injection and Filming

This part of the study is procedure specific and varies by institution and physician. Almost all angiographic procedures require the use of an automatic injection device to deliver the contrast agent at the desired flow rate. The image recording or filming will depend on the type of equipment available in the angiographic suite. Advances in the field have changed the filming process from film/screen to digital recording. Many physicians still feel that screen/film recording is the gold standard; however, more institutions are converting their conventional equipment for digital units.

If interventional radiology is to be performed, it is usually accomplished with diagnostic angiography as a mapping and planning procedure. Interventional techniques may require that the patient return to the department at a later time for a follow-up angiogram. In these cases, the documentation provided at the time of the original study is valuable in ensuring the safety of the patient during subsequent examinations.

Postprocedural Care and Instructions

When the study has been completed, the catheter is removed. If the catheter has a shaped tip, the guide wire must be reinserted to remove the catheter. Manual pressure is applied to the puncture site until bleeding has stopped. Any abnormal condition of the patient requires that notation be made on the chart and the physician be notified.

The patient is then moved to a designated location and remains on bed rest for a minimum of 4 hours. Continuous monitoring of the patient should be carried out during this period; this includes recording the pulse on the side of entry four times during the first hour at 15-minute regular intervals and twice an hour for the remaining 3 hours. Vital signs should be checked at these intervals and recorded on the patient's chart. The puncture site should be observed as part of the monitoring process for possible internal or external bleeding.

The patient should be urged to take fluids by mouth even if intravenous hydration is being applied. If the patient appears to be stable after the prescribed period of bed rest and has someone who can care for him or her for a 24-hour period, the patient can be discharged.

Risks of Catheterization

Angiography is a relatively safe procedure. The risks attendant with diagnostic and interventional procedures fall into two major categories—catheterization and contrast-related risks.

Complications that can occur as a result of the catheterization procedure include bleeding (internal and external), thrombus formation, cholesterol embolization, pseudoaneurysm, arterial dissection, and rupture of an aneurysm. The cardiac, renal, or neurologic blood flow can be compromised during the procedure, resulting in ischemia, permanent organ damage, or death.

Continuous monitoring of the patient's vital signs and pulse can result in an early warning of complications, and any abnormality should be immediately brought to the attention of the physician. Complications related to the administration of contrast agents are discussed in Chapter 6.

Patient Discharge

Discharge should be delayed until the patient has demonstrated the ability to drink and has voided at least once. He or she should be alert and oriented to the surroundings. The patient should also demonstrate the ability to walk, even though he or she will be discharged in the care of a competent adult. The vital signs should be stable and approach the benchmarks that were recorded prior to the study. There should not be any bleeding around the puncture site, and the patient should exhibit only minimal pain or nausea.

If the examination was done on an outpatient basis, the patient can be released if stability has been achieved after the 4-hour mandatory bed rest period. The patient should be advised to increase and maintain fluid intake, restrict movement for the following 24-hour period, and immediately report any difficulties such as fever, pain, or bleeding at the site of entry, coldness, numbness, or tingling of the extremities.

SUMMARY

Care of the patient extends from the preprocedural contacts through the discharge after the completion of the study. The health care professional should be somewhat familiar with obtaining a history, establishing baseline vital signs, pharmacologic awareness, and current privacy regulations. It is essential to possess good patient communications and observational skills in order to bring the patient safely through the procedure. The radiographer should become familiar with the proper conventions for the documentation of vital information.

The importance of obtaining a signed consent form cannot be overstressed. Patient cooperation can be secured by thoroughly educating the patient as to the study process and the procedures to follow both before and after the study.

The radiographer should also establish a standard operating procedure that should be followed for each case. This should include a check of the equipment prior to the introduction of the patient to ensure that problems or malfunctions will be identified before the procedure begins. This protocol will reduce the possibility of unwanted complications to the patient during the performance of the procedure.

Complications can occur as a result of the catheterization process, catheter manipulation, or contrast agent administration. These complications should be reported as soon as possible after the resolution of the incident. The appropriate protocols and forms should be used to document the type of situation, treatment, and follow-up care provided based upon observational data.

SUGGESTED READINGS

Aiken TD: *Legal and Ethical Issues in Health Occupations.* Philadelphia, 2002, WB Saunders.

Amatayakul M: Forms and documentation for HIPAA privacy—a closer look. *J AHIMA* 72(5):suppl 16A–16D, 2001.

Baris S, Karakaya D, Aykent R, et al: Comparison of midazolam with or without fentanyl for conscious sedation and hemodynamics in coronary angiography. *Can J Cardiol* 17(3):277–281, 2001.

Breese P, Burman W, Rietmeijer C, et al: The Health Insurance Portability and Accountability Act and the informed consent process. *Ann Intern Med* 141(11):897–898, 2004.

Elger BS, Harding TW: Avoidable breaches of confidentiality: a study among students of medicine and of law. *Med Educ* 39(3):333–337, 2005.

Graham DH: Are you guilty of unsafe documentation? *Emerg Med Serv* 29(6):81, 2000.

Larcher V: Consent, competence, and confidentiality. *BMJ* 330(7487):353–356, 2005.

Lightdale JR: Sedation and analgesia in the pediatric patient. *Gastrointest Endosc Clin N Am* 14(2):385–399, 2004.

Fundamentals of Special Radiographic Procedures

Martin ML, Lennox PH: Sedation and analgesia in the interventional radiology department. *J Vasc Interv Radiol* 14(9 Pt 1):1119–1128, 2003.

Nilsson I, Nilsson P: Medical documentation through the ages. *Lakartidningen* 100(51–52):4304–4306, 2003.

Quallich SA: The practice of informed consent. *Urol Nurs* 24(6):513–515, 2004.

Schiliro G, Di Cataldo A: Reflection about communication of diagnosis and informed consent in pediatric oncology. *Pediatr Blood Cancer* 44(4):429, 2005.

Tamparo CT, Lindh WQ: *Therapeutic Communications for Health Professionals*, 2nd ed. Delmar, 2000, Thompson Learning.

STUDY QUESTIONS

1. The normal range of blood urea nitrogen levels for an adult patient is:
   a. 1.0–2.2 mg/dl
   b. 10–22 mg/dl
   c. 100–220 mg/dl
   d. 1000–2200 mg/dl

2. The informed consent document must be:
   a. signed by the next of kin
   b. negotiated after the procedure
   c. negotiated prior to the procedure
   d. signed by the patient but not necessarily explained

3. At the end of the procedure the patient is usually moved to a recovery location until the sedation wears off. How often should the vital signs be taken in the first hour of recovery?
   a. once
   b. twice
   c. four times
   d. every 5 minutes

4. Conscious sedation is achieved by administering a combination of which of the following medications?
   a. Versed and midazolam
   b. Versed and Sublimaze
   c. fentanyl and lidocaine
   d. lidocaine and Versed

5. Prior to and after the procedure the patient is usually advised to:
   a. create a will
   b. drive himself or herself to the hospital
   c. drink plenty of fluids
   d. eat a hearty meal

6. Which of the following types of blood work is not commonly prescribed before the procedure?
   a. serum creatinine
   b. activated prothrombin time
   c. platelet count
   d. lipid panel

7. Which of the following is not a reason for discussing the procedure with the patient before the study?
   a. secure the patient's cooperation
   b. ensure that all aspects are covered for informed consent
   c. make the patient nervous
   d. prepare the patient for what the procedure will be like

STUDY QUESTIONS (*cont'd*)

8. It is reasonable to assume that under HIPAA it would be permissible to discuss the patient's status in the hospital elevator.
   a. true
   b. false

9. A civil conviction of an individual who has violated HIPAA is generally accompanied by a monetary fine of up to _____ per violation.
   a. $250
   b. $2500
   c. $25,000
   d. $250,000

10. Which of the following would be considered as a complication resulting from the catheterization procedure?
    i. thrombus formation
    ii. aneurysm rupture
    iii. ischemia
    a. i only
    b. i and ii only
    c. ii and iii only
    d. i, ii, and iii

8 *Principles of Angiography*

CHAPTER OBJECTIVES

After completing this chapter, the reader will be able to perform the following:

- Describe the historical background of angiography
- List and describe the methods of patient monitoring
- Define the principles of pulse oximetry
- Describe the basic principles of electrocardiography
- Identify the method for evaluating the electrocardiogram tracing
- Identify some common cardiac arrhythmias
- Identify and describe the various means for obtaining vessel access
- Describe the procedure for the Seldinger technique for vessel puncture
- Describe the various arterial and venous access approaches
- Describe the direct exposure of an artery or vein for vessel access
- Describe the various vessel puncture closure devices

CHAPTER OUTLINE

HISTORICAL PERSPECTIVE

MONITORING TECHNIQUES

    Physiologic Monitoring
    Pulse Oximetry (Oxygen Saturation)

BASIC PRINCIPLES OF ELECTROCARDIOGRAPHY

    Evaluating the Electrocardiogram Tracing
    Arrhythmias

ESTABLISHMENT OF VESSEL ACCESS

    Arterial Puncture Techniques
    Venous Puncture Techniques
    Direct Exposure of an Artery or Vein (Cut-down Procedure)

VESSEL PUNCTURE CLOSURE DEVICES

SUMMARY

Angiography is defined as "the x-ray visualization of the internal anatomy of the heart and blood vessels after the intravascular introduction of radiopaque contrast medium."[1] The contrast medium is introduced by an intravenous or intra-arterial injection or through a catheter that is inserted into a peripheral vessel and guided to the desired target area.

Before the discovery of x-rays, the injection of materials into the vessels of the body was performed primarily on cadavers. The procedure was limited to the injection of various vital dyes that stained the tissues of the body and facilitated the study of human anatomy after dissection. This practice was continued after Roentgen's famous discovery and extended to the introduction of radiopaque materials that permitted physicians and anatomists to record the anatomy with x-rays. The use of this technique was not successfully applied to live subjects until about 1920, when a contrast agent was developed that could be safely introduced into the vascular system.

Improvements in radiographic and ancillary equipment and the development of safer contrast agents fostered research in angiographic procedures. Angiography became a safe, reliable diagnostic technique. The angiographic catheterization procedure provided a springboard for the use of angiography for therapeutic purposes.

HISTORICAL PERSPECTIVE

Angiography is a general term for the radiographic examination of the blood vessels. These studies are used to image pathologic and physiologic changes in visceral, cerebral, peripheral, and cardiac anatomy by injecting a contrast agent into specific portions of the vascular system.

In 1844, Claude Bernard performed catheterization of both the right and left ventricles of the heart of a horse. This first step enabled investigators to develop innovative techniques that were ultimately used in human subjects. Angiography had its beginnings in the late 1800s when investigators injected radiopaque materials into the vessels of corpses to outline the anatomy. These early contrast agents were highly toxic and could not be used in living subjects.

During 1918 through 1919, Walter Dandy, a neurosurgeon at The Johns Hopkins University, developed a procedure that used air to image the ventricular system of the brain of living humans. The technique was called **pneumoencephalography**. This development created an interest in the exploration of other substances that could be used to image anatomic structures not easily visualized with conventional radiography.

In early 1920, sodium iodide, a radiopaque substance, was found to be safe for use in living subjects. Egas Moniz and J. P. Caldas began performing cerebral angiography. They used sodium iodide as the contrast agent and the radiocarousel to image the vascular system of the brain. The **radiocarousel,** which was invented by Caldas, could image at the rate of one image per second for a maximum of 6 s. Simultaneously, B. Brooks was investigating the use of sodium iodide in imaging the femoral arteries. This marked the beginning of the era of angiography.

Werner Forssmann searched for a method of delivering medication directly to the location of need and is credited with performing the first human cardiac catheterization. In 1929, at the age of 25, he passed a 65-cm catheter through his left antecubital vein into his right atrium. He documented this achievement with a chest x-ray demonstrating the placement of the catheter. His research was used as a foundation by many investigators for the study of cardiovascular physiology.

Various changes were made in contrast agents, equipment, and methods between these first attempts at angiography and the early 1970s. During the 1940s, rapid sequence cassette changers were further developed, and image intensifiers, generators, and x-ray tubes were beginning to be developed. In the 1950s and 1960s, automatic injection devices were used to deliver the bolus of contrast agent to the desired location. Rapid sequence imaging devices were improved, and the Schonander cut film changer was introduced.

Catheters were being investigated for the introduction of the contrast agents directly to a desired location. H. A. Zimmerman reported a successful cardiac catheterization in a human. The method of choice in the early years of angiography for the introduction of the catheter was by direct approach. This involved making an incision, exposing the vessel of interest, and placing the catheter directly in its lumen.

In 1953, S. I. Seldinger described a method for the introduction of the catheter through the percutaneous replacement of the needle. This technique improved the safety of angiographic studies and simplified the procedure. In 1959, J. Ross Jr. and C. Cope described the transseptal catheterization procedure. Cope was also perfecting a method for selective coronary arteriography, and he experimented with a variety of catheter shapes to achieve this goal.

Serial magnification techniques and subtraction were introduced during this period, and the use of computer systems in connection with radiographic equipment was beginning to be investigated.

Through the 1980s, refinements in digital techniques advanced the basic subtraction principles and launched digital subtraction angiography as the modality most often used for cardiac catheterization. The development of computed tomography and magnetic resonance as imaging tools further reduced the use of angiography as the primary tool for diagnosis. Interventional procedures were perfected during this period, and angiography shifted from a purely diagnostic tool to an adjunct to the nonsurgical intervention in many disease processes. Interventional radiography has become the primary focus of vascular and cardiac therapy. The basic principles underlying diagnostic angiography still apply to interventional studies, and although the discussion of these principles may refer to diagnostic procedures, a transfer to interventional radiography is just a small leap away.

The evolution of faster computed tomography units, magnetic resonance angiography, and positron emission tomography has made possible noninvasive diagnosis in the heart and vascular system. However, invasive advanced procedures are still used for diagnosis and have provided the basis for the field of interventional radiology. Each year heralds new interventional procedures. This poses a challenge for both the radiologist and the radiographer. An increased knowledge of pharmacology, communication, and an ever-changing array of technical skills are required to safely and effectively perform these procedures. Interventional radiology has overshadowed diagnostic angiography and become a specialty field in its own right.

In January 2003 the American Registry of Radiologic Technologists (ARRT) introduced two postprimary advanced level examinations to replace its existing cardiovascular–interventional technology examination: vascular–interventional and cardiac–interventional technology examinations. (See www.ARRT.org for content specifications and additional information.) Although the diagnostic portion of the procedures plays an important part of the total patient care, the field of interventional (therapeutic) radiology is rapidly becoming the primary focus of the radiographer's responsibilities in the advanced procedure field. The techniques learned and practiced in the diagnostic studies are critical to the understanding and practice of interventional procedures.

MONITORING TECHNIQUES

Physiologic Monitoring

During the procedure physiologic monitoring of the patient is essential. This involves the measurement of several factors, including blood pressure, renal output (if appropriate), heart rate and rhythm, respiration, and pharmacologic monitoring. The values and observations should be documented in the procedural notes, and the physician should be made aware of variations from the normal as they occur.

Pulse Oximetry (Oxygen Saturation)

The amount of oxygen that is bound to the hemoglobin contained in the red blood cell can easily be monitored throughout the procedure. It is accomplished noninvasively by means of a pulse oximeter and provides real-time information regarding the oxygen saturation. The physiologic process is the binding of hemoglobin and oxygen to form oxyhemoglobin (HbO_2). Pulse oximetry provides a measurement of the oxyhemoglobin saturation of the arterial capillaries (SaO_2). The measurements are made by means of a sensor that is attached to the patient's finger or toe. Figure 8-1 illustrates the TruSat pulse oximeter manufactured by Datex-Ohmeda. This system has a display range from 0% to 100% displayed on a highly visible backlit screen. It provides a measurement of the oxyhemoglobin saturation (SpO_2) value and pulse rate. This unit is also equipped with both audio and visual alarms for SpO_2 and pulse rate limits.

The most common type of sensor is the finger probe. It contains two light-emitting diodes (LEDs) and a silicone photodiode. The sensors transmit light through the capillary bed and receive the information on the opposite side.

When using this device it is important to follow the manufacturer's instructions for correct alignment of the digit and the sensors. If this is not accomplished, the readings will not be accurate. It is

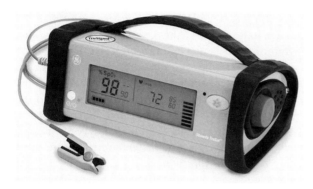

FIGURE 8-1. The TruSat Pulse oximeter by Datex-Ohmeda is used to measure the oxygen saturation of the blood.

also important that the location chosen be checked for adequate perfusion. If the circulation in the area is not sufficient, readings will also be inaccurate. A simple check can be performed by gently applying pressure on the area of interest by squeezing the distal end between the thumb and forefinger for several seconds. When the pressure is released there should be a rapid return of color to the digit. This is indicative of proper circulation. Other factors that can affect the readings are nail polish and excessive pigmentation. The readings should be documented throughout the procedure. The normal oxygen saturation range is between 90% and 100%.

BASIC PRINCIPLES OF ELECTROCARDIOGRAPHY

Electrical changes in the heart muscle taking place during systole can be led off from the surface of the body by electrodes to a recorder capable of producing an electrocardiogram (ECG) tracing. This tracing represents the pattern of electrical activity in the heart.

Standard locations on the body for these electrodes are the right and left arms, right arm and left leg, and left arm and left leg. Each segment of the ECG shows the electrical cycle of the heart (Fig. 8-2). The P wave initiates the cycle, and the excitation spreads from the **sinoatrial node** over the atrium to the **atrioventricular node**. Peaks Q, R, and S follow as the impulse spreads throughout the **atrioventricular bundle of His** over the ventricles. At this time, the heart is in ventricular systole. Finally, as ventricular excitation subsides, the T peak is recorded. The U wave is not usually attendant in the normal ECG; it is usually present when the serum potassium level is low and appears as a small upward wave.

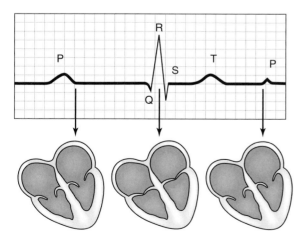

FIGURE 8-2. Electrocardiogram showing the location of the major waves. The P wave begins the cycle and represents the depolarization (contraction) of the atria when forcing the blood into the ventricles. The QRS complex represents the depolarization (contraction) of the ventricles when forcing the blood into both the pulmonary and systemic circulation. Relaxation of the heart occurs at the T wave. The cycle begins again with the new P wave.

A normal single heartbeat comprises five waves (P, Q, R, S, and T). The P wave occurs when the atria contract. The presence of the QRS complex indicates that the ventricles are undergoing contraction. The T wave is the electrical recovery from the ventricular contraction phase.

The small and large blocks on the ECG paper and tracing illustrate the interval in seconds (horizontal blocks) and the measurement of electrical activity in millimeters (vertical blocks) of the wave. Each of the small horizontal blocks represents 0.04 s on the horizontal line and 1 mm on the vertical line (Fig. 8–3). Because each of the large blocks comprises five horizontal and five vertical blocks, its value can be stated as 0.2 s (0.04 s × 5 = 0.2 s) horizontal and 5 mm (1 mm × 5 = 5 mm) vertical. The vertical height is correlated to the electrical activity. Five millimeters of height (one large block) is equal to 0.5 mV of electrical activity. Table 8–1 summarizes the normal ECG tracing and lists the wave, segment, or interval, the significant physiology, and how the normal pattern should be represented on the ECG paper.

Evaluating the Electrocardiogram Tracing

The ECG tracing should be systematically evaluated in the following categories:

1. **Rate of rhythm.** The rate of the cardiac rhythm should be categorized into one of the following.
   a. No rate. No waves present or any sign of electrical activity.
   b. Slow rate. Rates less than 60 beats/minute (**bradycardia**).
   c. **Normal rate.** Rates between 60 and 100 beats/minute.
   d. Increased rate. Rates in excess of 100 beats/minute (**tachycardia**).
2. **Regularity of the rhythm.** This is measured by the distance between the QRS complexes, which is sometimes referred to as the RR interval. This should vary by no more than three small squares (0.12 s).
3. **PR ratio.** This is the ratio of the number of P waves to QRS complexes. The normal PR ratio is 1:1.
4. **PR interval.** This is measured as the distance between the onset of the P wave and the onset of the QRS complex. It should not be any less than three small squares (0.12 s) or more than five small squares (0.20 s).
5. **QRS complex interval.** This is measured as the distance from the start of the QRS complex to the end of the same QRS complex. The normal QRS interval is about two and one-half small squares (0.10 s).

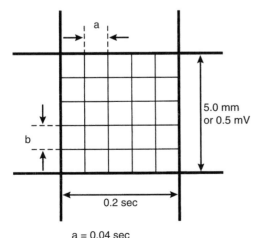

a = 0.04 sec
b = 1.0 mm or 0.1 mV

FIGURE 8-3. Time and voltage lines on ECG paper. Five large horizontal boxes (25 small squares) equal 1 s. Two large vertical boxes equal 1 mV or 10 mm.

TABLE 8-1   *Summary of the Normal Electrocardiogram*

Wave/Segment/Interval	Significance	Normal Pattern
P wave	Upward deflection. Begins with electrical discharge from sinus node. Electrical current flows in the atria. Depolarization of the atrial muscle produces the P wave.	Less than three small blocks wide. Less than three small blocks high.
PR interval	Interval between the beginning of the P wave and the beginning of the QRS complex. Electrical impulse spreads along the following route: Atrium Atrioventricular node Bundle of His Right and left bundle branches	More than three and less than five small blocks wide.
QRS complex	Three separate deflections: Q–Downstroke before the R wave (downward deflection) R–First upward wave (upward deflection) S–Downstroke after the R wave (downward deflection) Represents a depolarization of the ventricles. Electrical impulse travels along the following pathway: Purkinje fibers Ventricular muscle fibers	Less than 2.5 small blocks wide.
ST segment	Begins at the end of the S wave and ends at the beginning of the T wave. Point at which the tracing "turns" following the S wave.	The ST segment should not be elevated or depressed.
T wave	Repolarization of the ventricular tissue.	Normal wave less than 10 small blocks high in the chest leads and less than five small blocks high in the remaining leads.
U wave	Small upward deflection that follows the T wave.	Not normally present unless serum potassium level is low.

ECG tracing pattern changes in any of these areas should be noted on the patient's chart, and the information should immediately be transmitted to the physician performing the procedure. Any change from the normal ECG tracing pattern usually signifies the presence of an arrhythmia.

Arrhythmias

The recognition of cardiac arrhythmias is a skill that is acquired through experience or education. Many of the abnormalities that appear on ECG tracings can apply to more than one type of arrhythmia. A systematic analysis of the ECG tracing pattern can narrow the choices dramatically. The novice practitioner should be conversant with the normal ECG pattern and be able to recognize any deviation from it. During the procedure, any changes in the normal pattern should be noted and the physician alerted.

Arrhythmias are basically changes in the ECG tracing and denote a change in the rate of the impulses (automaticity), the conduction of the impulses, or both. Variations from the normal ECG pattern should be immediately pointed out to the physician during the procedure; careful observation of the patient in conjunction with monitoring of the regularity of the ECG pattern is important during a special procedure. Symptoms to watch for include chest tightness, pain, palpitations, rapid or distressed breathing, restlessness, loss of consciousness, pallor, and cool, moist skin. The physician should be alerted if any of these symptoms appear in conjunction with an abnormal ECG trace pattern. These symptoms can be invaluable in determining the exact diagnosis and treatment protocol to be followed subsequent to the event. Table 8-2 summarizes a variety of major arrhythmias and their general characteristics.

ESTABLISHMENT OF VESSEL ACCESS

Angiography is usually accomplished by accessing a vessel, introducing a catheter into its lumen, and manipulating it so that it arrives at the desired location. The arterial approach is used most often. Most studies performed today utilize the percutaneous puncture of the specific vessel following the **Seldinger method** of percutaneous vessel access.

In the early days of angiography, the vessel had to be surgically exposed to accomplish this task. In 1953, Ivan Seldinger developed a technique that has become the basis for modern angiographic catheterization (Fig. 8-4). The technique is applied to both arterial and venous catheterization techniques. The technique is accomplished through the Seldinger procedure as follows:

1. The arterial pulse is identified, and the puncture site is chosen.
2. The site is shaved, surgically prepared, and draped.
3. Local anesthetic is applied to the area, and a nick is made in the skin to facilitate needle access.
4. An 18-gauge Seldinger needle or its variant is inserted into the vessel, the stylet is removed, and pulsatile blood flow is sought.
5. A guide wire is inserted through the lumen of the needle.
6. The needle is withdrawn.
7. Depending upon the catheter size, the puncture site may have to be dilated. This is accomplished by means of a dilator sheath, which is placed over the guide wire and inserted into the vessel with a slight twisting motion. The sheath dilator is usually equipped with a valve to prevent leakage. The sheath serves several purposes, including the maintenance of vessel access if the guide wire is accidentally removed.
8. The catheter is then threaded over the guide wire and advanced into the lumen of the vessel. A catheter that is one size smaller than the sheath diameter should be used.
9. The guide wire is removed, and the catheter is advanced in the vessel to the desired location.
10. During the procedure, the catheter is flushed with heparinized saline, if not contraindicated, to prevent thrombosis.
11. At the conclusion of the study, the catheter is removed, and pressure is maintained at the site until hemostasis is achieved.

TABLE 8-2 *Summary of Major Arrhythmias and Their General Characteristics*

Type of Arrhythmia	Heart Rate	Pattern Regularity	PR Ratio	PR Interval	QRS Complex
Asystole	None	Regular "flat line" wave	None	None	None
Ventricular fibrillation	None	Irregular wavy line	None	None	None
Junctional rhythm	Slow	Regular	1:1 or 0:1	None or shortened	Within normal limits
Sinus bradycardia	Slow	Regular	1:1	Within limits	Within normal limits
Idioventricular rhythm	Slow	Regular	0:1	None	Increased
First-degree heart block	Normal to slow	Regular	1:1	Increased with regular pattern	Within normal limits
Mobitz 1 heart block (second degree)	Normal to slow	Irregular	Between 1:1 and 2:1	Increased with regular pattern	Within normal limits
Mobitz II heart block (second degree)	Normal to slow	Regular or irregular	1:1, 2:1, or greater	Constant for beats that are conducted	Within normal limits
Third-degree heart block	Normal to slow	Regular	1:1	Variable	Increased
Atrial fibrillation	Slow or fast	Irregular	0:1	None	Within normal limits
Atrial flutter	Ventricular rate normal / Atrial rate 250–300 beats/minute	Usually regular	2:1 or greater	Regular	Within normal limits
Sinus tachycardia	Fast (100–150 beats/minute)	Regular	1:1	Within limits	Within normal limits
Atrial tachycardia	Fast (150–350 beats/minute)	Regular	1:1	Within limits	Within normal limits
Ventricular tachycardia	Fast	Regular	0:1	None	Increased
Junctional tachycardia	Fast	Regular	1:1	None or shortened	Within normal limits

In actual practice, the procedure may undergo some minor variation depending on the type of needle used, whether an obstruction is encountered, whether the insertion is being done at the site of a previous graft, and whether vascular dilators or sheaths are needed.

Arterial Puncture Techniques

Several approaches are used for the arterial catheterization procedure—through the common femoral, brachial, or axillary artery. The most frequent approach is through the femoral artery. This approach to

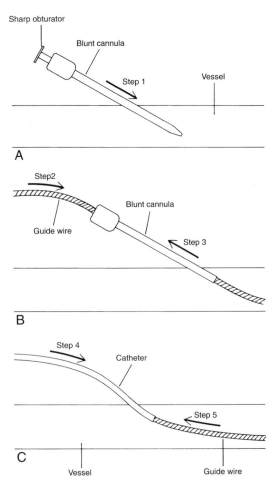

FIGURE 8-4. The Seldinger method of percutaneous puncture. **A,** The puncture needle has been inserted into the vessel (Step 1); **B,** the guide wire has been inserted into the vessel through the needle (Step 2); the needle is withdrawn, with the guide wire remaining in the vessel (Step 3); **C,** a catheter is threaded into the vessel over the guide wire (Step 4); the guide wire is then removed, and the catheter is advanced in the vessel (Step 5).

vessel access is one of the safest methods. It has been simplified through the use of the Seldinger puncture technique. It is easily accessible and can be compressed against the femoral head, which prevents leakage around the site and allows for the compression necessary to close the puncture site.

Femoral Artery Approach

The femoral artery can be approached both antegrade and retrograde. The antegrade approach is less desirable in obese patients owing to the difficulty in maneuvering the needle around large abdominal folds. The retrograde puncture method is accomplished approximately 1 cm below the inguinal ligament; the exact location can be determined by manually palpating for the best femoral arterial pulse. Once the skin is anesthetized both superficially and into the deep tissue a small skin incision can be made. Depending upon the approach, retrograde or antegrade, the position of the skin incision varies. For retrograde puncture the skin incision is made approximately 1 to 2 cm below the intended puncture site. Antegrade access is similar with the exception that the skin nick is usually 1 to 2 cm above the intended puncture site.

After the incision has been dilated to allow for access of the catheter, an 18-gauge needle with stylet is inserted toward the femoral head. The needle is inserted between the index and middle fingers at an angle of 25 to 30 degrees toward the midline (Fig. 8-5). This angle should correspond to the longitudinal axis of the vessel. Once the vessel is entered a guide wire is inserted through the needle into the vessel. This should be accomplished easily. Undue resistance may indicate an obstruction or subintimal insertion of the guide wire. If repositioning the angle of the needle does not solve the problem,

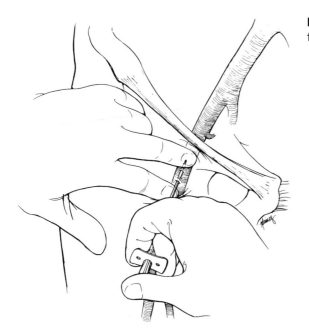

FIGURE 8-5. Method used for retrograde femoral artery puncture.

it may be necessary to withdraw the guide wire and repuncture the artery. If passage of the guide wire is not compromised, then the needle can be removed, leaving the guide wire in place in the vessel. A dilator is then threaded over the guide wire and introduced into the puncture site to create a path for the catheter. The dilator is then exchanged for the catheter, and the study can proceed.

Axillary and Brachial Approaches

The axillary and brachial approaches are used when both femoral arteries are compromised or in cases of aortic occlusion. These approaches are also reserved for procedures in which access from above is desirable. Brachial and axillary catheterization techniques pose the risks of cerebral embolization, neural injury, spasm, and arterial thrombosis. The risks of complications using these methods are twice those of the femoral approach.[2] The brachial approach is usually preferred over the axillary puncture because the potential for complication is somewhat reduced. The technique for the puncture is the same for either arm; however, the left arm is preferred for studies involving the abdominal aorta to lower extremities. This arm also poses less of a risk for embolic stroke than the opposite limb. The use of the right arm is reserved for studies involving the ascending aorta and cerebral vessels.

As with all of the studies, the pulse in both arms at the high and low positions should be accomplished prior to puncture. This is done to determine if there is stenosis present in either of the limbs. A difference of more than 20 mm Hg between the extremities would indicate the potential for stenosis, and the opposite arm should then be used. During the study it is important to ensure that there is adequate perfusion of the arm. This can be accomplished with the use of a simple pulse oximeter attached to one of the patient's fingers.

Axillary puncture is accomplished in the lateral axillary fold (Fig. 8-6). The arm can be fully abducted with the hand placed under the head. The needle is inserted into the artery at the point of maximal pulse. As in the other puncture techniques, the needle is inserted between the index and the middle fingers. Once cannulation is effected, a guide wire can be introduced. The catheter can then be introduced into the vessel over the guide wire to complete the procedure.

The brachial approach involves the introduction of the needle into the midportion of the humerus (bicipital sulcus). The arm is abducted 90 degrees, and the brachial artery is located by palpation. The needle is inserted in the same manner as for the previous approaches. The angle the needle forms with

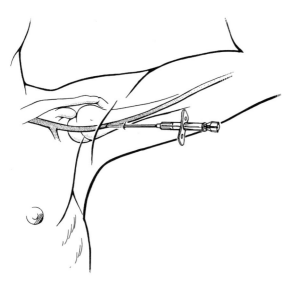

FIGURE 8-6. Technique used for an axillary arterial puncture.

the plane of the arm should be approximately 45 degrees. The brachial artery is a superficial vessel, and the needle does not have to be inserted very deep for cannulation.

Translumbar Approach

In cases in which there is suspected aneurysm or occlusion of the aorta, or in rare cases when the femoral and brachial routes are compromised, the translumbar approach can be used (Fig. 8-7). This procedure can be done at either of two levels—the high approach (lower border of T12) or the low approach (lower border of L2). This approach is not as desirable owing to its attendant risks. Patient selection is limited to individuals who have normal coagulation results.

The specific technique of direct puncture of the aorta differs according to the physician performing the procedure. There are two basic variations—high and low—and the approach chosen depends on the anatomic information desired. The procedure is accomplished with a specially designed 18-gauge catheter with a 6F sheath 18 to 24 cm in length. The patient is placed into the prone position. The insertion point can be slightly below the level of the twelfth thoracic vertebra (high approach) or at the third lumbar vertebra (low approach), and it is always made from the left flank approximately one hand's width from the spinous process.

In the low approach, the needle is directed in the axial plane at an angle of approximately 40 degrees. This approach provides opacification of the vessels of the lower extremity without superimposition of the vessels of the abdominal viscera.

The high approach is used when there is a suspected aortic aneurysm or occlusion. The needle is directed cranially to avoid accidental injury to the renal artery. The angle is similar to that of the low approach, but there is the added risk of inducing a pneumothorax through accidental puncture of the lung. This approach is less desirable than the low approach because of the opacification of the vessels of the abdominal viscera.

Once aortic puncture has been accomplished, a guide wire is inserted and advanced through the needle into the aorta. The sheath is then placed in the vessel over the guide wire. The injection of contrast agent is made through the sheath.

Venous Puncture Techniques

If angiography of the venous system is required, the catheter can be inserted into the lumen of the vena cava. This catheterization approach is usually through the femoral vein, but the study can be accomplished by using the right internal jugular vein or several veins in the upper extremity. Venous

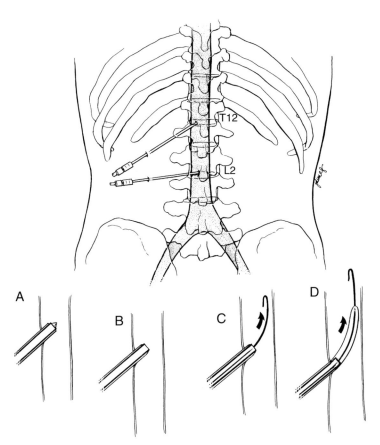

FIGURE   8-7. Translumbar puncture. The patient is placed in the prone position, and the needle is inserted in the left flank. **A,** The needle and obturator are inserted into the aorta. **B,** After successful insertion, the obturator is removed. **C,** A guide wire is then inserted through the needle into the aorta. **D,** A catheter is then threaded over the guide wire into the aorta.

access can also be achieved through translumbar or transhepatic puncture. In most cases it is advisable to incorporate either ultrasonography or fluoroscopic guidance for venous puncture. Unlike arteries the veins are soft and pliant. These characteristics can make cannulation somewhat difficult. These characteristics also render the veins adaptable to a variety of different catheters and accessories. The risks from venous puncture are limited and relatively rare.

These techniques are usually used during venous angiographic procedures. The choice of approach is determined by the patient's condition, purpose of the study, and the preference of the physician. Some physicians prefer the use of single-walled needles without a stylet when accessing the venous system.

The usual approach is through the femoral vein; however, it can be seen that a number of different approaches can be used. The basic technique is the same as that for arterial puncture and any of the arterial puncture needles can be used to gain venous access. After the vessel has been transfixed, the needle stylet is removed, and a flexible connector with a syringe is attached to the needle hub. As the needle is withdrawn, suction is applied using the syringe. When blood is seen in the tubing, the dilator sheath is advanced into the vessel. A guide wire can then be inserted into the vessel, and a catheter is threaded into the lumen of the vein in a manner similar to that used in arterial catheterization.

Femoral Vein Approach

The femoral vein can be found 1 to 2 cm below the inguinal ligament and 0.5 cm medial to the femoral artery. The area is anesthetized with a local anesthetic such as lidocaine. A small skin incision is made over the area, which lies somewhat lower than that for the femoral arterial puncture. The femoral artery is secured and moved away from the puncture site with the fingers before the needle is inserted. Throughout the puncture process the arterial pulse should be palpated with the fingers of the opposite

Fundamentals of Special Radiographic Procedures

hand to avoid inadvertent arterial puncture. A single-walled needle without a stylet is used to make the puncture. Suction is applied throughout the process, and vessel access will be confirmed when blood is drawn into the connector tubing attached to the needle. Just as in the arterial puncture, the femoral vein can be accessed either antegrade or retrograde, depending on the reason for the procedure.

Upper Extremity Approach

The median antecubital vein can be accessed via the antecubital fossa. The cannulation is usually accomplished with an angiocatheter sheath needle; specially designed needles are available for this procedure. The possible restrictions to this approach, especially on an inpatient, are that this is a commonly used vein and may be thrombosed or already in use when the patient arrives in the department.

The basilic vein is superficially located on the medial side of the arm. It is easily located slightly above the antecubital fossa and provides easy access. The upper extremity offers several sites for the puncture. The choice would be the physician's preference, the patient's condition, and the procedure being performed.

Internal Jugular Approach

Puncture of the internal jugular vein is usually made on the right side. This provides the best access to the superior vena cava for studies involving the thorax or the abdomen and in the treatment of dialysis patients. The right internal jugular vein approach is the method of choice for transjugular intrahepatic portosystemic shunt placement (TIPS). Ultrasound guidance for the puncture is generally recommended to ensure that the vessel has been accessed. The internal jugular vein is located lateral to the carotid artery, medial to the external jugular vein, and slightly lateral to the sternocleidomastoid muscle. A small skin incision is made in the area of the sternocleidomastoid muscle. A syringe is attached to an Amplatz needle, and suction is applied throughout the insertion procedure. The aspiration of blood into the syringe allows the physician to know when he or she has achieved successful cannulation of the vessel. A Valsalva maneuver can be used to distend the internal jugular vein for better visibility. When the vessel is cannulated, a catheter introducer sheath is inserted, and catheterization can proceed. The Valsalva maneuver should also be done when the needle, catheter, or sheath is open to air or removed.

Although complications are rare during the cannulation of the internal jugular vein, there is the possibility of introducing an air embolus. This can occur whenever a needle, catheter, or guide wire sheath is open to ambient air. Although a small amount of air generally will not cause a problem, larger amounts in excess of 20 ml can be dangerous. Treatment consists of careful observation of the patient's vital signs, sealing the source of the air, positioning the patient in a left lateral decubitus position, and administering oxygen until the air is absorbed. In extremely severe cases the physician may attempt to catheterize the right atrium to manually aspirate the air.

Translumbar Inferior Vena Caval Approach

This technique is similar to the translumbar aortic puncture. It is sometimes referred to as an infrarenal translumbar puncture technique. The access is from the patient's right side rather than the left. The patient should be placed in the left lateral decubitus position. The puncture needle is the same as is used for translumbar aortography. The insertion point is 3 cm above the iliac crest and 10 cm lateral to the spinous process of L3. The angle of insertion is approximately 45 degrees toward the head. Once the inferior vena cava has been punctured the stylet is removed, and the needle is positioned to achieve blood flow.

Transhepatic Inferior Vena Caval Approach

If both the thoracic and lower inferior vena cava are compromised, a transhepatic puncture can be performed. This approach, however, is usually limited to children requiring long-term parenteral nutritional supplement. Generally a long 21-gauge microaccess needle is used for the puncture, and the procedure is carried out under general anesthesia. The puncture is made with the patient in the supine position either below the rib margin or at the tenth intercostal space. The needle is advanced in a slight cephalic angle through the liver parenchyma toward the vertebral column. When blood is aspirated through the needle, a successful vascular puncture is indicated. This can be confirmed by the injection of contrast medium.

Subclavian Vein Approach

The subclavian vein is an extension of the axillary vein, which drains the arm. It extends from the lateral border of the first rib to the sternal end of the clavicle. The puncture is usually accomplished by inserting the needle at the point where the subclavian vein crosses the first rib. The needle is advanced until blood is aspirated into the syringe. Access to the subclavian vein can be confirmed by injecting a small amount of contrast agent into a vein of the distal arm.

Direct Exposure of an Artery or Vein (Cut-Down Procedure)

Sometimes it is desirable to directly expose the artery or vein to introduce the catheter. The technique is basically the same for any vessel. It begins with the isolation of the vessel of interest by palpation. Local anesthetic is introduced initially through a short 25- to 27-gauge needle to raise a superficial intradermal wheal. This is followed by deep introduction into the subcutaneous, deep fascial, and periosteal tissues using a $1\frac{1}{2}$-in 22-gauge needle. When the proposed catheter insertion site is anesthetized, a transverse incision is made in the area of interest. The tissues are separated using a blunt instrument to expose the desired vessel, which is then brought to the surface. The vessel is secured both proximally and distally with silk suture material, umbilical tape, or silicone elastomer tape.

If an artery has been exposed, the incision into it is made with a scalpel blade (cutting edge up); the catheter is then inserted and moved to the desired location. A vein can be incised using small scissors. The catheter is inserted and moved to the location of choice.

At the end of the procedure, the vessels are repaired, and the incision is closed and dressed.

VESSEL PUNCTURE CLOSURE DEVICES

At the conclusion of the procedure the puncture site must be sealed. In the case of venous access, simple manual compression of the puncture site for a minimum period of at least 10 minutes should be accomplished. The site should be visually inspected every 15 minutes for at least 4 hours to determine if any bleeding has or is occurring. Vital signs should be taken at 30-minute intervals for the same period, and IV fluids should be continued.

Arterial puncture sites can be sealed either through manual compression or mechanical means such as the use of collagen plugs or mechanical sutures. Manual compression should be done for a minimum period of 20 minutes. It is important to maintain the peripheral pulse throughout compression. If after 20 minutes bleeding is apparent, compression should be continued for another 20 minutes. Compression can be applied using compression cuffs, weights, or specially designed clamps.

The use of collagen plugs to provide vessel closure is a common method used today. It significantly reduces the time required to attain vessel closure. Other mechanical suturing devices are available; however, these are much more costly than the use of either of the two methods for vessel closure described here.

SUMMARY

Angiography requires the placement of a catheter into a vessel to inject a contrast agent to obtain the necessary information. The most common method of introducing the catheter is the Seldinger method. This is a percutaneous technique that can be accomplished easily and relatively safely.

A variety of approaches are used to gain vessel access. The arterial routes include femoral artery puncture, axillary puncture, brachial puncture, and the translumbar approach. The femoral routes can be either antegrade or retrograde. The brachial puncture is favored over the axillary and the left limb poses less potential for complication than the right. The translumbar approach is used only on rare occasions when all of the other access sites are compromised or if there is the presence of metal clips that would contraindicate magnetic resonance imaging.

Physiologic monitoring includes monitoring the patient's oxygen saturation levels, pulse rate, and electrocardiogram. A basic knowledge of these competencies is essential for the advanced practitioner. An understanding of the normal values for these areas is warranted.

REFERENCES

1. Seldinger SI: Catheter placement of the needle in percutaneous arteriography. *Acta Radiol (Diagn)* 39:368–376, 1953.
2. Hessel SJ, Adams DF: Complications of angiography. *Radiology* 138:273–281, 1981.

SUGGESTED READINGS

Abando A, Hood D, Weaver F, et al: The use of the Angioseal device for femoral artery closure. *J Vasc Surg* 40(2):287–290, 2004.

Applegate RJ, Rankin KM, Little WC, et al: Restick following initial Angioseal use. *Catheter Cardiovasc Interv* 58(2):181–184, 2003.

Aytekin C, Boyvat F, Firat A, et al: Portacaval shunt creation using the percutaneous transhepatic-transjugular technique. *Abdom Imaging* 28(2):287–292, 2003.

Cleveland G, Hill S, Williams S: Arterial puncture closure using a collagen plug. II. VasoSeal. *Tech Vasc Intervent Radiol* 6(2):82–84, 2003.

Inglese L, Lupattelli T, Carbone GL, et al: Axillary artery access for interventional procedures. *J Endovasc Ther* 11(4):414–418, 2004.

Kern MJ: Should vascular access closure devices be routine after interventional procedures? *J Invasive Cardiol* 12(8):400–401, 2000.

Kinney TB: Translumbar high inferior vena cava access placement in patients with thrombosed inferior vena cava filters. *J Vasc Interv Radiol* 14(12):1563–1568, 2003.

Levy EI, Boulos AS, Fessler RD, et al: Transradial cerebral angiography: an alternative route. *Neurosurgery* 51(2):335–340, 2002.

Madoff DC, Hicks ME, Vauthey JN, et al: Transhepatic portal vein embolization: anatomy, indications, and technical considerations. *Radiographics* 22(5):1063–1076, 2002.

Parry G: Trendelenburg position, head elevation and a midline position optimize right internal jugular vein diameter. *Can J Anaesth* 51(4):379–381, 2004.

Physician's Desk Reference. Montvale, NJ, 2004, Thompson Micromedics.

Quinn SF, Kim J: Percutaneous femoral closure following stent-graft placement: use of the Perclose device. *Cardiovasc Interv Radiol* 27(3):231–236, 2004.

Spector KS, Lawson WE: Optimizing safe femoral access during cardiac catheterization. *Catheter Cardiovasc Interv* 53(2):209–212, 2001.

Wallace MJ, Hovsepian D, Balzer C: Transhepatic venous access for diagnostic and interventional cardiovascular procedures. *J Vasc Interv Radiol* 7:579, 1996.

Yokoyama N, Takeshita S, Ochiai M, et al: Anatomic variations of the radial artery in patients undergoing transradial coronary intervention. *Catheter Cardiovasc Interv* 49(4):357–362, 2000.

STUDY QUESTIONS

1. During the procedure oxygen should be applied to the patient when the oxygen saturation level falls below:

    a. 50%   **c.** 75%

    b. 60%   **d.** 90%

STUDY QUESTIONS (*cont'd*)

2. Which of the following puncture techniques requires that the patient be placed in a left lateral decubitus position to insert the needle?
   a. femoral artery puncture
   b. axillary artery puncture
   c. translumbar aortic puncture
   d. brachial artery puncture

3. The individual responsible for the development of the percutaneous puncture technique was:
   a. Egas Moniz
   b. Sven Ivan Seldinger
   c. C. Cope
   d. J.P. Caldas

4. The symbol used to denote that oxygen has been bound to hemoglobin to form oxyhemoglobin is:
   a. HbO_2
   b. SbO_2
   c. SaO_2
   d. SpO_2

5. Which of the following measurements would represent a normal oxygen saturation level for an adult patient?
   a. 66%
   b. 78%
   c. 84%
   d. 97%

6. The basilic vein is located:
   a. high in the neck area
   b. next to the femoral artery
   c. flanking the aorta
   d. on the medial side of the upper arm

7. The local anesthetic that is used to infiltrate the potential puncture site is:
   a. lorazepam
   b. lidocaine
   c. Sublimaze
   d. Versed

8. A heart rate of less than 60 beats per minute would be considered to be:
   a. tachycardia
   b. normal
   c. bradycardia
   d. isocardia

9. The normal value for the ratio of the number of P waves to QRS complexes is:
   a. 1:1
   b. 2:1
   c. 1:3
   d. 3:1

10. Which of the following ECG deflections is *not* considered to be a part of the normal single heart beat:
    a. M
    b. Q
    c. S
    d. T

9 *Computed Tomography*

Computed tomography (CT) is a specialized modality that links the basic theory of body section radiography with a computer system to produce the anatomic images. The fundamentals of computer technology as it applies to radiography are presented in Chapter 2. The basic principles and terminology are similar for all computer-enhanced techniques, with minor variations applicable for CT and magnetic resonance imaging (MRI). The physical principles of CT are presented, but a detailed discussion is beyond the scope of this book.

STANDARD COMPUTED TOMOGRAPHY

Historical Perspective

CT appears to be a very recent innovation, but the theoretic principles were presented by Radon in 1917. This Austrian mathematician proved that it was possible to reconstruct a three-dimensional object from the infinite set of all of its projections. The actual breakthrough in making CT a useful diagnostic tool was made by Hounsfield in 1967. It was not until 1971, however, that the first working model was installed and ready for clinical trials. The transition from Radon's hypothesis to Hounsfield's breakthrough was aided by the experimental work of many researchers, including Oldendorf and Cormack. The use of CT has expanded since 1971, and new developments are occurring rapidly. Each major innovation heralds a new generation, or category, of CT scanners. These generations are identified primarily on the basis of the geometry of the mechanical scanning motions. Each successive generation has shown improvement in scanning mode, detection system, and rotational movement (degrees of rotation). The main result of the changes made to each of the successive generations of CT systems has been an increase in scanning speed. Scan times have been reduced from approximately 5 minutes for early slice by slice acquisition units to less than 0.4 s for current fourth-generation volume data acquisition (spiral or helical CT) scanners. The unique design of the electron beam CT (EBCT) systems, sometimes referred to as fifth-generation CT, has made possible scanning times of 50 to 100 ms. Figure 9-1 illustrates the beam geometry for the first four generations of CT scanners and the basic design of an EBCT system.

Mechanical CT Designs
Physical Principles

Tomography is the term used to describe body section radiography. The procedure produces a sectional image, or "slice," of the body part being examined. Traditional tomography uses the principle of blurring to remove unwanted superimposed structures while keeping the selected layer in focus. This can be accomplished by moving the x-ray beam and film through mechanical linkages or similar devices. Blurring can also be achieved by moving the patient and the film, the x-ray beam and the patient, or only the patient (**autotomography**). All these methods use conventional radiographic principles to produce the image, that is, to acquire diagnostic data. Conventional radiography and tomography, however, have several disadvantages. Superimposition of structures is one encountered problem. Conventional tomography can remedy this problem to some degree but not without a trade-off. With conventional tomographic methods, the blurring procedure can be somewhat distracting, and it cannot be completely eliminated from the final image produced by the scattered radiation.

CT is accomplished in three steps—scanning the patient (data acquisition), processing the data (image reconstruction), and displaying the image.

Data Acquisition

The first step, **scanning** the patient, is the radiographic portion of the study. The method used to scan is dependent upon the equipment.

CT equipment has undergone many changes since it was first used for diagnostic imaging. The geometry has evolved through four basic generational designs. A fifth-generation scanner, the **electron beam CT scanner**, allows physicians to produce high-resolution images of moving organs, free from motion artifacts.

The four basic generations of CT scanners incorporated the following geometric designs: First-generation CT scanners used a pencil x-ray beam, a single detector, and a **rotate-translate parallel beam** 180-degree geometric design. Second-generation scanners incorporated a fan x-ray beam with multiple detectors and a **rotate-translate** 180-degree geometric design. The first- and second-generation CT scanners required very long scan times to complete a study. The scan time was improved in the third- and fourth-generation designs to the range of 2 to 10 s. Third-generation scanners used the fan beam with 360-degree rotation of the x-ray tube and multiple detector array, considered a **rotate-rotate** design. Fourth-generation equipment incorporated a rotating fan beam with a 360-degree stationary ring of detectors, or a **rotate-stationary** geometric design. These scanners used two methods: rotation of the x-ray beam *within* the detector array or rotation outside a "tilting" (nutating) detector array. One disadvantage of this geometric design is that the system must be reset after only two complete revolutions of the x-ray tube. This is due primarily to the arrangement of the cables within the gantry. It can be seen that there is a time delay between periods when the x-ray tube is activated. This is referred to as the interscan delay (ISD).

All of the older generation methods use slice by slice scanning. In this process, the scan is made, followed by a delay while the scanner is reset, and then the patient is repositioned for the next slice. The sequence is repeated until the area to be scanned has been covered. Among the limitations of the slice by slice scanning method are the following:

1. Long examination times due to interscan delay
2. Omission of portions of the anatomy due to inconsistent respirations
3. Inaccurate reformatting of three-dimensional (3D) images due to inconsistent respirations
4. Only a few slices can be scanned during the maximum contrast enhancement phase

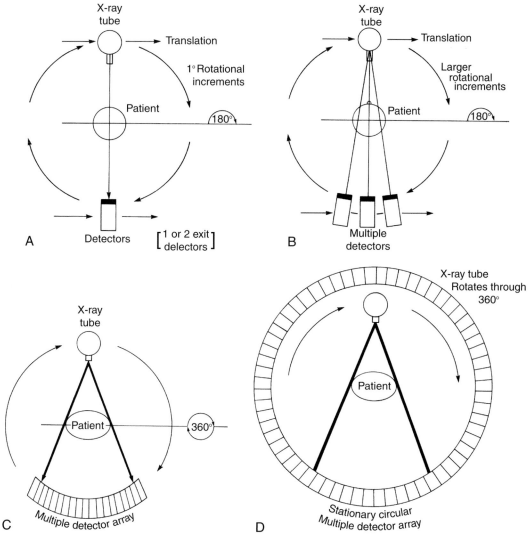

FIGURE 9-1. **A,** Rectilinear pencil beam scanning typical of first-generation CT scanners, based on the rotate-translate parallel beam design. **B,** Rectilinear multiple pencil beam scanning used in second-generation CT scanners, based on the rotate-translate design. **C,** Continuously rotating pulsed fan beam scanning with moving multiple detector arrays typical of third-generation CT scanners. **D,** Fourth-generation CT scanning design based on a rotating x-ray source and a 360-degree multiple detector array. *Continued*

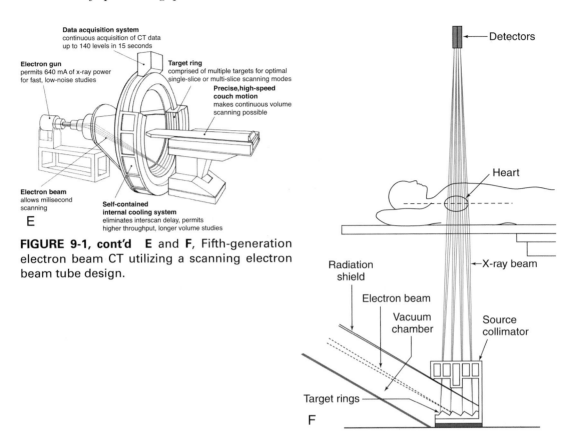

FIGURE 9-1, cont'd E and **F**, Fifth-generation electron beam CT utilizing a scanning electron beam tube design.

A change in the fourth-generation beam geometry led to a scanning technique known as **volume data acquisition scanning**, commonly referred to as spiral, or helical, CT scanning, depending upon the manufacturer of the equipment. In these systems, a continuous x-ray beam is used to produce the scan while the patient is continuously moved (transported) through the gantry. The continuous movement of the tube around a moving patient yields a spiral geometric path that allows for the collection of a large volume of data in a short period (Fig. 9-2). In fact, the scan times have been

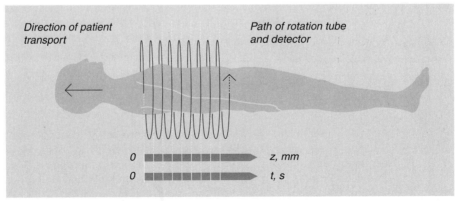

FIGURE 9-2. Illustration of spiral (helical) CT scanning. The patient is advanced steadily through the gantry as the x-ray tube and detectors rotate, creating spiral configuration. This is an example of volume data acquisition.

reduced to less than a second in this type of system. This type of scanning is made possible through the use of the slip ring geometric design in which there is a set of stationary conductive rings that allow the components of the CT system to continuously rotate by means of conductive brushes that serve as sliding contact points for the transmission of electrical current. Figure 9-3 illustrates the components of the spiral CT scanner within the gantry. This design eliminates the need for the electrical cables that restricted the movement of the x-ray tube in the previous generation of CT scanners.

Computed tomography has undergone a major change in the technology used to accomplish image acquisition. Initial helical scanners had the capability to acquire 4 slices per rotation. Manufacturers have been able to increase the number of slices acquired per rotation from this level through 8, 16, 32, and 64 slices per acquisition. This has also been accompanied by an increase in the resolution produced by the systems. This growth has been mainly attributed to improved detector materials and design.

The system is designed so that the x-ray tube is located opposite the detector system in a circular configuration. The detector is composed of several parts: a scintillator, photodiode, electric channels, and an analog to digital converter.

In earlier computed tomographic units xenon gas detectors were used. They operated by means of ionization of the xenon gas in response to the x-radiation. The ions collected on parallel plates connected to amplifiers to produce the signal. Today scintillators are primarily used to convert the x-rays to light. A photodiode is incorporated into the system to convert the light produced by the scintillator into an electrical signal that is collected and used to produce the image. Figure 9-4 illustrates the process by which the remnant radiation exiting the patient is converted into a digital signal that is used to produce the image. The detectors used vary with the manufacturer. Siemens has developed what they refer to as an ultrafast ceramic (UFC). This material has a very short afterglow, which improves the resolution of the finished image (Fig. 9-5). Note the chessboard pattern of the plate. The illustration shows 16 rows or lines. Older systems had only one detector line producing only one slice per

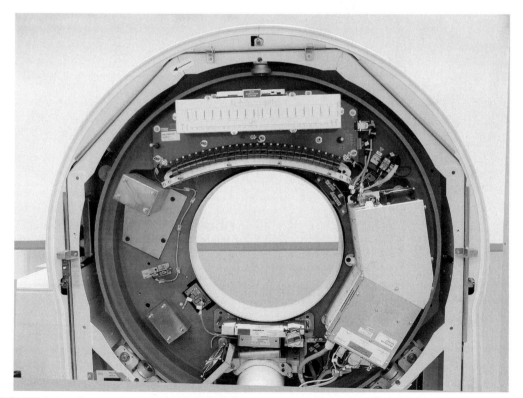

FIGURE 9-3.   Composite photograph showing the components of the system within the gantry.

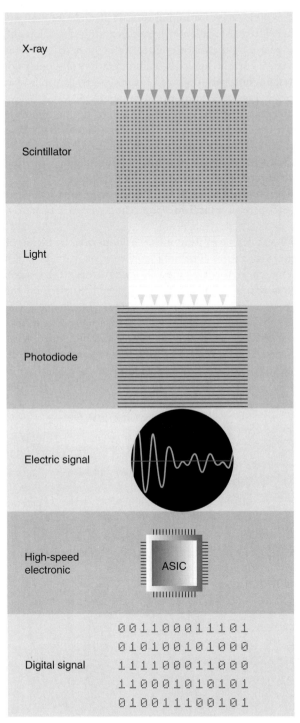

X-ray

Scintillator

Light

Photodiode

Electric signal

High-speed electronic

ASIC

Digital signal

00110001110 1
01010010100 0
11110001100 0
11000101010 1
01001110010 1

FIGURE 9-4. Steps involved in the transformation of the remnant radiation into a digital image.

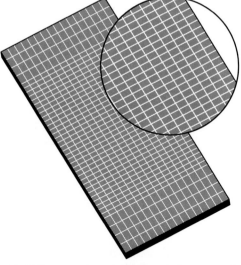

FIGURE 9-5. An example of the ceramic detector produced by Siemens for use in the Somatom Sensation 64 computed tomographic scanner. Note the magnified portion, which shows the checkerboard pattern of the detector.

acquisition. The multislice systems discussed here utilize detectors with multiple lines allowing a wider section of the patient to be imaged in the same acquisition period. Among the advantages of this technology is the reduction in examination time. Higher end systems are capable of imaging the entire body in less than 10 seconds. The advantage to this is that the patients are required to hold their breath for shorter periods. There is also a corresponding decrease in motion artifacts.

The multislice units, especially the 64 slice systems, allow for thinner tomographic sections. As we know from basic tomographic principles, the thinner slices will allow the physician to study extremely small anatomic details and increase the accuracy of the diagnoses.

Image Reconstruction

The scanning process produces the image by the attenuation of the x-ray beam; the patient absorbs the radiation in varying amounts depending upon its interactions with the various tissue types. The exit radiation is collected by the detector array and transmitted to the computer for processing. This process is termed **image reconstruction**.

The information (measurements) acquired from the scan is recorded in digital form by the computer. From this information, the computer reconstructs the image. The computer software that runs the image reconstruction procedure processes the data. The computer programs are generally referred to as **algorithms,** or more specifically, **reconstruction algorithms**. The processing procedure can affect both the quality and the appearance of the image—selection of the matrix size can affect the resolution. In general, the larger the matrix, the greater will be the resolution (and quality) of the image.

The algorithm is a part of the computer program and cannot be altered. Many different algorithms are used for processing the data; however, the algorithms are specific for the type of equipment and software options used.

CT is the production of reconstructed images from information acquired from the remnant radiation through one of the image reconstruction algorithms. These transmitted x-ray photons represent some amount of attenuation within the patient. They are compared with the intensity of the radiation from the x-ray tube, which is measured by a special "reference" detector, to give relative transmission values after digitization. The attenuation values of various tissues are related to the attenuation value of water and may be arranged as a scale (Fig. 9–6). These scale values are called EMI, or Hounsfield, numbers and represent the various CT digital numbers used to reconstruct the image. When

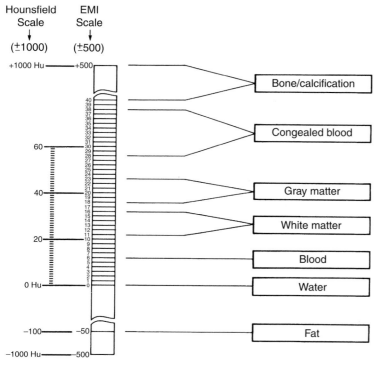

FIGURE 9-6. Absorption values common to clinical radiology. The values shown are for the EMI (±500) and Hounsfield (±1000) scales.

the image is produced, the scale (CT digital) numbers represent a certain brightness level. Figure 9–7 illustrates how the scale numbers and brightness level are related. The brightness level (gray scale) can be manipulated to demonstrate different structures in the image. This manipulation, or variation in the relation between the scale numbers and level of brightness, is often called **windowing, or setting a window**.

The window is controlled by the operator of the CT unit and usually set as a window width and window level. The window width represents the range of scale numbers used for the gray scale. Adjusting the window width is equal to adjusting the contrast of the image. The window level represents the midpoint of the gray scale and can be considered a density adjustment. When viewing an image, these values can be adjusted, usually by the radiographer, to enhance certain anatomic structures. The effect of varying window width and window level is illustrated in Figure 9–8.

Image Display and Storage

CT images are digitally captured and manipulated. The reconstructed image can be displayed on a cathode ray tube (CRT) monitor for viewing. The image can also be recorded and stored for future viewing. One common method for viewing and storage of the study is by producing hard copy images on medical x-ray film using laser cameras. The images can also be stored on discs, or optical storage media. The images can usually be manipulated through the use of various software packages.

Most institutions have added a digital centralized storage system that provides easy access to images which can be transmitted to any workstation on its network. The system is referred to as **PACS (picture archiving communications system)**. One advantage of the PAC system is that the physician has access to not only the patient's film but also the patient information data. PACS eliminates the need for processing facilities and allows the images to be transmitted and manipulated at

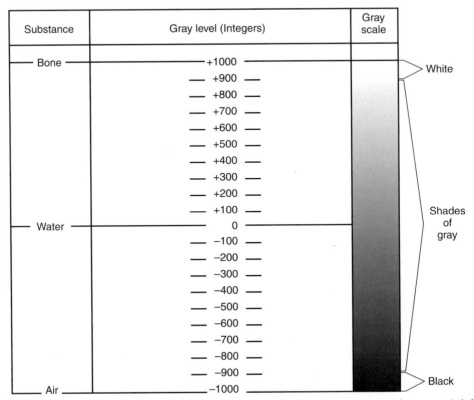

FIGURE 9-7. The relation between CT numbers and the brightness level (gray scale) for the ±1000 scale.

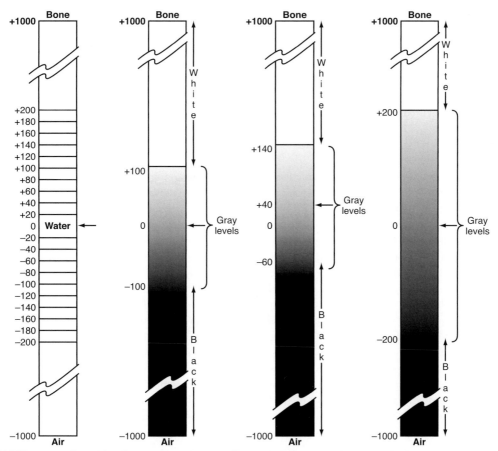

FIGURE 9-8. Graphic illustration of the effect of different window width and window level settings on the CT image.

any one of the network workstations without affecting the stored image. The system greatly improves communications and productivity. A full discussion of PACS is beyond the scope of this text; however, some resources have been included in the Suggested Readings at the end of the chapter.

Room Design

As in special procedure radiography, CT requires specialized construction specifications. The nature of the equipment requires that there be three separate and distinct areas—the scanning area, the control area, and the computer hardware area. The ultimate size and configuration of the CT suite are determined by the manufacturer's representative, the radiographer, the radiography administrator, and the architect. In general, a suite size of 600 ft² (55.74 m²) is necessary to house the CT components. About half of this space, or 300 ft² (27.87 m²), must be devoted to the scanning area, in which the imaging equipment is housed. There should be sufficient room around the scanning unit for stretchers or beds to be easily maneuvered. The doorway to the scanning area should be a minimum of 4 ft (1.2 m) wide to provide unobstructed access to the area.

The control area should have approximately 150 ft² (13.935 m²) of floor space. The control console, x-ray control unit, viewing equipment, and hard copy imaging recording devices are located in this room. Each manufacturer has different system configurations that may alter the room design. Some system designs provide for remote viewing stations in addition to the operating-viewing console station located in the main CT control area. The control area should allow a direct view of the scanning area so the radiographer can monitor the patient throughout the course of the procedure.

The entire CT suite should follow the same basic design and construction requirements as those for a special procedures suite in regard to radiation protection standards, concealed wiring, emergency equipment, and air conditioning. All equipment should be explosion-proof and should meet the requirements specified by the National Fire Code.[1]

Equipment

CT systems can be broken down into three main groups—the imaging group, the computer group, and the control group. A fourth group takes into consideration image reproduction and storage.

The **imaging group** contains all of the elements necessary to produce an image, including the x-ray generator, x-ray tube, and detector system. The generator, x-ray tube(s) and detector(s) are located in housing called a **gantry** (Fig. 9-9), which also contains the mechanics that provide the motion used in the CT unit. The gantry housing conceals the motion of the x-ray tube and detectors. The equipment will vary depending on the generation of CT equipment. (See Suggested Readings at the end of the chapter for references on the mechanics of the gantry.) Each CT gantry comes with a patient table or couch that is styled according to the individual manufacturer's specifications. The purpose of the table or couch is to support and move the patient through the central opening in the gantry. Movement of the patient couch can be controlled either by the computer or manually in a horizontal plane. The gantry can be angled with respect to the body axis before the scanning procedure. With the images collected from a series of axial scans, it is possible for the computer to combine segments of the images to create a new image in other planes.

The x-ray tubes used in CT units can be of either the stationary or rotating anode variety. These tubes should be relatively heavy duty to tolerate the production of many images in a short period of

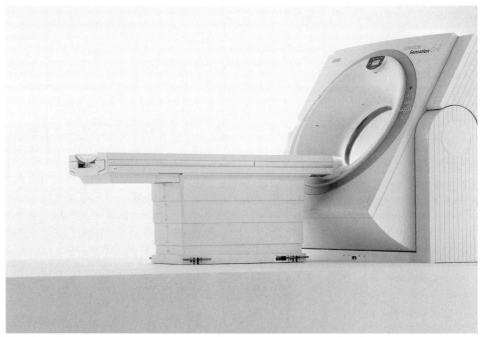

FIGURE 9-9. Photograph of the Siemens Somotom Sensation 64 CT unit showing the gantry and patient couch.

time. The focal spot size is usually determined by the type of tube used in the manufacture of the system; fixed anode x-ray tubes have larger focal spot sizes. The third- and fourth-generation scanners use the rotating anode x-ray tube, which can provide more intensity and power output for short exposure times than stationary anode tubes. These tubes have small focal spots and extremely high heat loading capacities. Siemens has developed a new x-ray tube design, the straton, that allows for a rapid (<0.4 s) gantry rotation time. This is accomplished through a direct anode cooling providing cooling rates of 5.0 million heat units per minute. This virtually eliminates cooling delays, eliminating the need for heat storage capacity. In fact, a whole body trauma examination using full tube current can be accomplished in under 20 s, demonstrating the design's ability to produce high-resolution scans in extremely short periods (Fig. 9-10).

Another component housed in the gantry is the detector system. There are two types of detectors in use today—the gas ionization and the scintillation detector. Each has advantages and disadvantages.

Scintillation detectors work by converting the x-ray photon energy into light. The light is then converted into electrical energy, which produces the output signal. These detectors originally consisted of a crystal of material connected to a photomultiplier tube. Early scintillation detectors used crystals of sodium iodide (NaI), calcium fluoride (CaF_2), and bismuth germanate ($Bi_4Ge_3O_{12}$). Modern scintillation detectors are actually photodiodes coupled with a scintillation crystal. The materials that are used today are cadmium tungstate ($CdWO_4$), yttrium gadolinium oxide, and other rare earth oxide ceramic crystals. This type of detector produces an output signal that is dependent upon the energy of the exit radiation that strikes the detector crystal (Fig. 9-11).

Gas ionization detectors rely on the ionization of pressurized xenon gas. The exit radiation strikes the detector cell and ionizes the xenon. The positively charged ions move toward the negatively charged side of the detector, and the negative ions move to the positive side of the detector; this creates a weak electrical signal that is directed through an amplification system. The output signal of the detector is proportional to the number of x-ray photons involved in the ionization. One problem with the gas ionization detector is its low absorption efficiency; many of the x-ray photons can pass through the detector cell without being ionized. The choice of detector depends on the manufacturer and equipment design specifications. The information produced by the detector system is transferred to the computer group for processing.

Filtration and collimation are two conventional radiographic principles that are also applied to CT. **Filtration** is used primarily to harden the x-ray beam, which, as in conventional filtration, is accomplished by absorption of the "softer," or less penetrating, photons. Filtration also provides a

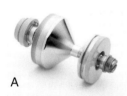 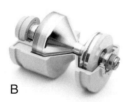 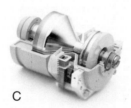 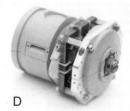

A   B   C   D

FIGURE 9-10. Siemens Straton CT x-ray tube. **A,** Tube insert. **B** and **C,** Insert shown in housing. **D,** X-ray tube insert shown completely enclosed in housing.

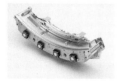

FIGURE 9-11. Image of the complete detector system of the Siemens Somatom Sensation 64 CT system.

uniform hardening effect across the entire x-ray beam (Fig. 9–12). In earlier head scanning units, water baths or bags were used to do this. Manufacturers supply different filtration systems with their units. Some units include selectable filtration modes, which have several different types of filters.

Collimation in CT is used to limit the patient dose and improve image quality. The collimation is accomplished at the x-ray source as well as at the detector. This type of system effectively limits the x-ray beam and reduces the scattered radiation that could reach the detector. Collimation in CT also determines the thickness of the scan section. Each generation of CT scanners has its own collimation design. (Many other factors are related to collimation, but they are beyond the scope of this discussion.)

The computer group is usually located in a room separate from the room that houses the gantry or scanner. The heart of the computer group is the central processing unit, which collects, reconstructs, and prepares the data for display. The central processing unit usually directs the movement of the patient table during the examination. It is equipped with short-term storage capabilities, which allow it to reconstruct and display an image in a relatively short period. This storage system is in the form of a digital disc.

The digital discs are used primarily for the storage of raw data and two- and four–dimensional volume data. The archival storage of images is accomplished with digital linear tape systems and optical disc storage systems. These are capable of large volume storage of compressed images. The digital linear tape archival system is capable of capacities of 3500 studies comprising static images or 700 studies of dynamic imaging clips. Another method of long-term storage is the use of digital videodiscs (DVD). The capacity of this type of archival storage is approximately 300,000 studies consisting of static images and 60,000 dynamic clip studies. Archiving is also accomplished through a multiple media system that moves the data from one type of mass storage device to another depending on the importance of the data.

The computer group can also contain peripheral system components, including the interface connection between the imaging group and the computer group, a line printer, and the disc storage system.

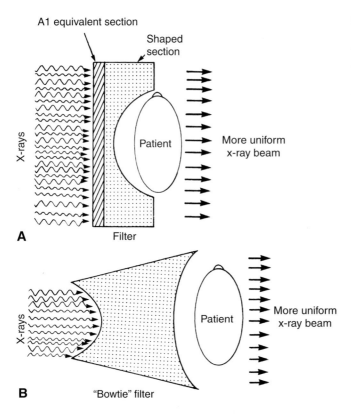

FIGURE 9-12. A and **B**, Filters may be placed between the x-ray tube and object to reduce the dynamic range of the electronics (analog-to-digital converters) by shaping the beam to produce uniform beam hardening.

The control group contains the display control console and keyboard. The display control console is similar to other x-ray machine consoles in that it has an on-off switch and a means of selecting the technical factors and section level. The CT control console resembles that of a computer system. The input devices include a keyboard for inserting data and a touch screen monitor that is used to select the different parameters for the scan. The keyboard is used to introduce information into the system. It resembles a standard computer system keyboard with the full complement of letters and numbers. There are also a number of keys dedicated to various functions specific to the type of CT system purchased. The touch screen monitor shows the various parameters that have been set on the system. These can be changed by touching the appropriate area on the screen. Each screen displayed highlights the next step in the procedure.

The scanning gantry is also energized and can be controlled from the console. In most CT room designs, the control group is stationed separate from the computer and imaging groups. The console workstation is usually located so that the scanning gantry and patient can easily be seen during the procedure.

Hard copy image reproduction is usually accomplished by means of a laser imaging unit. This is usually a self-contained unit, in which the CT image is transmitted to the laser, which in turn scans the unexposed film in a line by line fashion, exposing the film and thereby creating a latent image. The exposed film can then be either sent to a receiving magazine for remote processing or directed to a processing unit that is usually connected directly to the laser imaging system.

ELECTRON BEAM TOMOGRAPHY

In the third-generation mechanical CT systems using the slip ring architecture, the rotation speed is limited by the physical design of the equipment. As previously stated, the maximum speed that these units are capable of achieving is in the vicinity of less than 0.4 s. The slip ring design reduced the time required for the study, allowing for enhanced contrast opacification and improved slice registration for 3D imaging applications. Most areas of the body can be satisfactorily imaged using these mechanical slip ring systems, with the exception of those areas having a considerable amount of involuntary motion such as the chest.

Dynamic CT has been made possible by means of fifth-generation electron beam CT (EBCT). This system, manufactured and distributed by GE Imatron, Inc., reduces the scanning times to 50 to 100 ms, allowing the display of physiologic motion in real time. The original application for EBCT was in cardiac imaging, but this modality can be used for motion studies in other areas as well as all conventional CT applications.

Physical Principles

The component parts of the GE Imatron C-300 electron beam tomography (EBT) system are somewhat similar to those of a standard CT system. The major similarity is in the computer and operator control groups. Their function and appearance are comparable to those of conventional CT systems and do not require a detailed discussion. The gantry and patient couch also resemble those found in fourth-generation CT systems. The major difference is in the design of the imaging system. Conventional systems incorporate an x-ray tube as a functional part of the gantry as the radiation source. In a manner of speaking, the GE Imatron C-300 EBT unit actually functions as the x-ray tube.

Central to the design of the GE Imatron C-300 EBT system is the electron gun, which produces the electron beam. An electron particle beam is generated, then focused and deflected by a series of electromagnets. The electron beam is accelerated along the length of the scanner toward the four fixed tungsten target rings. These rings are located in the lower portion of the gantry and envelop a 210-degree arc. Radiation is produced as the electron beam is focused along the target area at a speed of 66 m/s. The focal spot, less than 4×2 mm, sweeps around each target ring to produce the image. The target rings can be scanned serially to provide rapid multislice volume studies. The electron beam can move along the target rings in rapid succession imaging up to 8 cm without moving the patient through the gantry. The imaging can be triggered by an electrocardiographic triggering device and can provide cine and flow study capabilities.

The unique design of the electron gun allows the heat generated by the production of x-rays to be dissipated quickly into the target structure. Because of the mass of the cone that supports the target rings, x-ray production can be increased to provide the high-output, short-term exposures necessary for ultrafast computed tomography (UFCT). When the electron beam strikes the target ring, an x-ray fan beam is produced. This is collimated to a 2-cm-thick fan-shaped beam, which is then used to produce the imaging information through attenuation. The remnant radiation strikes the detectors, which are arranged in two 216-degree arcs around the upper portion of the gantry. These are arranged as two contiguous rings to provide a pair of 8-mm-thick tomographic slices for each single scan.

The detector arrays are two stationary rings of crystals that convert the remnant radiation to a light signal. Each detector ring contains 1728 calcium tungstate crystal detectors. These crystals convert the x-rays to light and are linked to photodiodes, which convert the light signal into an electrical current that is proportional to the incident quantity of radiation. The electrical current is fed through an amplification system and directed to the computer group, which digitizes the signal in much the same way as in conventional CT systems.

The GE Imatron C-300 system is designed to operate in two different modes—single slice and multislice scanning. Continuous volume scanning (CVS) and step volume scanning (SVS) can be accomplished using the *single slice* mode. Continuous volume scanning is accomplished by moving the patient continuously through the scanner. The step volume scan technique involves moving the patient incrementally through the scanner during the acquisition.

Continuous volume scanning is similar to fourth-generation spiral/helical scanning; that is to say, the data are acquired continuously during rapid translation (movement) of the patient couch through the gantry. Continuous volume scanning (CVS) produces images without motion blurring. Some of the advantages of this mode are the reduction in the amount of contrast agent required, thereby decreasing patient risk and cost; the production of images with excellent slice registration, enabling the reformatting algorithm to produce high-quality 3D images; the acquisition of motion-free images within one breath hold; and enhanced detection of pathology and subtle focal lesions. Current fourth-generation spiral/helical scanners can scan continuously for 30 s, yielding from 30 to 60 contiguous slices. Reduced exposure values are required in order to scan continuously without damaging the x-ray source, and the longer exposure time tends to increase system noise and motion artifacts. In comparison, the GE Imatron C-300 electron beam scanner can accomplish each scan in 0.1-s intervals, which are averaged into either a 0.3-s or a 0.4-s slice. The unit can acquire data at the rate of nine scans per second to a maximum of 160 scans in 18.4 s. The short exposure time reduces motion artifacts, and breath holding is not usually required.

Scans can also be triggered by a time signal, typically derived from electrocardiographic input. The system will provide a diagnostic flow study with much better temporal resolution than that achieved by conventional or gated CT. This type of scan can demonstrate selected phases of the heart cycle by producing a dynamic sequence of images at a particular cardiac phase.

The **multislice mode** can be accomplished as either **cine** or **flow** scanning modes. In the cine scanning mode, the electron beam is directed across each of the target rings several times. The data thus acquired demonstrate motion in the body, including ventricular function, joint motion, and airway physiology. As its name implies, flow mode shows the flow of a fluid such as blood in an organ or region of the body. The data are acquired by directing the electron beam over each target ring in succession and repeating the procedure several times. The series of images produced show the movement of the fluid over a period of time, displaying physiologic motion in real time.

Used either individually or in combination, these modes have a wide range of applications. Table 9-1 lists some of the basic applications of electron beam tomography available with the GE Imatron C-300 Electron Beam CT (EBCT) scanner. The efficacy of electron beam CT using the GE Imatron C-300 scanner in demonstrating coronary heart disease in asymptomatic patients via noninvasive coronary

TABLE 9-1	*Summary of Clinical Applications of the GE Imatron C-300 Electron Beam Tomography Scanner*			
Mode	**Single Slice**	**Multislice**	**Scan Feature**	**Applications**
Continuous		X	Function study 17 scans per s 2 levels	Ventricular function Valve motion Systolic and diastolic volumes Ejection fraction Wall motion
	X		Function study 9 scans per s 1 level	Cardiac wall thickening Orthopedic joint motion Airway measurements
Triggered		X	Flow study ECG or timed trigger	Myocardial perfusion Cerebral perfusion Valvular regurgitation Blood flow
	X		Flow study ECG or timed trigger wih couch motion	CT angiography of coronary with couch motion arteries Coronary calcium Aortic dissection Bypass graft patency
Volume		X	Small volume 8-mm slices covering 8 cm	Localization Myocardial mass Pericardial disease
	X		Large volume 32.5 s of continuous scanning with table motion 1.5-, 3-, or 6-mm slices High acquisition speeds	Standard CT examination of the head, chest, abdomen Pulmonary nodules Pulmonary emboli Trauma studies Pediatric studies
	X		Large volume 1.5-, 3-, 6-, or 10-mm slices with table incrementation	Standard CT examinations
PreView	X		Concurrent Anteroposterior and lateral views	Localization Examination planning

Courtesy of Imatron, Inc.

artery scanning has been well documented.[2] Coronary artery scanning with this system can accurately document the progression of coronary atherosclerosis and measure lesion density and arterial plaque volume. The system is also capable of scanning for pulmonary emboli and is also useful in CT angiography.

Room Design

The basic room design considerations are similar to those required for conventional CT. An ideal setup includes a minimum of four rooms and should be large enough to house the scanner, control equipment, and computer hardware. The scanning area is divided into an examination and an equipment section. The examination area houses the gantry and patient couch, whereas the remainder of the scanner, high-voltage, couch control, and deflection systems are located in the equipment area.

The room size and specifications are determined by the type of hardware to be housed. The computer equipment can be housed in a separate room and can be adjacent to the radiologist's reading room. The total area encompassed by the suite should be a minimum of 789 ft^2 with an overall ceiling height of 9 ft.

Equipment

The EBCT system contains the same basic components as conventional CT. The imaging components' unique design has already been discussed. The gantry is similar in design to that of a conventional CT unit. The patient couch can support a weight of 136 kg (300 lb) and is designed to provide a wide range of positioning flexibility. The couch can be moved in longitudinal (forward and backward), vertical (up and down), and horizontal swivel (side to side) planes, up to 25 degrees in each direction. The couch can also be tilted at angles of up to 25 degrees from the horizontal. A bicycle ergometer can be attached to the couch to stress the patient during a study to reveal abnormalities. The patient couch can be controlled from the table side as well as from the operator's console in the control room.

The computer component digitizes and stores the data from the detectors at the rate of up to 14.4 mb/s. It has a short-term memory capability that retains as many as 80 slices in the multislice mode of operation or up to 2 s of continuous scan data before transfer to a long-term storage system. The image storage system contains a laser camera that can provide images on 14- × 17-in film in a wide range of formats. A magneto-optical disc storage system is also integrated into the computer component for long-term data storage.

The scanner console is designed to permit display of the images produced by the EBCT scanner. It has an alphanumeric keyboard for functional and operational control of the scanner and computer system. The system consists of the high-resolution display monitor, an alphanumeric monitor, a trackball, window and level control knobs, and function keys for data processing.

EBCT can be used to image all areas of the body, and it is especially useful for imaging areas in which involuntary motion is present. The primary region of interest involves cardiac scanning, where it has capabilities for demonstrating flow studies as well as volume measurements. It is also being used to diagnose early coronary heart disease in nonsymptomatic individuals utilizing the measurement of coronary calcium deposits. The procedure is noninvasive and correlates well with results obtained through coronary angiography. Other areas include the measurement of myocardial perfusion and cardiac output, gauging the amount of restenosis after PTCA and coronary bypass, and determining the location of pulmonary emboli. One advantage of the EBCT system is that contrast agent studies can be performed using a bolus injection or drip infusion of the radiopaque material. The following is a summary of the image display and range of image analysis of EBCT:

1. Real-time movie display
   a. Fixed level
   b. Fixed time
2. Measurement of blood flow and tissue perfusion with time-density graphs
   a. Heart
   b. Other organs
3. Quantitative measurement
   a. Motion of heart
   b. Thickening of heart wall

Continued

Continued

4. Quantitative volume measurements of any region of interest
5. Image enhancement
    a. Subtraction
    b. Averaging
6. Functional imaging
    a. Static
    b. Dynamic
7. Image reformation
    a. Movies
    b. Flow studies
    c. Oblique views
    d. Sagittal views
    e. Coronal views
    f. Parasagittal views
8. Region of interest
    a. Ellipse
    b. Rectangle
    c. Irregular
    d. Mean CT number
    e. Standard deviation
    f. Area
    g. Base value
9. Zoom function
10. Pan function
11. Identify
12. Save screen
13. Print screen

Technical Considerations

CT can be performed on any portion of the anatomy, and it is rapidly becoming the procedure of choice for the diagnosis of many disorders. There are many reasons for its popularity; the major advantages of performing CT examinations may be summarized as follows:

1. Precise demonstration of abnormalities, with minimal error
2. Ease of performance
3. Elimination of patient discomfort
4. Noninvasive procedure
5. Reduction in hospitalization cost
6. May be performed on an outpatient basis

Patient Preparation

Patient preparation for CT varies with the type of study. If the CT study involves the administration of a contrast agent, the guidelines are similar to those of most contrast examinations.

For most head studies, the patient is instructed to consume no food and water for 2 to 4 hours before the examination. CT of the body, including the abdomen and gastrointestinal system, requires food and water to be withheld from the patient from midnight before the examination. No special preparation is required for CT studies of the chest or extremities.

The procedure should be explained to the patient before the study begins. If iodinated contrast agents are to be used, a baseline of vital signs should be taken, and the patient should be questioned for a history of allergies and previous contrast reactions. The patient's blood work should be reviewed to determine the blood urea nitrogen (BUN) and creatinine levels prior to the injection. If the patient is extremely agitated or nervous, a sedative may be prescribed; this should be administered by the special procedure nurse or the physician responsible for the procedure. If contrast agents are to be used or the procedure involves an interventional technique, the patient is usually required to complete an informed consent form.

Postprocedural care depends on the type of study and medication, if any, received by the patient. If a sedative is administered, the patient should have someone drive him or her home. Iodinated contrast agent studies require that the patient increase fluid intake for 24 to 36 hours after the procedure. The patient should be monitored for 20 to 30 minutes after the procedure, especially if contrast agents are administered. If studies do not require the administration of a contrast agent, the patient will not need special care before discharge.

Three- and Four-Dimensional Imaging

The advent of the 64-slice scanner and advanced computer software and hardware has made true three- and four-dimensional imaging practical and with a comparative reduction in patient dose. Several companies have developed systems capable of producing this type of image. The Siemens Syngo In Space4D produces high-resolution image reconstruction that produces a true four-dimensional diagnostic study. This system can produce images that demonstrate the beating heart in real time allowing for the evaluation of functional defects.

SUMMARY

CT uses the basic fundamentals of radiography to produce the diagnostic image. During performance of these procedures, it is necessary to adhere to radiation safety practices identical to those for any radiographic examination to provide maximum protection for the patient and staff. Knowledge and proficiency come from observation and practical experience; the protocol for performing CT differs by institution. In addition, the radiographer must have a working knowledge of cross-sectional anatomy to position the patient properly and critique the images for diagnostic quality.

CT equipment and computer software now provide the physician with information in a timely fashion. Three- and four-dimensional imaging in real time allows the evaluation of not only anatomic pathology but also functional defects.

REFERENCES

1. National Fire Codes: NFPA 99, Standard for Health Care Facilities, Quincy, MA, 2002, National Fire Prevention Association,.
2. Arad Y, Spardo LA, Goodman K, Newstein D, Guerci AD: Prediction of coronary events with electron beam computed tomography. *J Am Coll Cardiol* 36:1253–1260, 2000.

SUGGESTED READINGS

Arad Y, Spardo LA, Goodman K, Newstein D, Guerci AD: Prediction of coronary events with electron beam computed tomography. *J Am Coll Cardiol* 36:1253–1260, 2000.

Baumgartner F, Brundage B, Bleiweis M, et al: Feasibility of ultrafast computed tomography in the early evaluation of coronary bypass patency. *J Cardiac Imaging* 10:170, 1996.

Budoff MJ: Prognostic value of coronary artery calcification. *J Clin Outcomes Manage* 8(11):42–48, 2001.

Budoff MJ: Atherosclerosis imaging and calcified plaque: coronary artery disease risk assessment. *Progr Cardiovasc Dis* 46(2):135–145, 2003.

Budoff MJ, Achenbach S, Duerinckx D: Clinical utility of computed tomography and magnetic resonance techniques for noninvasive coronary angiography. *J Am Coll Cardiol* 42:1867–1878, 2003.

Foley WD, Karcaaltincaba M: Computed tomography angiography: principles and clinical applications. *J Comput Assist Tomogr* 27(Suppl 1):S23–30, 2003.

Frohwein S, Chronos N: The use of electron beam computed tomography in the primary care setting. *J Med Assoc Ga* 90(4):23–26, 2001.

Gerber TC, Kuzo R, Karstaedt N, Lane G, Morin R, Sheedy P II, Saffard R, Blackshear J, Pietan J: Current result and new developments of coronary angiography with use of contrast enhanced computed tomography of the heart. *Mayo Clinic Proc* 77:55–57, 2002.

Huang HK: Some historical remarks on picture archiving and communication systems. *Comput Med Imaging Graph* 27(2–3):93–99, 2003.

Kalra MK, Maher MM, Toth TL, et al: Techniques and applications of automatic tube current modulation for CT. *Radiology* 233(3):649–657, 2004.

Lefkovitz Z, Shapiro R, Koch S, et al: The emerging role of virtual colonoscopy. *Med Clin North Am* 89(1):111–138, viii, 2005.

Mitchell TL, Pippin JJ, Devers SM, Kimball TE, Gibbons LW, Cooper LL, Gonzalez-Dunn V, Cooper KH: Incidental detection of preclinical renal tumors with electron beam computed tomography: report of 26 consecutive operated patients. *J Comput Assist Tomogr* 24(6):843–845, 2000.

Nallamothu BK, Saint S, Bielak LF, Sonnad SS, Peyser PA, Rubenfire M, Fendrick AM: Electron-beam computed tomography in the diagnosis of coronary artery disease: a meta-analysis. *Arch Intern Med* 161(6):833–838, 2001.

Nawa T, Nakagawa T, Kusano S, Kawasakiv Y, Sugawara Y, Nakata H: Lung cancer screening using low-dose spiral CT: results of baseline and 1-year follow-up studies. *Chest* 122:15–20, 2002.

Park R, Detrano R, Xiang M, Fu P, Ibrahim Y, LaBree L, Azen S: Combined use of computed tomography coronary calcium scores and C-reactive protein levels in predicting cardiovascular events in nondiabetic individuals. *Circulation* 106:2073–2077, 2002.

Pickhardt PJ, Choi R, Hwang I, Butler JA, Puckett ML, Hildebrandt HA, Wong RK, Nugent PA, Mysliwiec PA, Schindler WA: Computed tomographic virtual colonoscopy to screen for colorectal neoplasia in asymptomatic adults. *N Engl J Med* 349:2191–2200, 2003.

Pilling JR: Lessons learned from a whole hospital PACS installation. Picture Archiving and Communication System. *Clin Radiol* 57(9):784–788, 2002.

Pilling JR: Picture archiving and communication systems: the users' view. *Br J Radiol* 76(908):519–524, 2003.

Raggi P, Cooil B, Callister TQ: Use of electron beam tomography data to develop models for prediction of hard coronary events. *Am Heart J* 141:375–82, 2001.

Ritman EL: Cardiac computed tomography imaging: a history and some future possibilities. *Cardiol Clin* 21(4):491–513, 2003.

Seeram E: *Computed Tomography: Physical Principles, Clinical Applications, and Quality Control*, 2nd ed. Philadelphia, 2001, WB Saunders.

Shaw LJ, Raggi P, Schisterman E, Berman DS, Callister TQ: Prognostic value of cardiac risk factors and coronary artery calcium screening for all-cause mortality. *Radiology* 228:826–833, 2003.

Thali MJ, Braun M, Buck U, et al: VIRTOPSY—scientific documentation, reconstruction and animation in forensic: individual and real 3D data based geometric approach including optical body/object surface and radiological CT/MRI scanning. *J Forensic Sci* 50(2):428–442, 2005.

Weintraub WS: Electron-beam tomography coronary artery calcium and cardiac events, accompanying editorial. *Circulation* 107:2528–2530, 2003.

Weiss DL, Hoffman J, Kustas G: Integrated voice recognition and picture archiving and communication system: development and early experience. *J Digit Imaging* 14(2 Suppl 1):233–235, 2001.

Wisnivesky JP, Mushlin AI, Sicherman N, Henschke C: The cost-effectiveness of low-dose CT screening for lung cancer. Preliminary results of baseline screening. *Chest* 124:614–621, 2003.

STUDY QUESTIONS

1. The use of a continuously rotating pulsing fan beam was incorporated in the design of _____ generation computed tomography systems.
   a. first
   b. second
   c. third
   d. fourth

STUDY QUESTIONS (*cont'd*)

2. The CT system that utilizes a continuous x-ray beam while the patient is being continuously moved through the gantry has been referred to as _____ computed tomography:
   - **i.** spiral
   - **ii.** translation
   - **iii.** helical
   - **a.** i only
   - **b.** i and ii only
   - **c.** i and iii only
   - **d.** i, ii, and iii

3. The term algorithm is defined as:
   - **a.** the detector array of the second-generation CT system
   - **b.** the computer program that processes the data obtained from the scan
   - **c.** the type of CT study that requires the patient to continuously move through the gantry during the exposure
   - **d.** another name for volume data acquisition

4. Water has a value of _____ on the Hounsfield and EMI number scale.
   - **a.** 0
   - **b.** 10
   - **c.** 100
   - **d.** 1000

5. Adjusting the window width is comparable with adjusting the _____ of the image.
   - **a.** size
   - **b.** contrast
   - **c.** density
   - **d.** shape

6. In a CT scanner, which of the following houses the x-ray tube, detectors, and the mechanics that provide the motion?
   - **a.** slip ring
   - **b.** couch
   - **c.** gantry
   - **d.** scintillation system

7. Which of the following is the result of using collimation at the x-ray source and the detector of the CT scanner?
   - **i.** improve image quality
   - **ii.** limit patient dose
   - **iii.** reduce scattered radiation
   - **a.** i only
   - **b.** i and ii only
   - **c.** i and iii only
   - **d.** i, ii, and iii

8. Scintillation detectors convert the remnant x-ray photons into _____.
   - **a.** light
   - **b.** electric signals
   - **c.** digital images
   - **d.** a shaped beam

9. The type of electron beam scanning accomplished in the single slice mode in which the patient is moved incrementally through the scanner is referred to as _____.
   - **a.** continuous volume scanning
   - **b.** rotation/translation scanning
   - **c.** step volume scanning
   - **d.** longitudinal imaging

10. If iodinated contrast agents are required for the scan, the following should be accomplished during the patient preparation.
    - **i.** the patient's vital signs should be taken
    - **ii.** a history of allergies should be taken
    - **iii.** food should be withheld for 24 hours before the examination
    - **a.** i only
    - **b.** i and ii only
    - **c.** i and iii only
    - **d.** i, ii, and iii

10 *Magnetic Resonance Imaging*

CHAPTER OBJECTIVES

After completing this chapter, the reader will be able to perform the following:

- Describe the history of magnetic resonance imaging (MRI)

- Explain the elements of room design in MRI

- Identify the types of magnets used in MRI

- Identify the common equipment groups in MRI systems

- Describe the basic physical principles behind MRI

- Define the term *precession*

- Describe the physical principle of excitation in MRI

- Define the term *relaxation* as it applies to MRI

- Explain the process of imaging gradients in MRI

- Describe the use of MRI in vascular imaging

Magnetic resonance imaging (MRI), formerly called nuclear magnetic resonance (NMR), is not a new concept. The basic principles were proposed in the early 1920s, and investigations continued throughout the 1930s and 1940s, during which the application of the technique was relegated primarily to investigating the principles of physics. Felix Bloch described magnetic resonance in a solid and continued his experiments to place the foundation for future discoveries that led to the use of magnetic resonance in medicine. In 1950, it was shown that chemical shifts could be detected. This discovery led to the use of this technique in chemistry and biochemistry. Investigations were made into the properties of biologic fluids as well as a variety of chemical compounds. The technique was commercialized in 1953 and marketed as NMR spectroscopy. By the middle of the 1960s, there was widespread application of NMR spectroscopy by the chemical and pharmaceutical industries in analyzing the structure of compounds.

In 1973, it was suggested by P. Lauterbur that the technique could be applied to imaging. However, it was not until 1977 that images of human anatomy were produced; this was accomplished almost simultaneously by W. S. Hinshaw, P. A. Bottomley, and G. N. Holland and R. Damadian, M. Goldsmith, and L. Minkoff.

By 1981, clinical trials of MRI as an imaging modality were under way. Various advances in equipment and techniques have made the modality a viable diagnostic tool that not only yields anatomic information but also distinguishes between healthy and diseased tissue. Unlike computed tomography (CT), MRI can provide information about the functional and physiologic conditions as well as the anatomic structure of the body's tissue without the use of x-radiation. This chapter presents an overview of the basic theory behind MRI, the hardware, and the potentials for its use in medical diagnosis.

MAGNETS

There are basically two types of magnets used in the manufacture of MRI equipment—the permanent magnet and the electromagnetic or superconductive magnet. Permanent magnets are constructed from permanent magnetic materials enclosed in a massive steel frame. Electromagnets create a magnetic field by circulating electric currents through wire coils. Each type of magnet has its own specific requirements and limitations.

Permanent Magnets

Permanent magnets do not require the use of an electrical current to create the magnetic field. A familiar example of a permanent magnet is the small magnet commonly used to hold items onto a metallic surface, such as a refrigerator. Once magnetized, they require no special care. When these are used in MRI, they are usually encased in a special steel frame, which guides the lines of magnetic force and contains the magnetic field. This type of system is advantageous because the magnetic field is contained, so there is essentially no "fringe" magnetic field that requires extensive shielding to protect either the static magnetic field uniformity or the mechanical or electrical equipment located in the surrounding environment. The major disadvantage to the use of permanent magnets is their weight. A typical permanent magnet installation with steel frame can weigh more than 100 tons. This would not be a problem in a new installation in which the design could be adjusted to accommodate the weight. In an existing situation, however, construction expenses could be greater than those for a resistive or superconductive type magnet. Permanent magnets also have the disadvantage of having limited field strength.

Electromagnets
Superconductive Magnets

Superconductive magnets use specialized wire coils made from materials that lose their electrical resistivity when they are exposed to very low temperatures. The type II superconductors are usually alloys, such as niobium-titanium. Because this type of system requires operating temperatures of almost absolute zero, an elaborate cooling and insulating system must be provided; this system is called a *cryostat*. It cools the magnet and maintains it at the proper temperature for extended periods. The system uses both liquid nitrogen and liquid helium to provide the cold operating temperatures required. The superconductive system is considerably more complex than either of the other types of magnets discussed. It requires a high capital and operating investment to control and monitor the devices for the use of liquid helium and nitrogen.

One major disadvantage to the use of the superconductive system is the large area of "fringe" magnetic field (Fig. 10-1). This fringe field can cause mechanical and electrical disturbances within a diameter range of 20 to 60 ft. Any ferromagnetic material or object within 20 ft of the units could become magnetized and disturb the homogeneity of the static magnetic field. The system has to be placed in an environment shielded from such materials. The manufacturers of superconductive equipment have architectural specifications designed to eliminate this hazard. Care should be taken when working around this type of magnet system to remove any ferromagnetic object from the patient or staff; these objects could act as projectiles and create a dangerous "missile effect." Another disadvantage to the use of superconductive magnet systems is the possibility of the helium boiling off, causing the magnet to lose its superconductive capability. This problem is called *quenching,* and it can cause the unit to become inoperative for the length of time it takes to cool and readjust the system.

ROOM DESIGN

MRI systems depend on the use of magnetic fields, which necessitate specific requirements for room designs. The major constraints are that the magnetic field created by the static magnetic source can be affected by the wide variety of ferromagnetic materials present in the surrounding areas, and there is the possibility of interference with other mechanical and electrical devices in the facility. The type of magnet used determines the necessary architectural modifications required.

Room size varies according to the type of magnet system used and the manufacturer's specifications. The scanning-control room can be from 325 to 900 ft^2 in area. The rooms should be climate controlled to provide a comfortable atmosphere for the patient and staff. There should be an adequate amount of room for a patient dressing room as well as a waiting room. If superconductive magnets are used, these areas must be away from the fringe magnetic field.

The MRI scanning room must also be shielded from radio frequency (RF) interference. This is accomplished by using nonferrous modular panels that are constructed by laminating aluminum or copper sheets onto a suitable base, such as particle board. These panels are then applied to the interior surfaces of the room and joined together with clamping devices that effectively shield the joint spaces between the panels. Special shielded door designs are also available that provide total RF shielding. RF interference testing should be carried out after the rough shielding is in place and the interior of the room has been surfaced and finished.

The type of magnet used determines the amount and variety of architectural modifications that are necessary.

Safe practices should be established in order to ensure the safety of all patients undergoing a MRI study. A detailed history should be taken to identify if there are any implants or foreign bodies that would be contraindicated in MRI. The radiographer must be knowledgeable about the different types of implants and devices that could be affected by the magnet. The *Reference Manual for Magnetic Resonance Safety: 2003 Edition* is an excellent resource for recommendations on MR safety. This text references safety guidelines, information on implants, devices, and materials that have been tested for safety in the MR suite. The book also contains MR screening guidelines for patients and other personnel.[1]

Many patients exhibit emotional anxiety and distress prior to the study. The radiographer should have a sufficient level of education, training, and skill to effectively interact with these individuals. This is important for the safety of the patient as well as for the quality of the MR study.

Fundamentals of Special Radiographic Procedures

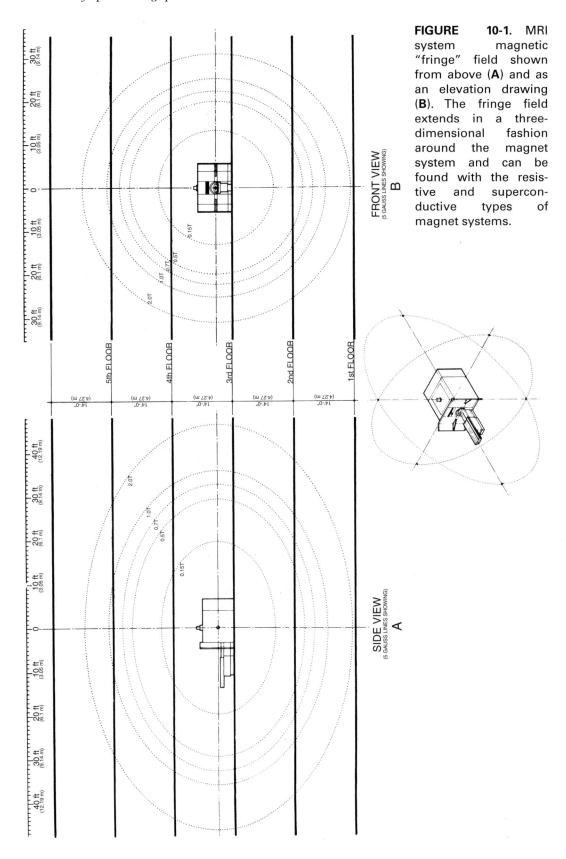

FIGURE 10-1. MRI system magnetic "fringe" field shown from above (**A**) and as an elevation drawing (**B**). The fringe field extends in a three-dimensional fashion around the magnet system and can be found with the resistive and superconductive types of magnet systems.

EQUIPMENT GROUPS

There are several equipment groups common to all types of manufactured MRI systems—the magnet, RF synthesizer, gradient coil system, shimming coil system, and computer and control-display group.

The magnet system group has already been discussed. Use of the different types of magnets necessitates a variety of design specifications for the gantry and patient couch elements. The Fonar open MRI system has many advantages over the tunnel or bore type system (Fig. 10-2). Among these is the reduction in the claustrophobic feeling that certain patients experience when placed in the scanner. The upright MRI system by Fonar also allows for a variety of patient positions during scanning (Fig. 10-3).

The open sky system by Fonar presents the illusion that the patient is in a landscaped scene rather than a medical device. Open systems are being considered for use in the operating theater and are suited for MRI guided surgical and interventional procedures as well as diagnostic scanning. Fonar has developed a small unit that can be used for extremity MRI. The patient can be placed in a variety of positions that will enable the imaging of the extremities. This unit also has the capability to perform weight-bearing studies and is small enough to be utilized in a physician's office. One of the more innovative designs is the upright MRI system. This unit has the capabilities to scan patients in the erect, sitting, or recumbent positions. It also allows for flexion, extension, rotation, and lateral bending. This means that the patient can be scanned in the position that produces their pain or symptoms, providing a more accurate diagnosis. The size of the patient opening will vary by vendor. When using permanent magnets, the magnetic field lines will pass vertically through the patient's body.

To perform MRI, an RF synthesizer or probe must be included in the design. This system provides the RF pulses necessary to change the direction of the net magnetization vector (Mv). The RF synthesizer or probe is essentially a coil of wire that can accommodate a high-frequency alternating current. It is designed to act as both a transmitter and receiver of the RF signal. The coil that produces the RF signal can also be used to detect the echo from the magnetic nuclei. The RF pulse is produced by an RF generator located some distance away from the imaging system.

There are two basic configurations for the RF coils—volume coils, which can be used for the total body or the head, and local or surface coils.

Volume coils, as their name implies, are used to image the head or the entire body. Another type of volume coil is the **quadrature** coil, which can detect the magnetic resonance signal from many different directions. The signal is transmitted and received by a pair of these coils, allowing for "stereo" viewing. Quadrature coils can be found in several different designs and are referred to as either "saddle" or "bird-cage" coils, depending on their basic design. The "bird-cage" quadrature coil is commonly used.

Surface or **local coils** are placed in the vicinity of the anatomic area being imaged, and the signal that is received comes only from the area around the coil itself. Although surface coils can transmit and receive signals from smaller body parts, they are used only to receive the signal because the tip angle is a function of the distance from the coil as well as the length and strength of the RF pulse. Surface coils furnish very high signal-to-noise ratios (SNRs) in the local area; however, they exhibit a high degree of nonuniform sensitivity. These coils can be configured in a variety of ways: simple loops, half saddle coils, solenoidal, intracavity, and phased array coils. Local coils provide a high SNR and high-resolution images. Local coils are now being manufactured that are hybrids of the volume and local coil; they have increased uniformity, but it still does not approach that of the volume coils.

Because of their smaller size, surface coils detect less noise. It can be said that the smaller the coil, the greater the SNR, which in turn can either decrease scan time or increase the resolution. These coils are usually tuned for specific anatomic locations. Figure 10-4 illustrates some commonly used radio frequency coils.

Because the surface coils are positioned close to the patient, there is a possibility of RF burns. Stringent safety measures are necessary when these accessories are used. These coils are manufactured by a variety of companies and designed to work with specific magnet configurations. Operating and safety instructions should be carefully followed.

Fundamentals of Special Radiographic Procedures

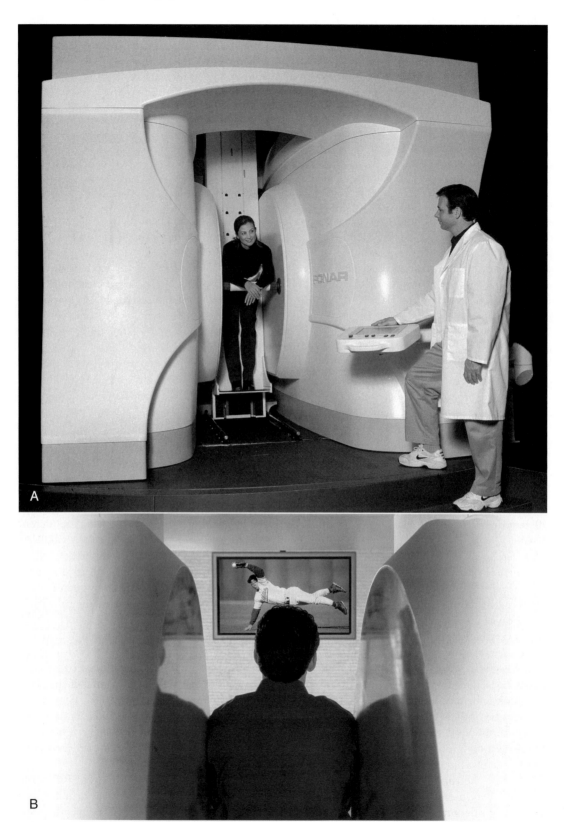

FIGURE 10-2. The Fonar upright open MRI system. **A,** The system from the operator's point of view. **B,** The patient's view from inside the unit.

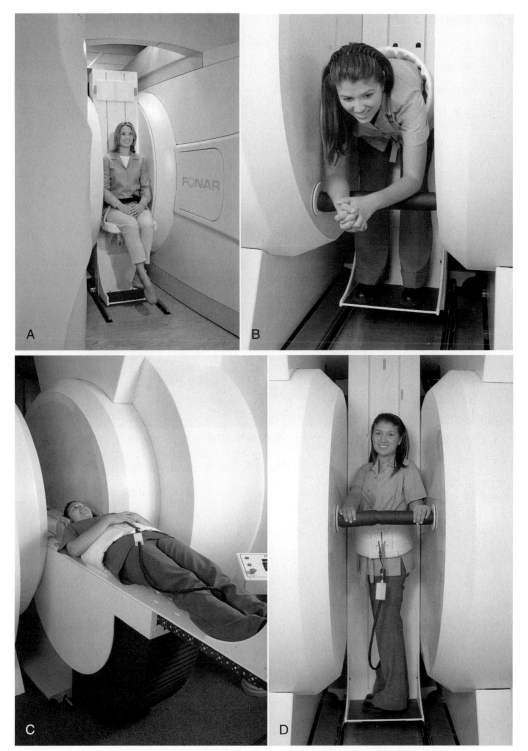

FIGURE 10-3. **A** to **D,** Various positions that a patient can assume while inside the Fonar upright open MRI system.

Fundamentals of Special Radiographic Procedures

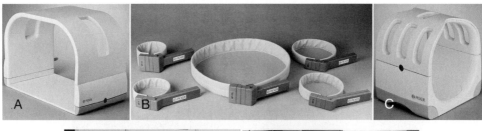

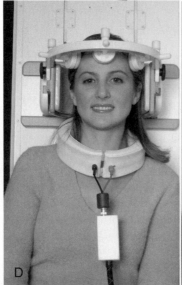

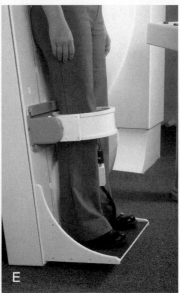

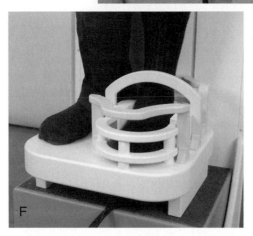

FIGURE 10-4. **A**, Body and spine coil. **B**, Multi-purpose flexible coils. **C**, Head coil. **D**, Head and neck coil. **E**, Knee coil. **F**, Ankle coil.

Gradient coil systems are necessary for the selection of the imaging plane. There are usually three sets of gradient coils, each corresponding to one of the axis lines—x, y, and z. The plane can be selected by applying a preselected field gradient over the patient. In this method, only some of the nuclei are stimulated—those perpendicular to the direction of the applied gradient. (The effects of using the gradient coil system have been discussed.)

The shimming system is necessary to provide homogeneity of the magnetic field. Two types of shimming are used—passive and active. Passive shimming is done at the time of the magnet's installation. The technique involves the placement of ferromagnetic materials around the magnet site. Active shimming is accomplished by manipulating an induced current in coils that surround the magnet. In some units, the active shimming is accomplished automatically through the computer system.

The computer units linked to the MRI system function in much the same way as those used in computer technology. These systems convert the analog information provided from the MRI scan to digital information that can be analyzed and manipulated by the computer. The computer system used is based on the type supplied by the manufacturer of the MRI equipment. The computer system will have short-term memory systems, but long-term storage should also be provided, such as the magnetic tape or floppy disc method.

The control-display system varies depending on the types of software packages that are purchased with the imaging system. Some other peripheral equipment that could be added to the imaging system includes a printer and a multiformat imaging camera for hard copy reproduction of the MRI.

PHYSICAL PRINCIPLES

MRI does not involve the use of radioisotopes or x-radiation to secure diagnostic information. The theory of MRI is based on the magnetic properties of certain atomic nuclei. The nucleus of the atom is composed of two types of particles, also called *nucleons*: *protons* and *neutrons*. The atomic weight of an atom is found by adding the sum of these particles. Currently only certain atoms exhibit activity with magnetic resonance.

It is well known that the atomic nucleus spins on its axis, similarly to the planet earth. The nucleons (protons and neutrons) each possess a **spin**, or **angular momentum**. If the number of protons and neutrons in the nucleus are equal, the resultant positive charge is balanced by the negative charge of the orbital electrons. In these cases, the nucleon spins tend to cancel each other out to produce a net spin of zero. In atoms having an uneven atomic number, the spins are unbalanced and a "net" spin is produced. Because of this uneven pairing, there is also an associated net electrical charge, and a magnetic field, known as the **magnetic moment (μ)**, is generated that acts like a bar magnet. These small nuclear magnets have a north and a south magnetic pole commonly referred to as a **magnetic dipole**. The nucleus of these types of atoms acts as a small magnet and as such can interact with other magnetic fields. These types of atoms are considered to be MRI active.

The following are some elements with MRI-active nuclei:

Element	Atomic Number
Hydrogen	1
Carbon	13
Nitrogen	15
Oxygen	17
Sodium	23
Phosphorus	31
Calcium	43

There is a common thread evident in this list of elements; they all have uneven atomic numbers.

If we were to look at the nucleus of one of these atoms, we would see that the magnetic moments (μ) of these small nuclear magnets are oriented in a number of random directions, resulting in a total, or net, magnetization of zero. When an external magnetic field is applied, the protons align themselves in one of two possible orientations or states: **spin-up** or **parallel** (in line with the direction of the external magnetic field) or **spin-down** or **antiparallel** (parallel but in the opposite direction of the external magnetic field).

Because it takes more energy to line up antiparallel with the external magnetic field, these nuclear magnets are considered to be at a higher energy level than those lined up parallel to the external field (Fig. 10-5). In general, the nuclei prefer to be in the lower energy level state parallel with the external magnetic field, and there are usually more nuclear magnets in this "spin state."

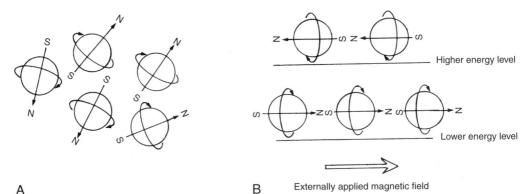

FIGURE 10-5. **A,** A sample of nucleons with net spins, showing the random orientation of the dipoles. **B,** The same sample of nucleons placed in a magnetic field. Some of the nuclei line up in opposition to the direction of the external magnetic field; these represent nucleons with a higher energy level.

It is difficult to measure the magnetic moment (μ), the magnetic field, of each nucleon individually. However, the total magnetic field of a group of nucleons can be represented by a symbol called a vector.

A **vector** represents a quantity which possesses a direction and a value that can be described by a real number. This number is referred to as the **magnitude**. A vector can therefore be defined as a quantity having direction and magnitude. Vectors are usually expressed as arrows. The length of the arrow indicates the magnitude, and the point of the arrow represents the direction.

The direction of the vector represents the relationship of the position of the magnetic moments with the external magnetic field. The length of the vector is a representation of the sum of the magnetic moments. The **net magnetization vector (Mv)** is the sum of the magnitudes and directions of the magnetic spins.

When the nuclear spins are oriented either with or opposed to an external magnetic field, they can be made to undergo a transition from one energy level to another. The transition is actually a change in the orientation of the net Mv. In other words the net Mv can be tipped from its longitudinal (parallel) orientation with the external magnetic field to another plane.

For this to occur, the nuclei must either absorb a definite amount (quantum) of energy to move to a higher energy level or release a quantum of energy to return to a lower energy level. The transition from one energy state to another is called **resonance**. The process of supplying the additional energy to effect the transition is called **excitation**. If a subject is stimulated (excitation), a change in energy states occurs (resonance), causing it to emit an electromagnetic signal. This signal is detected and an image is produced.

When the external magnetic field is applied to the nuclei, their dipoles (north and south poles) do not line up with it exactly (Fig. 10-6). This causes a **torque** (a turning or twisting force), which creates a motion similar to that produced on the axis of a spinning top when it begins to slow down. The spinning top rotates and wobbles about the former vertical axis in a motion similar to that of a cone (Fig. 10-7). This motion is called **precession**.

When the nuclei in a sample are exposed to an external magnetic field, their magnetic moments precess together in the direction of their spin state (spin-up or spin-down). The result can be visualized as two cones placed tip to tip (Fig. 10-8).

The **Larmor frequency** is the frequency that will cause a transition between two spin energy levels of a nucleus. The Larmor frequency is different for the nuclei of different atoms. When a radiofrequency pulse specific to the atom is applied to the nucleus, the protons will change their alignment from the direction of the main magnetic field to the direction opposite the main magnetic field.

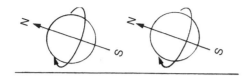

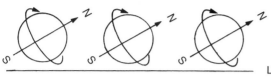

Higher energy level

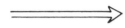

Lower energy level

Externally applied magnetic field

FIGURE 10-6. When an external magnetic field is applied, the magnetic dipoles of the nucleons are not lined up in exactly the same direction.

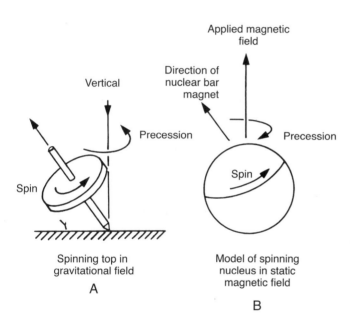

Spinning top in gravitational field

A

Model of spinning nucleus in static magnetic field

B

FIGURE 10-7. **A,** A spinning top is precessing around the vertical field of gravity. **B,** A spinning nucleus with the direction of its magnetization: its precession around the direction of the applied magnetic field is shown.

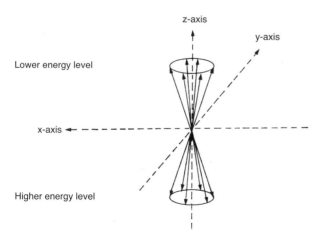

FIGURE 10-8. Configuration of a sample of nuclei precessing in both spin states.

Fundamentals of Special Radiographic Procedures

The rate of frequency of the precession is proportional to the strength of the externally applied magnetic field and is related to the type of atomic nucleus. Hydrogen protons, for example, will have a natural resonance frequency of 42.58 MHz in an externally applied magnetic field of 1000 G (0.1 T) or 42.58 MHz/T. The precessional frequency given earlier for the hydrogen proton is also known as the Larmor frequency.

The resonance frequency is directly proportional to the strength of the main magnetic field. This resonance frequency can be calculated using the Larmor equation:

$$\omega_0 = \gamma\, B_0$$

where the symbol ω_0 (omega zero) represents the resonance frequency or frequency of precession, γ represents the **gyromagnetic ratio** (a constant value dependent upon the characteristic of the nucleus, 42.56 MHz/T for protons), and B_0 represents the strength of the external or induction magnetic field in teslas (T).

It has already been stated that when an external magnetic field is applied to a group of nuclei, there are two potential energy states, **spin-up** (following the direction of the magnetic field) and **spin-down** (opposite to the direction of the magnetic field). The overall effect of these two energy states is usually a weak net Mv in the direction of the externally applied magnetic field. This orientation is associated with the lower energy state. The direction of this net Mv is usually considered to be the **axis** of the magnetic field.

The net Mv is aligned parallel with the external magnetic field and is dependent upon the type of magnet that is used. In the case of superconducting magnets, the orientation of the magnetic field is considered to be horizontal. In permanent magnets this orientation is usually vertical. In either case convention refers to it as the **Z-axis**. Figure 10-9 is a schematic representation of a group of nuclei precessing and producing a net Mv. The illustrations use vector diagrams that follow the Cartesian coordinate system named after René Descartes. This is the most common coordinate system for representing positions in space. It is based on three perpendicular spatial axes generally designated x, y, and z. The origin of the plane is the point at which the three planes intersect.

When the pulse is terminated, the precessional motion of the net Mv decays and a signal can be monitored; this is called the **free induction** or **free induction decay (FID) signal**. This signal decays to zero with a characteristic time constant. When the zero state is reached, it is in the equilibrium or normal state.

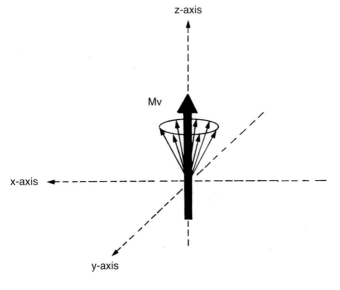

FIGURE 10-9. Individual precessions of the nuclei and their net magnetic moment (Mv).

Excitation

The net magnetic moment (μ) along the z-axis is insignificant when compared to the strength of the external magnetic field. In order to measure this phenomenon it is necessary to move the net Mv away from the direction of the external magnetic field. The nuclei can be made to undergo a transition from one energy level (state) to another, thereby shifting the Mv. In order to do this, the nucleons must absorb a definite amount (quantum) of energy to move to a higher energy level. The net Mv created by the magnetic nuclei will precess when a resonant magnetic field of the proper frequency is applied to the transverse plane (xy plane) (Fig. 10-10). The amount of the precession will vary with the strength (amplitude) and duration of the resonant magnetic field.

The transition to the higher energy state is made using a short, intense pulse of RF energy. The RF energy pulse supplying the additional energy is from the low end of the electromagnetic spectrum. Figure 10-11 shows the electromagnetic spectrum and location of the RF energy used to change the energy levels of the nucleons.

The RF pulse must have a specific frequency to accomplish the transition. This pulse of RF energy is the same as the frequency of precession of the nucleons. The frequency is dependent upon the strength of the external magnetic field. For a 1.0 T field, the RF pulse should be 42.6 MHz. Gauss and teslas are commonly used units that denote magnetic field strength. One tesla (T) is equal to 10,000 gauss (G). A 1.5 T external magnetic field would require an RF energy pulse of 63.9 MHz. This represents the amount of energy required to produce a transition. It is the difference between the

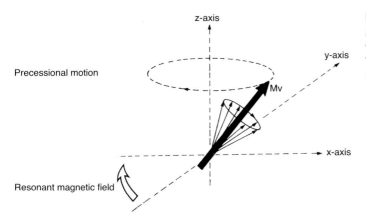

FIGURE   10-10. Result   of applying a resonant magnetic field in the transverse (xy) plane. The net magnetic moment of the nucleons will precess.

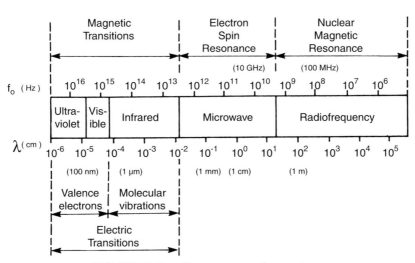

FIGURE 10-11.   Electromagnetic spectrum.

spin-up (parallel) and spin-down (antiparallel) energy states. As mentioned, the transition from one energy state to another is called **resonance**.

Excitation is the process of transmitting the RF energy pulse in order to change the orientation of the net magnetic vector. Two events occur as a result of excitation:

The nuclear spins get into phase with each other. Phase can be defined as the location or starting point from which a waveform begins. The RF energy pulse also changes the orientation of the net Mv. This can be considered as a tipping of the net Mv from its longitudinal (parallel) orientation with the external magnetic field into another plane. The result is movement of the net Mv from a longitudinal (parallel) position along the z-axis into a transverse position along the xy plane at right angles from the z-axis.

The amount of tipping caused by the RF energy pulse is described in degrees; if the net Mv were tipped halfway between the spin-up and spin-down states, the RF energy pulse that was applied would be referred to as a 90-degree RF pulse. If the Mv was already in the transverse position when the 90-degree RF pulse was applied, it would return to its longitudinal (parallel) position. Because the RF magnetic pulse affects the angle at which the magnetic nuclei are shifted, they are classified as either 90-degree or 180-degree pulses. The change in angle is dependent upon the length and amplitude of the pulse.

A **transition** will also occur when the nuclei release an amount (quantum) of energy to return to a lower energy level. When the RF energy pulse is stopped, the spins of the nucleons return to their equilibrium state. The nucleons lose energy as they spiral around the z-axis until the Mv is once again at its original longitudinal (parallel) position.

As the net Mv spirals around the z-axis, an electrical voltage signal is induced in a receiver coil which can be measured. This loss of energy and subsequent return to the equilibrium or lower energy spin state is called **relaxation.** In general, the same equipment that is used to produce the resonant RF magnetic field can act as the detector of the energy loss. This can be accomplished because the RF magnetic field is applied as a pulse.

Immediately after the RF pulse, the magnitude of the free induction decay (FID) signal can indicate the number of protons that are affected, thus yielding information about the proton density. This represents quantitative information about the overall concentration of specific nuclei in a sample of a certain type of tissue or about the numbers of specific nuclei in a sample of different types of tissue. In general, the greater the proton density, the stronger the MRI signal and the greater the image intensity. This does not have much effect in imaging most tissues because there is not much difference between proton densities. In brain imaging, however, there is enough proton density difference between gray and white matter to provide a contrast between these tissues during imaging.

The return of the net Mv to its position before the application of the RF pulse can demonstrate the composition of a particular sample. It can be characterized by two related time constants, or *processes,* called the spin-lattice relaxation process (T_1) and the spin-spin relaxation process (T_2).

The **spin-lattice relaxation process (T_1)** follows the time constant required for the net Mv to return to the original state, parallel to the external magnetic field. The time required depends on the nuclei giving off the extra energy quantum to their surroundings, which is usually called the lattice.

Spin-spin relaxation process (T_2) occurs while the individual nuclei are oriented in the xy plane. These nuclei are precessing in phase with each other throughout the duration of the RF pulse. When the RF pulse is terminated, the surrounding magnetic nuclei exert an influence on the precessing nuclei and cause them to be out of phase, or to "dephase." After time, this influence tends to cancel out the net Mv in the transverse (xy) plane. The time required for this to occur is the spin-spin relaxation time.

The time constants, spin-lattice relaxation process (T_1) and spin-spin relaxation process (T_2), derived from the MRI signal can provide qualitative information about tissue condition; the information can help to determine whether the tissue or area of anatomic interest is healthy or diseased. The RF pulses that are applied to shift the magnetic nuclei are varied to increase the contrast between different tissue areas. The conventional imaging sequences are saturation recovery, inversion recovery, spin echo, gradient echo, and steady-state free precession.

Saturation recovery is accomplished by sending the RF pulses with constant time spacing between each pulse. This time constant must be longer than the spin–spin relaxation time (T_2) and approximately the same length as the spin-lattice relaxation time (T_1). In this sequence, the received signal decays to zero between each successive pulse. By making several images with different constant time spacing, T_1 values can be obtained for each image pixel. In effect, a map of T_1 values is generated. This type of sequence can demonstrate differences between adjacent areas of soft tissues.

Inversion recovery is accomplished by applying a 180-degree pulse that inverts the net Mv. The 180-degree RF pulse is followed by a short delay, which again approximates the spin-lattice relaxation time (T_1). A 90-degree RF pulse is then applied to provide a decay signal. This 90-degree RF pulse can be referred to as a **read pulse**. This sequence also generates a T_1 map when the delay period is varied across the tissue sample. Inversion-recovery sequences can produce a better contrast in the tissue sample, but the imaging time is longer than in the saturation-recovery sequence.

Spin echo involves the application of a 90-degree RF pulse, which produces a signal in the detector coil. After a certain period, which approximates the spin–spin relaxation time (T_2), a 180-degree RF pulse is applied. This in effect brings the individual precessions through the 90-degree plane, creating what appears to be a double-sided FID signal. It can be seen that the time delay after the 180-degree RF pulse should be twice that of the 90-degree time delay (Fig. 10-12*A*). The echo signal produced will be reduced in size because any distortions produced in the 90-degree RF pulse decay by molecular interactions, which are nonreversible, will be eliminated. If subsequent 180-degree RF pulses are applied at twice the 90-degree RF pulse delay ($2T_2$), the echo signals are progressively reduced in size (Fig. 10-12*B*). A true spin–spin relaxation time can be derived by following the signal peaks in the sequence. The spin-echo sequence is usually used to measure the spin–spin relaxation times (T_2) free from imperfections.

Gradient-echo sequences are similar to spin-echo sequences except that the 180-degree pulse that induces the formation of the spin-echo is absent and the repetition time is kept short, which has the effect of increasing the MR signal strength. These sequences try to maintain the transverse magnetization in a steady state. The gradient-echo sequence features RF pulses that provide tip angles of less than 90 degrees. It has been demonstrated that reduced RF tip angles can affect the image intensity and contrast. In general, the intensity of liquids (structures with larger T_2-to-T_1 ratios) is enhanced with this type of sequence.

There are several advantages to using the gradient-echo sequence—there is less heat build-up in the patient, which results in a more comfortable study, and the imaging times are faster. Two-dimensional

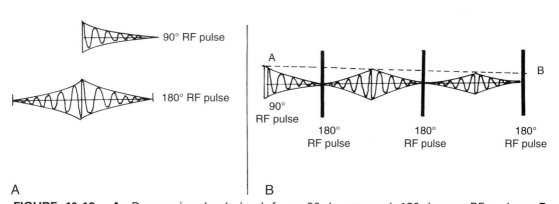

FIGURE 10-12. **A,** Decay signals derived from 90-degree and 180-degree RF pulses. **B,** Schematic of a spin-echo sequence showing the subsequent reduction in the size of the echo caused by nonreversible changes from molecular interactions. The dotted line *AB* represents the true spin-spin relaxation time (T_2).

BOX 10-1	*Gradient Echo Imaging Techniques*
Acronym	**Gradient Echo Imaging Technique**
FLASH	**F**ast **L**ow **A**ngle **Sh**ot
FISP	**F**ast **I**maging with **S**teady **S**tate **P**recession
ROAST	**R**esonant **O**ffset **A**cquisition into **S**teady State
GRASS	**G**radient **R**ecalled **A**cquisition in the **S**teady **S**tate
CE-FAST	**C**ontrast-**E**nhanced **FAST***

*Fourier Acquired Steady State.

slices can be produced in seconds rather than minutes, whereas three-dimensional imaging can be accomplished in minutes rather than hours. This decreased imaging time reduces the need for the patient to hold his or her breath for exceptionally long intervals during imaging. The shorter times result in the elimination of motion artifacts usually caused by breathing. A technique called **gradient moment nulling** (gradient moments of a pulse sequence are made to vanish) makes it possible to reduce or eliminate the artifacts produced by both vascular and cerebrospinal fluid effects.

There are many proprietary varieties of the gradient-echo sequence (rapid imaging technique), and they are known by various acronyms (e.g., GRASS, FISP, FLASH, ROAST, and CE-FAST) (Box 10-1). The acronyms are manufacturer-specific and a discussion of the various gradient echo sequences is beyond the scope of this text.

Steady-state free precession provides a signal that does not decay before the next RF pulse is applied. This type of sequence can improve the signal-to-noise (SNR) ratio of the signal. Steady-state free precession sequences can produce signals of greater intensity because contributions are made from both spin-spin (T_2) and spin-lattice (T_1) relaxation times. When using this sequence, high-quality images can be produced, but the individual contributions of spin-spin (T_2) and spin-lattice (T_1) relaxations cannot be determined.

GRADIENT SYSTEM

Spatial Encoding

This is the process by which the MR signals are assigned to distinct volume elements (voxels) in the image. Gradient coils are used to produce a linear increase in the magnetic field along one spatial axis. There is a gradient coil for each of the three spatial axes. During the procedure, one of the gradient coils is activated so that the RF pulse flips the net Mv from the structures in a particular slice. This gradient coil is sometimes referred to as the "slice select" gradient. The strength of the gradient system determines the minimum field of view, slice thickness, and echo time. The z gradient is used for spatial encoding along this axis and is responsible for the linear gradation of the main magnetic field.

Two processes are used to encode (identify) the MR signals of the shapes and positions of structures located within the selected slice—frequency encoding and phase encoding. Each of these processes involves the application of gradients while the MR signals are measured.

Frequency Encoding

The frequency encoding gradient, also called the read or readout gradient, makes the Larmor frequency vary along one direction in a plane. This gradient is usually applied along the x-axis and is responsible for the left-to-right gradation and spatial encoding in this plane. Structures at different locations in the plane contribute signals that oscillate at different rates. The variations in the frequency denote the position of the structures along the read axis. The frequency encoding gradient is applied while the MR signal is received.

Phase Encoding

The phase encoding gradient (y gradient) measures the anterior-to-posterior direction in the plane. It uses a third gradient coil that provides a phase change in the signals collected. The phase encoding gradient is applied for a short period of time and then terminated before collection of the data. The phase encoding sequence is repeated many times and is increased in amplitude after each successive MR signal. The number of different pulse sequences required is dependent on the spatial resolution desired and can vary from 128 to 256 phase encoding sequences.

The signals collected from these processes are subjected to computer processing to produce the completed image.

Three-Dimensional Imaging

Three-dimensional imaging is facilitated through manipulation of the gradient system during imaging. When this technique is used, data are collected from the entire imaging volume. The use of one of the varieties of the "fast imaging," gradient-echo sequences listed previously is within practical limits. Three-dimensional imaging provides images in all three planes—axial, coronal, and sagittal—from a single set of data. The data can be reformatted by the computer to rearrange the digital information to provide multiplanar imaging.

TECHNICAL CONSIDERATIONS

The MRI technique has proved its value as a diagnostic modality by providing greater contrast sensitivity than x-ray CT techniques, yielding a greater range of tissue discrimination. The information gained from the relaxation times T_1 and T_2 is representative of the local interactions of the nuclei. MRI has been used to image almost all areas of the body. Figure 10-13 depicts various portions of the human body as imaged using MRI technology. Currently, MRI is being used in the area of proton imaging because hydrogen nuclei are the easiest to image as they are relatively abundant in tissue and they give a measurable MRI signal.

One significant advantage to the use of MRI is that bone can be virtually eliminated from the image. When bone is imaged, it is actually the bone marrow that is being detected. This can be important when imaging areas of the spinal cord and brain, which are surrounded by bone. It has also been demonstrated that there is a difference in the relaxation times of the protons of cancerous and noncancerous tissue. Current research studies are incorporating MRI into the investigation of the chemistry and function of various tissues.

MAGNETIC RESONANCE ANGIOGRAPHY

Magnetic resonance angiography (MRA), which allows imaging of the cardiovascular system without the invasive introduction of a contrast agent, is made possible by adjusting the type of imaging sequence that is used. Although this sounds simple, the theory behind the procedure is rather complex and a detailed explanation is beyond the scope of this text. Two processes are important in understanding how blood flow in the body is imaged: these are **flow–related signal loss** and **flow-related dephasing.**

Flow-Related Signal Loss (Flow Void)

When spin-echo sequences are used, a 90-degree excitation RF pulse defines the image slice, and a second 180-degree RF pulse is applied at the echo time divided by 2 (TE/2), which produces a second echo. When flowing blood is in the image slice, the blood originally excited by the first 90-degree excitation RF pulse will have moved and the second 180-degree RF pulse will not be seen, resulting in a signal loss, or "flow void."

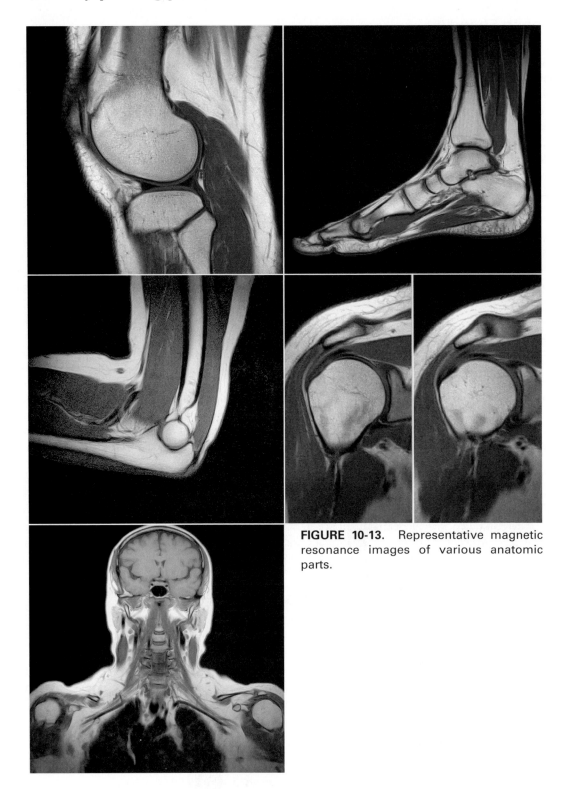

FIGURE 10-13. Representative magnetic resonance images of various anatomic parts.

Flow-Related Dephasing

Because the nuclear spins have somewhat different frequencies, which are determined by the type of tissue and its location, their spins tend to get out of phase with each other. In this process, the signal is greatest when the spins are in phase. Over time the spins lose phase with each other, creating a partial dephasing and ultimately complete dephasing. At this point, there is little or no signal. In the imaging sequences, a rephasing magnetic field gradient is applied a short time after the excitation RF pulse. This magnetic field gradient is in the opposite direction and results in the rephasing of the nuclear spins, which forms what is called a gradient echo, improving the sensitivity of the imaging sequence. This increase in the sensitivity works well if the spins are stationary. However, if the spins are moving, as in the case of flowing blood or cerebrospinal fluid, the spins will be out of phase and produce marked signal loss. The amount of dephasing is dependent upon the velocity of the blood flow: the greater the velocity, the greater the signal loss.

Time of Flight MR Angiography

This type of MRA depends upon the enhancement of the spins entering the image slice. In time of flight (TOF) imaging, spin–echo sequences are applied in different planes. A 90-degree RF pulse is applied that excites the spins in one plane while the 180-degree RF pulse excites them in a different plane. If there is no motion, no signal is produced because none of the spins will have the benefit of both pulses. Angiography can be accomplished because the blood from the 90-degree RF pulse flows into the plane that has experienced the 180-degree RF pulse, producing an echo. The slice plane of the 180-degree RF pulse must match the location of the blood that has had the 90-degree pulse applied to it in order to have only the blood contribute to the signal. An image produced using TOF MRA is shown in Figure 10-14.

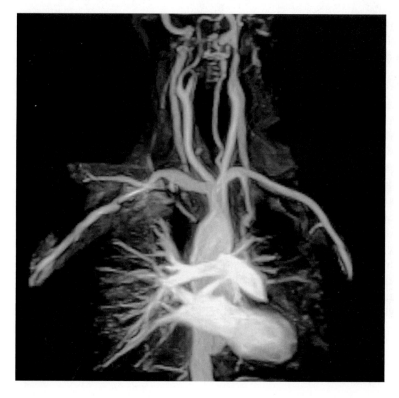

FIGURE 10-14. Representative magnetic resonance image of time of flight vascular study.

Phase Contrast MR Angiography

As mentioned, a phase shift occurs in spins that are moving in the same direction as a magnetic field gradient, and this shift is proportional to the velocity of the spins. This principle is the basis for phase contrast MRA. The pulse sequence utilizes a **bipolar gradient pulse** to encode the velocity of the spins. The bipolar gradient pulse consists of two pulses with equal magnitudes. The first pulse is applied in one direction and the second in the opposite direction. If no motion or flow is involved, there is no net change in phase following the bipolar pulse. In the case of flowing blood or cerebrospinal fluid, a net phase change will result because the spins having motion will experience a different magnitude of the second gradient in relation to that of the first gradient. The faster the spins are moving, the greater the net phase shift. Utilizing subtraction and a postprocessing technique known as **maximum intensity projection (MIP)**, the angiogram can be obtained.

Magnetic Resonance Perfusion and Diffusion Imaging

This type of MR imaging has made possible the process of functional studies. The imaging of the blood flow through the capillary network is termed **perfusion imaging**. It can be accomplished using a contrast agent that is administered through an injection or through the use of the patient's blood as the contrast agent. When a contrast agent is used the study is referred to as exogenous MRI. The term **exogenous** refers to originating from outside the body. This type of study has some disadvantages. The primary consideration is that it can be considered an invasive study. The patient is also at risk from a possible contrast agent reaction.

During endogenous (within the body) MRI the venous blood (deoxyhemoglobin) acts as the contrast agent. It is considered to be paramagnetic and therefore influences the signal intensity.

Diffusion studies can image the movement of water across the cell membranes and between various tissue compartments.

SUMMARY

MRI is a minimally invasive modality that can be used to image the anatomy of the body without the use of x-radiation. The basic principle behind MRI is the use of a magnetic field and radiowaves coupled with a sophisticated computer system to produce the images. State-of-the-art MRI systems also provide the means for biomedical and physiologic spectroscopic analyses during the imaging session.

Three different magnet configurations can be used to produce the main magnetic field—permanent, superconductive, and hybrid magnets. Each has advantages and disadvantages relating to its design. All MRI systems have certain equipment groups in addition to the magnet—the RF coil system, gradient coil system, shimming coil system, and computer system. Current magnets vary in strength depending on the manufacturer as well as the design. Magnet strengths are available in the 0.2 – 3.0 T range for human imaging (1 T = 10,000 gauss). Siemens is currently working with New York University (NYU), Massachusetts General Hospital (MGH), and the Center for Magnetic Resonance Research (CMRR) in Minnesota with magnet strengths from 7 T. It is anticipated that this will allow magnetic resonance to image not only the human anatomy but also its metabolic activities.

MRI is still in the growth stage. New techniques and equipment are being developed at a rapid rate, and existing techniques are being improved. The ultimate potential of MRI in imaging is still unknown, as are the potentials of its use as a diagnostic tool. The theory presented here is a simplified explanation of the basic technical principles underlying MRI.

REFERENCES

1. Shellock FG: *Reference Manual for Magnetic Resonance Safety: 2003 Edition.* Amirsys, Inc, 2003.

SUGGESTED READINGS

Bongartz GM: Contrast media in magnetic resonance angiography. *Eur Radiol* 13(9):2065–2066, 2003.

Brown MA, Semelka RC: MR Imaging Abbreviations, Definitions, and Descriptions: A Review. *Radiology* 213(3):647–662, 1999.

Byrdie A, Raby N: Early MRI in the management of clinical scaphoid fracture. *Br J Radiol* 76(905):296–300, 2003

Choyke PL, Yim P, Marcos H, Ho VB, Mullick R, Summers RM: Hepatic MR angiography: A multiobserver comparison of visualization methods. *AJR Am J Roentgenol* 176:465–470, 2001.

Gibby WA: Basic principles of magnetic resonance imaging. *Neurosurg Clin North Am* 16(1):1–64, 2005.

Golay X, de Zwart JA, Ho YC, et al.: Parallel imaging techniques in functional MRI. *Top Magn Reson Imaging* 15(4):255–265, 2004.

Goldman JP: New techniques and applications for magnetic resonance angiography. *Mt Sinai J Med* 70(6):375–385, 2003.

Hutter A, Kedan I, Srokowski TP, et al: Coronary magnetic resonance angiography. *Semin Roentgenol* 38(4):330–341, 2003.

Kircher MF, Mahmood U, King RS, Weissleder R, Josephson L: A multimodal nanoparticle for preoperative magnetic resonance imaging and intraoperative optical brain tumor delineation. *Cancer Res* 63(23):8122–8125, 2003.

Lee CE, Ng HB, Yip CW, et al: Imaging collateral circulation: magnetic resonance angiography and perfusion magnetic resonance imaging at 3 T. *Arch Neurol* 62(3):492–493, 2005.

Nitz WR: Fast and ultrafast non-echo-planar MR imaging techniques. *Eur Radiol* 12(12):2866–2882, 2002.

Perrin RL, Ivancevic MK, Kozerke S, et al: Comparative study of FAST gradient echo MRI sequences: phantom study. *J Magn Reson Imaging* 20(6):1030–1038, 2004.

Yim PJ, Choyke PL, Summers RM. Grey-scale skeletonization of small vessels in magnetic resonance angiography. *IEEE Trans Med Imaging* 19(6):568–576, 2000.

Zeh H, Choyke PL, Alexander HR, Bartlett DL, Libutti SK, Chang R, Summers RM: Gadolinium-enhanced 3-D magnetic resonance angiography prior to isolated hepatic perfusion for metastases. *J Comput Assist Tomogr* 23:(5):664–669, 1999.

STUDY QUESTIONS

1. The nucleons in certain atoms possess a property known as :
   a. charge
   b. angular momentum
   c. isotope
   d. electromagnetic energy

2. When the external magnetic field is applied to the nuclei, it creates a motion similar to that produced on the axis of a spinning top when it begins to slow down. This motion is known as:
   a. ionization
   b. relaxation
   c. precession
   d. the gradient

3. 1000 gauss is equivalent to _____ tesla(s).
   a. 0.1
   b. 0.15
   c. 1.0
   d. 10

4. Which of the following is representative of the Larmor equation?
   a. $\omega_0 = \gamma B_0$
   b. $\gamma = B_0 \omega_0$
   c. $B_0 = \gamma/\omega_0$
   d. $B_0 = \gamma \omega_0$

STUDY QUESTIONS (*cont'd*)

5. When the radio frequency (RF) energy pulse is stopped, the spins of the nucleons return to their equilibrium state. This process is termed:
   a. precession
   b. excitation
   c. gradient overflow
   d. relaxation

6. The symbol T_1 relates to the process known as:
   a. spin-lattice relaxation
   b. phase decoding
   c. spin-spin relaxation
   d. resistivity

7. Which of the following is not an advantage to using a gradient echo sequence?
   a. fewer motion artifacts
   b. increased body heat
   c. a more comfortable study
   d. reduced need to suspend respiration

8. Manipulating an induced current in coils that surround the magnet to provide homogeneity of the magnetic field is called:
   a. passive shimming
   b. active shimming
   c. precession
   d. gradient cohesion

9. The two basic designs for radio frequency coils are:
   i. surface
   ii. volume
   iii. resistive
   a. i only
   b. ii only
   c. i and ii only
   d. i and iii only

10. Which of the following types of magnets do not require electricity to produce the magnetic field:
   i. superconductive
   ii. permanent
   iii. resistive
   a. i only
   b. ii only
   c. iii only
   d. i and iii

11 Nuclear Medicine—SPECT, PET, and Fusion Imaging

CHAPTER OBJECTIVES

After completing this chapter, the reader will be able to perform the following:

- Describe how nuclear medicine is used as a diagnostic tool
- Explain the indications and contraindications for nuclear medicine studies
- Identify the various types of radiopharmaceuticals used in nuclear medicine
- Differentiate between SPECT, PET, and fusion imaging
- Describe the equipment used in each of these modalities

CHAPTER OUTLINE

NUCLEAR MEDICINE

    Indications and Contraindications
    Radionuclides
    Equipment
    Single Photon Emission Computed Tomography
    Positron Emission Tomography
    Fusion Imaging

SUMMARY

I t is not the intent of this book to present an in-depth explanation of nuclear medicine technology. The discussion will include only a brief introduction into the world of nuclear medicine and the use of single photon emission computed tomography (SPECT) and positron emission tomography (PET).

The term **fusion imaging** or fusion technology describes a hybrid of both computed tomography (CT) (transmission) and PET or SPECT (emission) scanning to present a complete picture of both the anatomic features and the metabolic information of a pathologic process. Imaging fusion occurs best in an advanced integrated system rather than having the patient undergo a CT scan and a PET or SPECT scan separately and attempting to correlate both studies manually. The integrated system uses software that aligns the images of the two scans to provide a more accurate diagnosis than individual PET/SPECT and CT scans.

The combination of PET and CT allows the physician to demonstrate not only anatomic information but also the functional activity of the tissue being studied. PET/CT is being used in the detection of a wide variety of pathologic processes including breast, lung, esophageal, thyroid, and head and neck cancers. Brain imaging and myocardial function studies are also being performed.

The integration of the two modalities reduces the time it requires to make a diagnosis as compared with performing each of the studies at different times. The patient must still have both examinations, but the fusion units have the advantage of integrating the images from both. The patient handling is effortless, and the improved data acquisition and registration of the information are improved because of the fusion of the images from the two separate examination. The procedure is extremely accurate in predicting location and pathologic condition of the tissues under investigation.

NUCLEAR MEDICINE

Nuclear medicine is a diagnostic tool that utilizes a radioactive substance to help diagnose a disease process from inside the body. These radiopharmaceuticals are organ-, tissue-, or even cell-specific in providing information about the pathologic process. The modality not only provides anatomic information but can assess the function of the organ, bone, or tissue that it is designed to identify. In fact, because the amounts of radioactive material are so small and the duration of the radioactivity so limited, it can provide a diagnosis without harm to nontargeted areas. In most cases the amount of radiation that a patient receives is no more than that received during CT scan or fluoroscopy.

Some of the disease processes that have been identified through nuclear medicine are ovarian, endocrine, colon, prostate, pancreatic, breast, bone, and lung cancers; diagnosis of heart disease is another area that has benefited from this modality through stress testing. Nuclear medicine has also been effective in the diagnosis of rheumatoid arthritis, joint disease, and meningitis, to name a few.

Indications and Contraindications

The indications using nuclear medicine imaging techniques are wide and varied. Each anatomic area has its own set of indications that apply to the type of organ study and the reasons for its performance. Some indications for the use of nuclear medicine studies are as follows:

- Demonstrate kidney function
- Scan lungs for respiratory and blood flow problems
- Investigate upper abdominal pain
    - Acute cholecystitis
    - Jaundice (obstructive vs. nonobstructive)
- Evaluate skeletal pathology
    - Bones
    - Joints
- Identify the presence or spread of cancer
- Locate the presence of infection
- Detect the function and disorders of the organs in the endocrine system
    - Pituitary
    - Thyroid
    - Adrenal
    - Pancreas
    - Gonads
- Image the heart
    - Coronary artery disease
    - Congestive heart failure
    - Atrial/ventricular septal defects
- Perform radionuclide angiography

This list is by no means complete; it is only a representation of the range of indications for nuclear medicine studies using SPECT and PET scanning. A nuclear medicine study can image any organ tissue or cell type that a radiopharmaceutical has been designed to target in the body.

The contraindications are grouped into three major categories: pregnancy, allergic reactions, and other.

Pregnancy

Because nuclear medicine depends upon the introduction of a radioactive material into the body, exposure to the fetus is possible. This can happen if the radiopharmaceutical can cross the placenta. Women who are breast feeding will also pose a possible risk to the infant. As in any other radiographic study, these contraindications are not absolute; however, the physician and the patient should consider the risks versus the benefits, fetal age, and type of study being performed before making a decision.

Allergic Reactions

When performing advanced radiologic studies, a foreign substance is usually introduced into the body to provide the necessary contrast to visualize the structures being examined. These contrast agents can produce allergic reactions. This premise will hold true for any nuclear medicine study as well. Reactions to the radionuclides are very rare; however, the technologist should always be alert for any signs of reaction. The symptoms will be similar to those listed for contrast agents in Chapter 6. If it is determined that the patient has had a reaction during a previous nuclear medicine study, the physician should be alerted to the potential for contraindication to use of the substance or performance of the examination.

Other Contraindications

As in routine radiography, it is well known that some radiologic procedures can affect the results of another procedure if they are not performed in the proper sequence. Some radiologic procedures can affect the result of the nuclear medicine procedure as well. Previous surgical procedures can also affect the outcome of the nuclear medicine study. Because of the potential adverse effect on the nuclear medicine procedure, these factors are considered as contraindications to performance of the examination. There is also the possibility that medications the patient is taking may affect the uptake of the radiopharmaceutical. In some cases the medications can be suspended prior to the examination, or if it is not possible this may become a contraindication for the procedure. The technologist should be aware of these situations and must alert the physician if the potential for contraindication exists.

Radionuclides
Terminology

It is important to understand some of the terminology associated with radionuclides. As in radiography, the radiation produced by the radionuclide is expressed by certain units. These units are the **curie (Ci)** and the **becquerel (Bq)**. Unlike units in radiography, these represent units of activity. Activity (radioactivity) is defined as the number of disintegrations per unit time. The curie represents a radioactivity equal to 3.7×10^{10} disintegrations per second (dps). The term *curie* was derived from the name of the individual, Madame Marie Curie, who was a pioneer in the field of radioactivity.

The **curie** is generally expressed in very small units such as millicuries (3.7×10^7 dps), microcuries (3.7×10^4 dps), nanocuries (3.7×10 dps), and picocuries (3.7×10^{-2} dps). Obviously, the curie is a very large number, and the smaller units are used for expressing radioactivity in curies.

In the International System of units, activity is represented by the **becquerel**. One becquerel is equal to 1 dps or 27.03×10^{-11} Ci. This unit was named after Henri Becquerel, who in 1896 was the first to discover radioactivity.

As a radionuclide ages over time its activity is dependent upon the number of atoms of the radionuclide present at a specific time and a **constant (k)** that is specific to the radionuclide. This constant represents the probability that a single atom of a particular radionuclide will decay (the disintegration of the nucleus of an unstable radionuclide). It can also be referred to as the decay constant. The actual calculation of the decay constant is beyond the scope of this text and is referenced here expressly to the discussion of the concept of half-life.

The concept of **half-life** is an important one when dealing with radionuclides. This is the time interval for a specific number of unstable nuclei to decay (disintegrate) to one half their original number. Half-life can be considered in a physical and biologic sense. The **physical half-life** of a radionuclide is the amount of time it takes for one half of the activity to decay. The **biologic half-life** refers to the amount of time it takes for one half of the radionuclide to physiologically clear from the body. Both types of half-life are important in nuclear medicine. Radionuclides with long half-lives would not be very useful because of the radiation dose that would be given to the patient over the course of the examination. Long biologic half-lives also create the same danger. Of course, radionuclides that have too short a half-life would not be useful either. This is the same as the characteristic of persistence in the use of contrast agents in radiography. The substance must remain long enough for the examination to be completed but be eliminated from the body within a reasonable amount of time to avoid adverse effects. In the case of nuclear medicine the half-life must be long enough to provide for an adequate study but limit the patient dose to its as low as reasonably achievable (ALARA) levels.

Basics of Radionuclide Production

Radionuclides are produced utilizing a number of different methods. Two major processes are used: **reactor-produced substances** (fission from heavier nuclides) and **accelerator-produced radionuclides**.

Neutrons are essential to the fission process. Fission is the splitting of a heavier radionuclide into several different radionuclides having mass numbers smaller than the target nuclide. Naturally occurring radioactive substances are excellent sources of alpha particles. These alpha particles produce neutrons when they react, and neutrons are responsible for initiating the fission process.

Fission requires that the neutron is captured by the heavier nuclide. One result of this process is that more than one neutron are produced in the process. The neutron is the initiator of the fission process, so the more neutrons produced, the greater the number of fissions. These additional fissions produce more neutrons, and the process continues until the supply of fissionable material is used up.

Reactor-produced radionuclides are possible because the neutrons released create an environment that is self-propagating. The reaction is controlled by the use of "moderators" and "neutron absorbers" to reach a state of equilibrium. The controlled production of these neutrons is the theory behind the working of a nuclear reactor. We are familiar with these systems as a means of creating power (electricity) under controlled conditions and as an atomic bomb in an uncontrolled chain reaction.

Once a controlled environment is accomplished, radionuclides can be produced in one of two ways. The radionuclide can be created by irradiating a substance (bombarding a target atom with neutrons having very small amounts of kinetic energy), referred to as a **thermal neutron reaction**. The neutrons are easily captured by stable nuclides, which at times become radioactive. Depending upon the method that the reaction follows, the result can be either beta or gamma emitters. It is the gamma emitter type of nuclide that is used in the nuclear generator to produce daughter products with short half-lives.

The second method of creating the radionuclide in the reactor is through **fission**. This is a process that occurs in a nuclear reactor and can produce a radionuclide that is formed from the fission of uranium (^{236}U) rather than from the bombardment of a target atom of another substance. In the nuclear reactor, neutrons interact with ^{235}U to form ^{236}U, which is unstable. This substance, ^{236}U, undergoes a fission reaction in the reactor producing various products, some of which can be used in nuclear medicine. The fission-produced radionuclides are usually considered to be "carrier-free" (containing no stable isotope of the same element) radionuclides and can be used to generate shorter lived radionuclides.

Radionuclides can also be produced by **accelerating** charged particles to interact with a specific target. The interactions of these high-energy charged particles (in the MeV range) and the target form high specific activity, carrier-free radionuclides. These interactions are dependent upon the energy of the charged particle and the threshold energy required by the target. If the energy is below the threshold, there will be no reaction. The charged particles that are commonly used in accelerators are protons, deuterons, helium–3, and alpha particles.

The radionuclides produced by the processes just discussed generally have relatively long half-lives. The radionuclides used in nuclear medicine are usually short-lived. This could pose some positive benefits and also some limitations. The short half-life of these radionuclides is beneficial to the patient in respect to the reduction in patient dose. Generators allow for the production of these short-lived radionuclides close to or at the site where they will be used.

A radionuclide generator is in fact a process whereby the long-lived radionuclide (commonly referred to as the parent) decays into a short-lived radionuclide (commonly called the daughter). Generators are devices that contain a glass column filled with a substance called alumina (Al_2O_3). The bottom of the glass column is sealed with a porous glass filter to prevent the alumina from passing from the column. The parent radionuclide and its daughter are in equilibrium at the top of the column. The daughter radionuclide is produced by separating it from the parent. This can be accomplished by a process called **elution**. Separation will occur when a suitable eluting solution is passed through the column, which dissolves the daughter radionuclide, carrying it past the porous glass and into a collecting or eluting vial. The process is also termed **milking** the generator. Some of the eluting solutions that can be used are 0.1% physiologic saline or methyl ethyl ketone (MEK). Depending on how the parent radionuclide was created, either by bombardment with neutrons or by fission, the amount of impurities that can be present will vary. Remember that radionuclide produced by fission produces substances that have a high specificity (low number of contaminants) and will produce a purer daughter radionuclide.

This is a rather simplified description of the operation of a radionuclide generator. There are other factors that should be considered when selecting a generator for use in nuclear medicine; it should be convenient to use and function rapidly to produce the daughter radionuclide and be highly efficient. The type of radiation shielding is also a consideration as well as the amount of parent radionuclide that comes through with the eluting solution. The larger the amount of parent radionuclide, the greater will be the patient dose without adding to the information garnered through the study. The specific concentration of the daughter radionuclide is also a major consideration in the use of a particular generator. The specific concentration, the number of millicuries per milliliter, should be high, especially when performing dynamic studies that require highly concentrated smaller boluses of radionuclide.

Radiopharmaceuticals

A **radiopharmaceutical** is a radionuclide that has been modified by chemically combining it with various biochemicals that may have physiologic or metabolic properties that would be beneficial in a particular study. This is similar to the concept of selective localization that was discussed in Chapter 6. The biochemical component of the compound is incorporated with the radionuclide to bring it to a specific anatomic location or to participate in a metabolic process. In most cases in nuclear medicine the radiopharmaceutical is used to gather diagnostic information and is rarely used in a therapeutic fashion.

One major consideration in the development of radiopharmaceuticals is that the radionuclide must emit a specific energy gamma (γ) ray. This type of emission occurs when there is greater than 100 KeV of energy in the excited nucleus. Almost all the radionuclides that are made into radiopharmaceuticals are created using a cyclotron (Fig. 11-1). This process will produce radionuclides with high specificity, or in other words purer samples.

When a gamma (γ) photon with an energy level at or above 1.02 MeV approaches a nuclear field, it is converted into two particles—a positive electron (positron) and a negatron (electron). When this occurs as part of the decay process, the positron can travel only a few millimeters. The positrons are attracted to an orbital electron of an atom, and a process called "annihilation" occurs. In the annihilation process the mass of the positron and negatron is converted back into energy. The energy from each of these particles is .511 MeV (Fig. 11-2). They are also given off at an angle of 180 degrees from each other, and the resultant radiation can be acquired by detectors in the unit. This process becomes the basis for positron emission tomography (PET) scanning (Fig. 11-3).

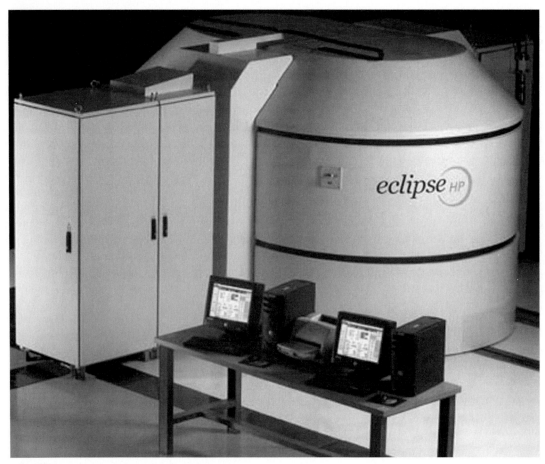

FIGURE 11-1. Photograph of a cyclotron.

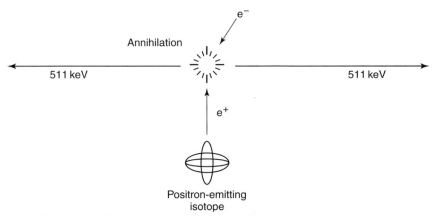

FIGURE 11-2. Schematic illustration of the annihilation event. A positron-emitting isotope produces a positive electron (positron), which interacts with a free electron to cause two 511 keV gamma photons to be emitted at 180 degrees to each other.

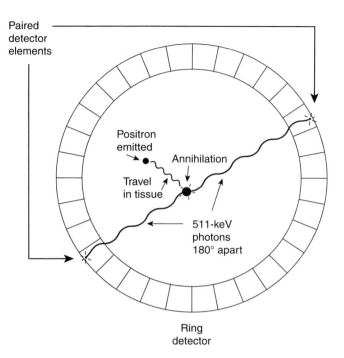

Paired detector elements

Positron emitted

Annihilation

Travel in tissue

511-keV photons 180° apart

Ring detector

FIGURE 11-3. Illustration demonstrating how the annihilation process produces an image during the PET scan. This is simplified only to show that there are two detector elements on opposite sides to record the annihilation events.

Equipment

Diagnostic imaging can be accomplished in two ways, by either **transmission** or **emission.** Imaging by transmission is done with an external x-ray source and is accomplished by the attenuation of photons as they pass through the body. This is the basis for radiography. Simple radiography produces an image of a three-dimensional structure represented in two dimensions. This type of image is made up of information gathered as a result of the x-ray photon passing through the body part. The information gathered by this imaging technique represents a projected image that includes the superimposition of structures above and below the **plane** of interest. The superimposition of structures can hinder an accurate diagnosis and can be considered as a disadvantage of this type of imaging. In planar imaging images must be made in more than one plane in order to make a diagnosis by allowing the separation of the structures that have been superimposed in the planar imaging process.

Nuclear medicine imaging is accomplished by the **emission** of photons from within the patient. Unlike transmission imaging, which demonstrates the location and view of a structure, the emission of the photon in nuclear medicine represents the location of the radionuclide within the structure. This information emitted from the structure is captured by a detector. (The scintillation detector is a commonly used means of capturing the emissions from the body. The theory behind the production of images using scintigraphy is beyond the scope of this text.) The image is produced as the detectors collect the emissions. An image can then be recorded by either analog or digital means.

The Anger camera is the most commonly used equipment for imaging in nuclear medicine. It was developed by Hal Anger[1] in 1957 and is still used today as the basic means of performing nuclear medicine studies. The Anger camera consists of a lead collimator and a means of detecting the emission. The collimator basically functions like a lens, eliminating any gamma photons that diverge substantially from the vertical or that fall below a specific energy. The detector is made up of a scintillation crystal coupled to a photomultiplier tube.

Scintillation occurs in certain substances when they are stimulated by ionizing radiation. These substances will give off (emit) light. The amount of light emitted is directly proportional to the amount of radiation that strikes the substance. The light photons emitted by the substance must then be converted into an electrical signal that can be projected as light on a cathode ray tube. This is similar in principle to the interactions of the crystals in an image–intensifying system in radiography.

The scintillation substance commonly used is thallium-activated sodium iodide. Pure sodium iodide is not used because it requires an impurity to produce light at room temperatures. Thallium provides such an impurity. Some of the newer units utilize solid state technology to collect and convert the emissions from the scintillations substance. These systems use thallium-activated cesium iodide as the scintillator and a silicon photodiode instead of the photo multiplier tube to collect the light emitted by the cesium iodide scintillator. The construction and operation of the Anger camera are much more complex than the simple description provided here. Simply put, the Anger camera basically creates an image illustrating the amount and location of the radioactivity that has collected inside the patient.

The images formed by the information gathered by the detectors of the Anger camera can be formed either through analog (photographic) means or primarily, today, by digitally collecting the information directly into a computer system. In both cases the image is formed during the time the data are gathered by the detectors.

The images collected by the scintillation camera are planar and require that images be produced in more than one plane for proper diagnosis. Images produced by transmission CT, after reconstruction, avoid the superimposition of structures that are above and below the plane of interest. The image produced can be considered as dimensional imaging. When a reconstructed computed tomographic image is viewed each point of information represents an individual volume of material without the disadvantage of the superimposition of other structures. This eliminates the need for imaging in multiple planes in order to make a diagnosis.

The principle of tomography can also apply to images produced by the emission of ionizing radiation from the patient. Currently, this is accomplished either by SPECT or PET.

Single Photon Emission Computed Tomography

Single photon emission computed tomography (SPECT) produces the image from the emissions of a **single photon** from the decay process of the radiopharmaceutical. There are several advantages to SPECT imaging. SPECT equipment is not as expensive as PET systems. Standard radiopharmaceuticals are used, eliminating the need for a cyclotron to produce the short half-life radiopharmaceuticals, such as fluorine-18 (^{18}F), oxygen-15 (^{15}O), and nitrogen-13 (^{13}N), necessary for PET imaging. This factor alone can reduce the capitalization and operating costs when comparing SPECT and PET imaging. SPECT units also require less space and consumables such as electricity and air conditioning. It is possible to utilize positron-emitting radionuclides in SPECT imaging using either type of system previously described. There are advantages and disadvantages to the use of the positron emitting radio-pharmaceuticals and some equipment design considerations must be given in order to maximize both system resolution and sensitivity.

In SPECT, the emissions are collected in one of two ways. First, the system may have the detectors surround the patient during the study by using a specialty ring detector system. Second, systems are also designed using rotating Anger cameras to collect the data. The information is acquired in a similar manner to transmission tomography. It is then processed in a computer by a special algorithm which reconstructs the layers or slices using the principle of **back projection**. This process is similar to that used in CT. The data is then filtered to remove any artifacts (streaks) that result from areas of high activity. When filtration is used in conjunction with reconstruction it is usually referred to as filtered back projection. Newer versions of the reconstruction algorithm are being used to produce images superior to those reconstructed by the filtered back projection algorithm called iterative reconstruction. Specific detailed explanations of reconstruction and filtering are beyond the scope of this text.

Positron Emission Tomography

The radionuclides used for **positron emission tomography (PET)** characteristically emit positrons that ultimately result in what is referred to in radiography as **annihilation radiation**. Radiographers should be familiar with the process of pair production, which occurs at energies above 1.02 MeV. A portion of the energy of the positron emitted by the radionuclide that exceeds 1.02 MeV represents the kinetic energy of the positron. This kinetic energy is deposited in the patient as the positron moves through the tissue. The distance traveled is not very great and ultimately the positron comes to rest. At this point it will combine with an electron in an annihilation process that produces two photons, each with energy of 0.51 MeV. The annihilation reaction is representative of Einstein's theory of the conversion of matter to energy. The annihilation photons move in opposite directions and can be collected by detectors in the system.

The equipment is designed so that there is a ring of detectors around the patient. Because the photons that are produced travel in opposite directions (180 degrees apart) it can be seen that they will be

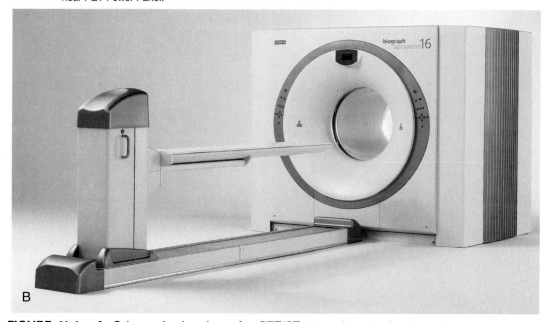

FIGURE 11-4. **A,** Schematic drawing of a PET/CT room layout showing the scanner room, operator S room, and the utility area as well as the minimum size requirements. **B,** Photograph of the Siemens Biograph 16 PET/CT system.

collected on opposite sides of the patient. The location of the annihilation reaction can be determined easily because it occurred along the line of travel (coincidence line) of the annihilation photons.

The radiopharmaceuticals used in PET make possible the imaging of physiologic and biochemical processes with an excellent quantitative accuracy as well as a high level of precision. The disadvantages to PET imaging are those which make SPECT imaging attractive. These include the cost of the equipment, the need for a cyclotron, imaging space requirements, and the increased operating expenses.

Fusion Imaging

As the name implies, **fusion imaging** is the combination of two different modalities to produce the final image. Manufacturers are producing systems that contain CT and SPECT or PET in a single unit. Figure 11-4 shows representative layouts for a PET/CT room configuration that enables the combination of the two modalities into one system. The images produced demonstrate not only structure (anatomy) but also function (physiology) in such a way as to eliminate the mismatching of images that would occur if the two examinations were performed at different times. Imaging times are also reduced when the two modalities are combined in the same system. The use of advanced computer systems and algorithms provides a high correlation between the two images. This allows for a more precise localization of the pathologic process and subsequently the ultimate diagnosis. Accurate localization also enables the physician to determine effective treatment plans. Figure 11-5 illustrates some representative images showing the differences between the modalities.

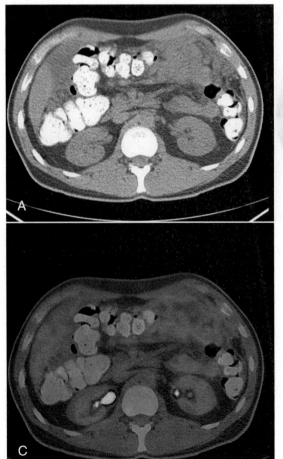
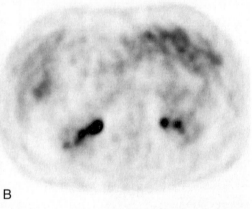

FIGURE 11-5. **A** to **C,** Sample SPECT/CT images showing the anatomic (CT) rendering (**A**), the physiologic (SPECT) image (**B**), and the fused SPECT/CT image (**C**) in the transaxial and coronal plane. Study demonstrates a unilateral stress fracture in the fourth lumbar vertebra. *Continued*

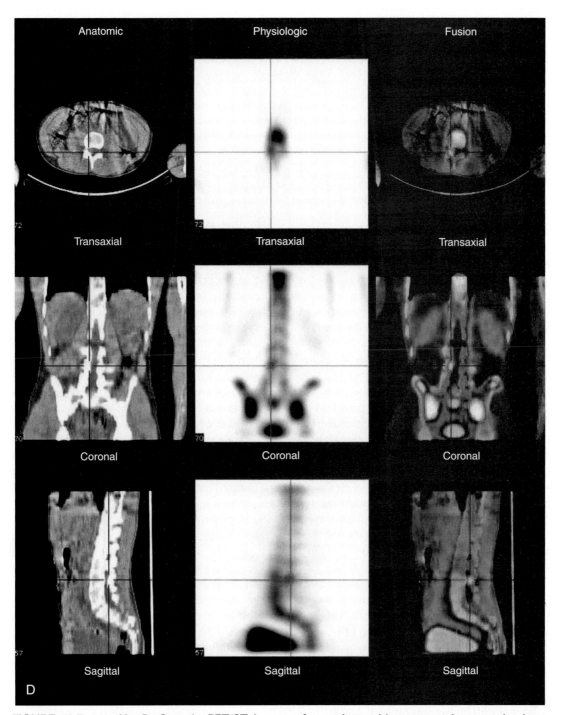

FIGURE 11-5, *cont'd.*   **D,** Sample PET/CT image of a patient with suspected omental adeno-carcinoma. The left column represents the CT scan image, the center column demonstrates the PET scan image, and the right column shows the combined image (PET/CT) showing the pathology.

The fusion process is not without disadvantages, such as the ultimate cost of the system and the controversy regarding the necessity for dual modality personnel. As fusion imaging becomes more available the cost associated with it will necessarily be reduced. The personnel issue is currently under discussion, and dual certifications have been discussed. Changes in educational programs and the certification process have also been discussed and are in the process of being implemented.

Fusion imaging is being used in the areas of cardiology, neurology, and oncology at the present time. In cardiology the detection of coronary artery disease and congestive heart failure can be accomplished by means of an injection rather than angiography. Neurologic studies are being performed to demonstrate physiologic changes in the brain to aid in the early diagnosis of Alzheimer's disease. The oncologic use of fusion imaging enables the early detection of cancer as well as more precise tumor detection and localization. This relatively noninvasive diagnostic tool provides the potential for the early diagnosis of pathologic conditions and the benefit of more precise treatment regimens.

SUMMARY

Nuclear medicine technology is gaining more importance as a diagnostic tool in diagnostic imaging. It utilizes radioactive emissions from a patient to produce an image that can be used to diagnose a variety of disease processes both functionally and structurally. Emission imaging relies on the production (generation) of various radiopharmaceuticals that when injected into the patient will collect in specific locations and produce radioactive emissions during its decay process. The units of activity are expressed as the curie and the becquerel.

The half-life of the radionuclide is determined when one half of its activity is left in the decay process. Effective half-life is both the biologic and physical half-life of a radiopharmaceutical. The biologic half-life is used when discussing the elimination of the radionuclide from the body. The physical half-life is the amount of time that it takes for one half of the radionuclide to decay.

Acquisition of the data is accomplished using a variety of tools. The most common system is the Anger camera. This system uses scintillation crystals coupled to photomultiplier tubes or solid state detectors. The radioactive emissions striking the scintillation crystal stimulate them to produce light that is collected by the photomultiplier tube or detector and converted to an electrical signal. This signal is then reconverted to light and captured either on film or collected directly by a computer. The computer then generates the image.

Single photon emission computed tomography uses standard radionuclides and either a series of detectors that surround the patient or rotating Anger cameras to produce images that represent layers or slices within the subject. The computer reconstructs the data using a specific algorithm to produce the image. As the name implies, this type of system uses radionuclides that will produce a single photon as the decay process progresses.

Positron emission tomography, unlike SPECT, requires the use of specialized radionuclides that produce positrons. These positrons then undergo an annihilation reaction with a resting electron to produce two opposing photons, each possessing 0.51 MeV of energy (energy that is equivalent to the rest mass of an electron). A PET system with a series of ring detectors then collects the data, and the computer manipulates the data to produce a more accurate image than either of the systems already discussed. The disadvantages of this type of system are the higher initial cost, the necessity for a cyclotron if specialized, the short half-life radionuclides used, and the higher operational costs.

Fusion imaging is the combination of more than one modality into a single system. This provides both structural and functional information to the physician to aid in the detection and treatment planning of a variety of disease processes.

REFERENCE

1. Wagner HN: Hal Anger: nuclear medicine's quiet genius. *J Nucl Med* 44:11, 2003.

SUGGESTED READINGS

Chandra R: *Nuclear Medicine Physics: The Basics*, 5th ed. Baltimore, 1998, Williams & Wilkins.

Cherry S, Sorenson JA, Phelps M: *Physics in Nuclear Medicine*, 3rd ed. Philadelphia, 2003, Elsevier.

Mettler FA, Guiberteau MJ: *Essentials of Nuclear Medicine Imaging*, 4th ed, Philadelphia, 1998, Elsevier.

RSNA 88th Scientific Assembly: Abstracts 383, 388; presented Dec. 2, 2002.

RSNA 88th Scientific Assembly: CT/PET Fusion Imaging Special Focus session; presented Dec. 4, 2002

Sandler MP, Coleman RE, Wackers FJ, et al: *Diagnostic Nuclear Medicine*, 4th ed. Baltimore, 2002, Williams & Wilkins.

Thrall JH, Ziessman HA: *Nuclear Medicine: Requisites Series*, 2nd ed. Philadelphia, 2001, Elsevier.

STUDY QUESTIONS

1. The type of emission tomography that utilizes the single photon emitted during the decay of a radionuclide is called:
   a. PET
   b. CT
   c. PET/CT
   d. SPECT

2. The measurement that is used to describe the fact that one half of the radionuclide has been eliminated from the body is the:
   a. half value layer
   b. biologic half-life
   c. physical half-life
   d. physical half value layer

3. Which of the following is not a contraindication for the performance of a nuclear medicine study:
   i. previous allergic reaction
   ii. pregnancy
   iii. hormone imbalance
   a. i only
   b. iii only
   c. i and ii only
   d. i and iii only

4. The unit of measurement that represents a radioactivity equal to 3.7×10^{10} disintegrations per second is referred to as a:
   a. roentgen
   b. becquerel
   c. sievert
   d. curie

5. Which of the following are methods used to generate radionuclides?
   i. reactor generated
   ii. milked and filtered
   iii. fission
   a. i only
   b. i and ii only
   c. i and iii only
   d. i, ii, and iii

6. _____ imaging requires that images be made in more than one plane in order to make a diagnosis by allowing the separation of the structures that have been superimposed.
   a. Planar
   b. Emission recording
   c. Tomography
   d. Scintillation

7. A _____ is a radionuclide that has been modified by chemically combining it with various biochemicals that may have physiologic or metabolic properties that would be beneficial in a particular study.
   a. contrast agent
   b. radiopharmaceutical
   c. metabolic isotope
   d. fission product

Fundamentals of Special Radiographic Procedures

STUDY QUESTIONS (*cont'd*)

8. When certain substances are stimulated by ionizing radiation, they can emit light. In nuclear medicine this is referred to as:
   a. scintillation
   b. solid state crystallization
   c. phosphorescence
   d. luminescence

9. In an annihilation reaction two photons are emitted in opposite directions, each having an energy equal to _____ MeV.
   a. 10
   b. 511
   c. 1.02
   d. 0.511

10. In PET imaging _____ emitting radionuclides are used to create the image.
    a. negatron
    b. positron
    c. back projection
    d. Anger photon

12 *Cardiac and Thoracic Procedures*

CHAPTER OBJECTIVES

After completing this chapter, the reader will be able to perform the following:

- Discuss vascular pathology
- Discuss the anatomy of the heart and its vasculature
- Discuss the anatomy of the thoracic aorta
- Discuss the anatomy of the pulmonary circulation
- List the indications and contraindications for angiography in these areas
- List the various procedures that can be performed in these areas
- Discuss vessel access for these procedures
- Discuss hemodynamics and the various calculations performed during cardiac catheterization
- Discuss the contrast agents used in cardiac catheterization
- List the specialized equipment found in the cardiac catheterization suite
- List the patient positions for cardiac angiography
- Identify common complications of these procedures

CHAPTER OUTLINE

NORMAL BLOOD VESSEL STRUCTURE

COMMON VASCULAR PATHOPHYSIOLOGY

ANATOMIC CONSIDERATIONS

- Heart
- Thoracic Aorta
- Coronary Vasculature
- Left Main Coronary Artery
- Right Main Coronary Artery
- Venous Drainage
- Pulmonary Circulation

INDICATIONS AND CONTRAINDICATIONS

DIAGNOSTIC PROCEDURES

- Aortography
- Cardiac Catheterization
- Coronary Arteriography
- Pulmonary Arteriography
- Vessel Access
- Vessel Closure

HEMODYNAMICS AND CALCULATIONS

- Calculation of Stenotic Valve Area—Gorlin Method
- Cardiac Output Calculation
- Shunt Detection and Calculation

CONTRAST AGENTS

Numerous **diagnostic** studies can be performed on the vasculature of the heart, lungs, and thoracic aorta. In most cases these diagnostic procedures are done with the intent of performing interventions, if possible, in order to correct any pathophysiology that might be identified. The common cardiac and vascular interventions that can be performed will be discussed in Chapters 17 and 18. The interventional studies usually involve the same parameters as the diagnostic procedures, and the basic principles from the diagnostic chapters will not be repeated in the discussion about interventions.

Generalized vascular pathology will be discussed in this chapter. The pathophysiology of the vasculature spans the entire circulatory system. The following discussion will serve to lay the groundwork for the various disease processes that will be treated in the interventional section of this book.

The thoracic cavity contains the heart, great vessels, aorta, and pulmonary circulation. Some of the procedures that are performed in this area are aortography, cardiac catheterization, coronary arteriography, and pulmonary arteriography. Discussion of the studies performed on the abdominal aorta and its associated vessels can be found in Chapters 13 and 14 .

The circulatory system is responsible for moving the blood throughout the body in order to bring oxygen and nutrients to the various tissues and remove any waste products for elimination. It consists of a pump (the heart), conduits to move the blood from place to place (arteries and veins), and locations where the nutrients and wastes are transferred (lungs, kidneys, and gastrointestinal system). As in any closed system, problems can occur that compromise its normal function. The common situations that cause malfunction of the system are leaks, reduced or increased flow, and directional anomalies that can cause flow in the wrong direction. The purpose of diagnostic and interventional angiography is to identify and possibly correct these problems.

Before a discussion of the gross anatomy of the circulatory system can be held it is important to understand the structure of the blood vessels, one of the important components of the circulatory system. The gross anatomy of the heart, location of the blood vessels, and operations of the transfer stations (lungs, kidneys, and gastrointestinal system) will be discussed in each of their representative chapters.

NORMAL BLOOD VESSEL STRUCTURE

Normal blood vessels are muscular tubes that consist of three layers: the tunica intima (interna), tunica media, and tunica adventitia (externa). The tunica intima is essentially a lining of endothelial cells over a layer of connective tissue separating the blood from the vessel proper. This layer is important for maintaining homeostasis in the circulatory system and subsequently is the site of much of the vascular pathology. It gets its nutrients from direct diffusion from the lumen of the vessel. Small arterioles (vasa vasorum) that permeate the adventitia and media provide the vessels with a supply of nutrients and oxygen.

The endothelial cells secrete a variety of hormones that allow the vessel to react to a variety of stressors and are vital in the vessel's response to injury. The endothelial cells also help to prevent clotting by secreting chemicals that inhibit the aggregation of platelets. Substances are also secreted by the endothelial cells that help control the relaxation (vasodilation) and contraction (vasoconstriction) of the vessels.

The media is the next layer of the blood vessels. This layer is composed of smooth muscle cells, elastic fibers, and connective tissue. The muscle cells and connective tissue of this layer provide support for the vessel walls, while the elastic fibers give it the capability to respond to the pressure changes from the systolic and diastolic action of the heart by changing the diameter of the vessel. Arteries have a larger muscular layer than do veins because they are subject to the direct pressures from the contractions and relaxation phases of the heart. The movement of blood in the veins is controlled by pressure gradients, folds in the endothelial layer that act in a similar manner to the valves of the heart (preventing the backflow of blood) and the contraction of the muscles surrounding the veins. The amount of elasticity depends upon the vessel. Larger arteries such as the aorta have a greater response than do smaller less elastic arteries.

The outer layer of the vessels is composed primarily of a thin layer of connective tissue, irregular elastic, and collagen fibers. This is the means by which the vessels are attached to the local body tissues. The tunica adventitia (externa) of the larger veins and their tributaries has a thicker layer of collagen and elastic fibers than do the arteries. Overall, the veins have relatively thin walls when compared to the arteries because they do not have to withstand the types of pressure changes that occur in the arteries. It is because of this factor that the veins do not have a similar pathophysiology to the arteries.

The arteries and veins of the circulatory system are connected by means of the capillary bed. As the vessels get smaller and smaller they form many branches that create the capillary network. The arteries become arterioles (very small vessels), which give off many smaller vessels called capillaries. These capillaries then collect into a group of venules (very small vessels that resemble the arterial capillaries). The capillary beds are where the diffusion of materials takes place across the walls of these small vessels.

COMMON VASCULAR PATHOPHYSIOLOGY

The arteries are subjected to a number of pathologic situations because of their structure and function. The endothelial lining of the vessel is designed to provide a smooth surface for the blood cells and platelets to move easily through the lumen. Just as in home plumbing, the action of the materials passing through the pipes can cause a narrowing of its inside diameter, restricting the flow of water. The arteries are similar in that some of the materials (platelets) passing through the vessel may become lodged on the interior wall of the vessel, and the prolonged exposure to the high pressures from the heart, trauma, or infection can trigger a response from the cells of the intima. The normal physiology of the cells of the tunica intima can cause the deposition of new endothelial cells over the area, reducing the vessel lumen and ultimately the flow of blood. The narrowing can be the result of arterial stenosis (atherosclerosis), thrombosis, or intimal hyperplasia. Stenosis is also found in veins, although not as often because the pressures are lower in the system.

Blockage of the vessel can occur if some material (embolus) dislodges and travels through the circulatory path until it becomes lodged in one of the vessels. The blockage effectively stops the flow of blood to the distal vessels and over time the blockage increases on the proximal side of the vessel. This type of pathophysiology lends itself to treatment utilizing interventional techniques.

Another common pathophysiologic process results from the constant expansion and contraction of the artery due to the pulsations from the heart. Exposure to a high level of pressure change can cause the vessel to lose its elasticity, causing an abnormal enlargement of the vessel (greater than 50% of its original diameter) accompanied by a thinning of the media and adventitia due to the loss of collagen, muscle, and elastic fibers. Veins, on the other hand, are not as prone to aneurysms (abnormal enlargement with vessel weakness) as arteries; however, they can lose the capacity for normal valve action, creating a condition of reversed blood flow.

Various congenital arteriovenous malformations can result in the increased flow of blood. These are generally present at birth and can increase in size and complexity as the child develops, making interventional treatment difficult. Malformations can occur in the venous system as well; however, these defects are not high flow disorders and are easier to treat by means of interventional radiographic procedures.

Fundamentals of Special Radiographic Procedures

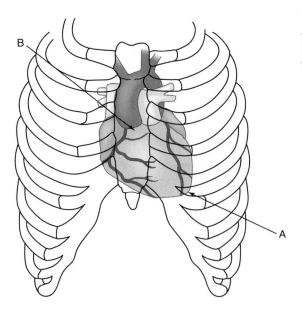

FIGURE 12-1. Schematic of the heart within the thoracic cavity showing the apex (A), the base (B), and their relationship to the bony thorax.

ANATOMIC CONSIDERATIONS

Heart

The heart is a hollow muscular organ that lies obliquely in the left median portion of the lower thoracic cavity. It adjusts the circulation of the blood to the metabolic rate of the tissue cells; in essence, it is a pump.

The heart has an apex and a base. The apex is located approximately 8 cm from the median plane at about the level of the fifth or sixth interspace; this level is approximately 2.5 cm inferior to the left nipple. The base of the heart is the most superior portion. It faces up and to the right, and from it emerge the greater vessels (Fig. 12-1).

An obliquely placed septum divides the heart into right and left halves. Each half consists of two chambers—an *atrium* and a *ventricle* (Fig. 12-2).

The atria receive blood from the veins, and the ventricles propel blood into the arteries. Blood from the heart flows in two circuits—a short circulation (lesser circuit) called the *pulmonary* and a longer, more extensive one (greater circuit) called the *systemic*.

The anatomy of the heart is easily understood if it is related to the flow of blood through it. Therefore, the anatomy of the heart is presented in relation to the blood flow, beginning with the drainage from the systemic circulation.

Blood returning from the systemic veins drains into the venae cavae. These great veins—the superior and inferior venae cavae—empty into the right atrium of the heart (Fig. 12-3). A small amount of venous blood drains from the myocardium directly into the right atrium; however, in general, the greatest portion of venous blood from the systemic circulation drains into the superior and inferior venae cavae.

With the contraction (systole) of the right atrium, the blood is forced into the right ventricle through the right atrioventricular aperture. This aperture is equipped with a valve, the tricuspid valve, that prevents the backflow of blood to the right atrium during systole of the ventricle. As the ventricle contracts, the blood is forced past the pulmonary semilunar valve into the pulmonary trunk and the lesser circulation. The arterial, or outflowing, portion of the right ventricle is called the conus arteriosus.[1] The pulmonary artery divides into right and left sides, which take the blood through the lungs. Here, the blood gives off carbon dioxide and becomes oxygenated. It is then transported by the four pulmonary veins to the left atrium (Fig. 12-4).

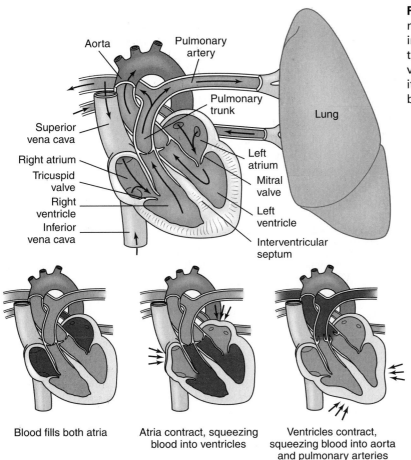

FIGURE 12-2. Schematic of the heart showing the four chambers, the valves, the great vessels associated with it, and the flow of blood through it.

Blood fills both atria

Atria contract, squeezing blood into ventricles

Ventricles contract, squeezing blood into aorta and pulmonary arteries

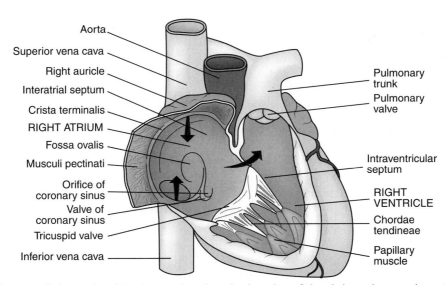

FIGURE 12-3. Schematic of the heart showing the interior of the right atrium and ventricle. The arrows indicate the flow of blood from the venae cavae to the right atrium and from the right atrium to the right ventricle.

Fundamentals of Special Radiographic Procedures

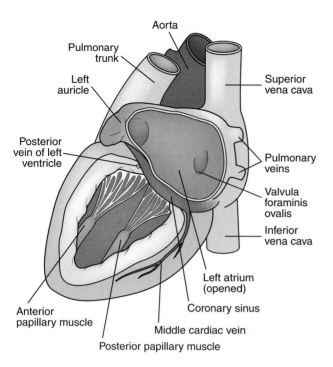

FIGURE 12-4. Schematic of the heart showing the left atrium and ventricle. The blood flows from the pulmonary veins to the left atrium, through the mitral valve into the left ventricle, and from there into the systemic circulation.

As the left atrium contracts, it forces the blood through the left atrioventricular valve into the left ventricle. This is the largest chamber of the heart, and its walls are considerably thicker than those of any other chambers. The thicker walls and larger capacity are necessary to offset the arterial pressure in the aorta. The upper anterior portion of the left ventricle is called the aortic vestibule.[1] As the left ventricle contracts, the blood is pushed through the aortic semilunar valve into the aorta and through the systemic circulation (Fig. 12-5). The blood returns from the body tissues through the systemic veins, which ultimately drain into the superior and inferior venae cavae; then the cycle begins again.

The cardiac cycle is repeated about 75 times per minute, and the time required for each cycle is about 0.8 s. The cycle consists of three phases—*atrial contraction (systole), ventricular contraction (systole),* and *complete rest (diastole)* (Fig. 12-6).

Thoracic Aorta

The aorta can be subdivided into four parts — the aortic root, ascending aorta, aortic arch, and descending aorta.

The aortic root or bulb begins at the level of the aortic semilunar valve. The three leaflets of the aortic valve form the aortic sinuses, right, left, and posterior. The right and left aortic sinus house the openings to the coronary arteries, which provide the heart muscle with the necessary nutrients for survival.

The ascending aorta originates at the base of the heart with the root of the aorta. The aortic sinuses are found in the wall of the root of the aorta. These are related to the cusps of the aortic valve and are named for them—right, left, and posterior. Two of these sinuses—the right and the left—contain the orifices of the coronary arteries. The ascending aorta extends anterosuperior from the base of the heart and slightly to the right for approximately 5 cm and terminates by becoming the arch of the aorta, which is usually at the level of the sternal angle (Fig. 12-7).

The aortic arch courses from right to left as well as from anterior to posterior. It lies in almost a true sagittal plane (Fig. 12-8). From the sternal angle, the aortic arch ascends toward the left. As it ascends, it is directed posterior. The upper portion of the arch courses posterior to the left of the

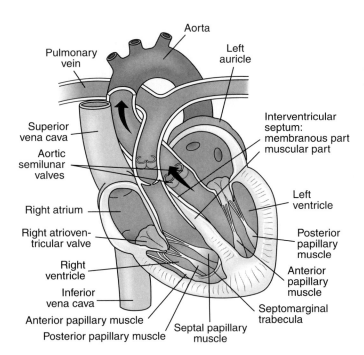

FIGURE 12-5. Schematic of the internal anatomy of the heart. The blood from the left ventricle passes through the aortic valve and into the general circulation.

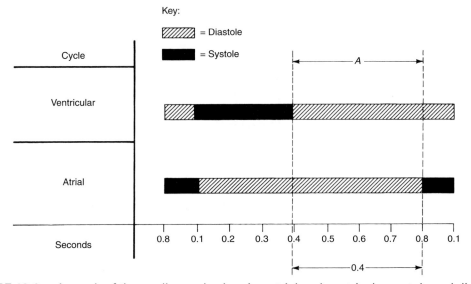

FIGURE 12-6. A graph of the cardiac cycle showing atrial and ventricular systole and diastole. It can be seen that the actual period of diastole is 0.7 s for the atria and 0.15 s for the ventricles. These periods overlap, giving the heart a period of 0.4 s of complete quiescence (A).

trachea and esophagus. At about the level of the fourth thoracic vertebra, it turns inferior and runs a short distance before becoming the descending aorta.

There are three major branches given off by the aortic arch—the brachiocephalic trunk, the left common carotid artery, and the left subclavian artery (Fig. 12-9). These branches supply the head and upper extremities with blood.

The descending aorta is a continuation of the aortic arch. It can be divided into a superior **thoracic** descending and an inferior **abdominal** descending portion. The thoracic descending aorta

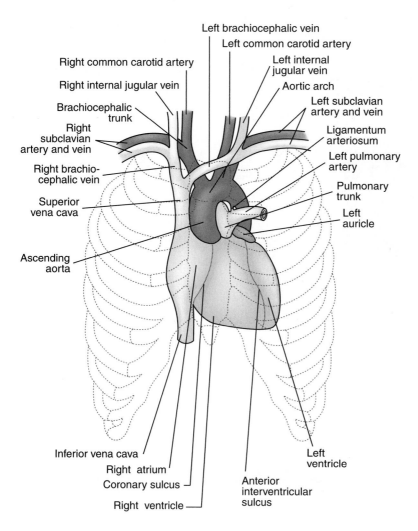

Left brachiocephalic vein

Left common carotid artery

Right common carotid artery

Left internal jugular vein

Right internal jugular vein

Aortic arch

Brachiocephalic trunk

Left subclavian artery and vein

Right subclavian artery and vein

Ligamentum arteriosum

Right brachio-cephalic vein

Left pulmonary artery

Superior vena cava

Pulmonary trunk

Left auricle

Ascending aorta

Inferior vena cava

Left ventricle

Right atrium

Coronary sulcus

Anterior interventricular sulcus

Right ventricle

FIGURE 12-7. The heart and great vessels within the bony thorax. Note that the ascending aorta changes to the aortic arch at the level of the sternal angle.

extends from its origin at the level of the intervertebral disk between the fourth and fifth thoracic vertebrae to the point at which it traverses the aortic hiatus in the diaphragm (Fig. 12-10), which is about the level of the twelfth thoracic vertebra. As the thoracic aorta passes through the opening in the diaphragm, it becomes the abdominal portion of the descending aorta.

The branches of the thoracic descending aorta can be classified as either parietal or visceral and may be summarized as follows:

Parietal branches

    Posterior intercostal arteries

    Subcostal arteries

    Superior phrenic arteries

    Vas aberrans artery

Visceral branches

    Bronchial arteries

    Esophageal arteries

    Pericardial artery

    Mediastinal artery

The parietal branches supply the body wall of the thoracic cavity, whereas the visceral branches supply the organs contained within the thoracic cavity.

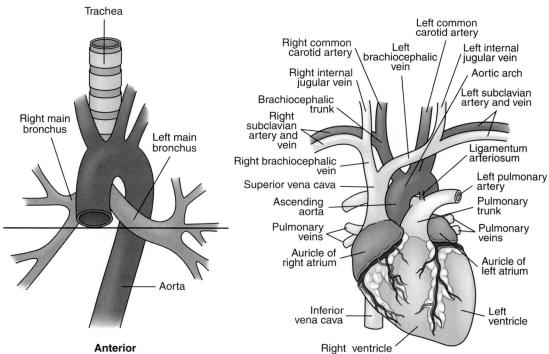

FIGURE 12-8. The aortic arch in the anterior view. From this aspect, the aortic arch is almost in a direct sagittal plane.

FIGURE 12-9. The aortic arch and its major branches.

Coronary Vasculature

The coronary arteries are the source of blood supplying the heart. The aorta is the origin of the two main coronary arteries (Fig. 12-11). Three small dilations, or sinuses, are located in the root of the aorta. They lie opposite the corresponding cusps of the aortic valve. The coronary arteries arise from two of these, so they are considered coronary sinuses. The third sinus is considered a noncoronary sinus because it does not connect directly with any coronary arteries.

The *left main coronary artery* arises from the left posterior aortic sinus, and the *right main coronary artery* originates from the anterior, or right, aortic sinus. These sinuses are called the aortic sinuses, or *Valsalva's* sinuses.

Left Main Coronary Artery

This artery originates in the left aortic sinus. It arises from a single opening in the upper portion of the sinus, and its length can vary from 2 to 3 mm to 3 to 4 cm. It divides to form the anterior interventricular branch (left anterior descending artery) and the left circumflex branch (Fig. 12-12). These branches occupy the anterior interventricular sulcus and the atrioventricular sulcus, respectively. This oversimplification of the bifurcation of the left main coronary artery is provided because usually no more than two large branches of this artery can be found.[1]

The anterior interventricular branch is considered a direct continuation of the left main coronary artery. It courses toward the apex of the heart in the anterior interventricular sulcus. In the frontal view, the left anterior interventricular branch plus the left main coronary artery form a gently reversed "S" curve. After reaching the apex of the heart, the left anterior interventricular branch continues up into the posterior interventricular sulcus and anastomoses with the terminal branches of the posterior interventricular branch of the right coronary artery. Along its route, the left anterior interventricular

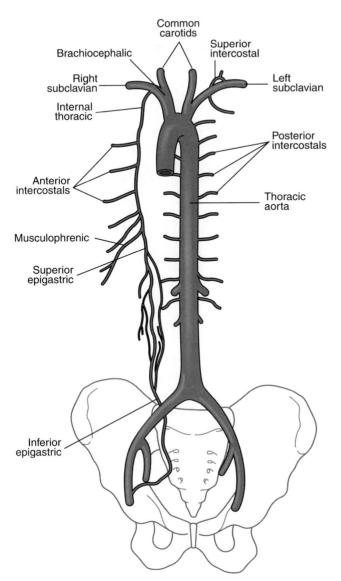

FIGURE 12-10. Route of the descending aorta.

branch gives off a variable number of arteries that course into the interventricular septum. At the level of the pulmonary valve, smaller branches are given off that supply the right ventricle. One or more of these branches form a curve around the heart and meet similar branches of the proximal right coronary artery. This circle is called Vieussens' ring, and it is an important means of collateral circulation between the right and left coronary arteries. Some larger branches are given off to supply the free wall of the left ventricle. At times, one or more of these branches arise at the point of division of the left main coronary artery; these are usually called the diagonal left ventricular arteries.

The left circumflex coronary artery, which is the second major branch of the left main coronary artery, courses at a sharp angle from its origin toward the left atrioventricular sulcus. It travels in this groove around to the back of the heart toward the right coronary artery, where anastomosis of these arteries frequently occurs. The circumflex artery gives off a large branch called the left marginal artery. The left marginal artery courses along the left margin of the heart to supply the left ventricle. Branches of the left marginal artery course over the free wall of the left ventricle somewhat parallel to those given off by the left anterior interventricular branch (left anterior descending artery).

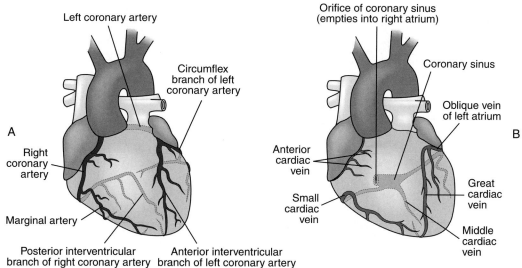

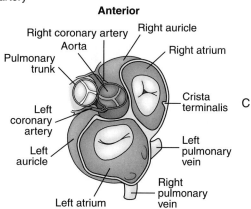

FIGURE 12-11. The coronary arteries. **A**, An external view of the heart, showing the course of the left and right coronary arteries from their origin at the root of the aorta. **B**, An external view of the heart showing the venous vasculature. **C**, Schematic of the three aortic sinuses at the root of the aorta, the origin of the coronary arteries, and their relation to the surrounding cardiac anatomy.

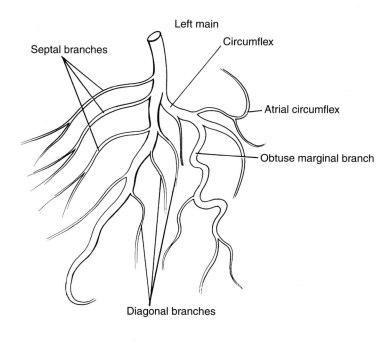

FIGURE 12-12. Left coronary artery in left anterior oblique projection with cephalad angulation.

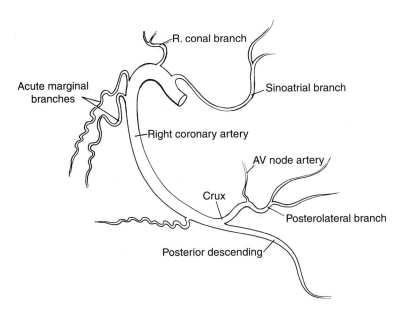

FIGURE 12-13. The right coronary artery in left anterior oblique projection with cephalad angulation. Note that the crux is well visualized.

Right Main Coronary Artery

Frequently, the right main coronary artery has two aortic ostia, which may arise from the anterior aortic sinus and from a smaller adjacent ostium. When present, the second ostium is very small—about 1 mm in diameter. This is called the conus artery of the right coronary system (Fig. 12-13). It is this artery that frequently anastomoses with an opposing branch from the left anterior interventricular artery, forming Vieussens' ring. When the right main coronary artery arises from a single ostium in the aortic sinus, the first ventricular branch is considered the conus artery.

From its origin in the aortic sinus, the right main coronary artery courses in the right atrioventricular sulcus (coronary sulcus) to the diaphragmatic surface of the heart. At the acute margin of the heart, the right coronary artery gives off an artery called the right marginal branch, which courses almost to the apex of the heart. On the diaphragmatic surface of the heart, the right coronary artery makes a U turn and courses toward the apex of the heart in the posterior interventricular sulcus. This terminal portion of the right coronary artery is called the posterior interventricular branch (posterior descending artery).

The U turn of the right coronary artery is located at the crux of the heart. This is the point at which the right and left atrioventricular sulci cross the posterior interatrial and interventricular sulci. It is also here that the atrioventricular node artery originates from the right coronary artery.

On reaching the apex of the heart, the posterior interventricular branch frequently anastomoses with the anterior interventricular branch of the left coronary artery.

Venous Drainage

The venous drainage of the heart is considered to consist of three separate groups, rather than one.

The first group from the area of the left ventricle drains into the coronary sinus. Some prominent veins in this system are the anterior interventricular, posterior interventricular (middle cardiac), and left marginal veins. As it enters the atrioventricular sulcus, the anterior interventricular vein becomes the great cardiac vein, which in turn becomes the coronary sinus. The posterior interventricular vein usually drains directly into the right atrium; however, it often joins the coronary sinus just before entering the atrium. The left marginal vein and associated smaller vessels drain from the left ventricle into the great cardiac vein and coronary sinus.

In the second group, several large veins called the anterior cardiac veins transport venous blood from the area of the right ventricle and drain directly into the right atrium. The most prominent of these veins—the right marginal vein—drains the lower margin of the heart.

The third group consists of many very small veins, thebesian veins, which are often found on the right side of the heart but seldom on the left side. These small venous tributaries begin in the myocardium and drain directly into the cardiac chambers. They are found primarily in the right atrium and right ventricle.

Pulmonary Circulation

The right portion of the heart receives oxygen-poor blood via the superior and inferior venae cavae and directs it to the pulmonary circulation for oxygenation. Some blood is also sent to the bronchial arteries to supply the trachea, bronchi, esophagus, and posterior mediastinum. The pulmonary vasculature is also supplied with nutrients by the small vessels called the vasa vasorum. The pulmonary circulation can be divided into three portions: the pulmonary arteries, the alveolar capillary system, and the pulmonary veins. The right atrium propels the blood through the main pulmonary artery (pulmonary trunk), which branches off into a right and left main pulmonary artery. Each of these arteries services its respective lung, entering at the level of the hilum.

Right Pulmonary Artery

Upon entering the lung the right main pulmonary artery branches into three lobar branches. Each of the three lobes of the right lung is supplied by its respective branch of the right pulmonary artery. The branches supplying the lobes give off a number of smaller vessels to provide a blood supply to the bronchopulmonary segments. The segmental branches continue to subdivide and are reduced in size until they terminate as small arterioles, which terminate in capillary beds in the walls of the alveoli.

Left Pulmonary Artery

As the left pulmonary artery enters the hilum it gives off two branches corresponding to the upper and lower lobes of the lung. These branches also subdivide, corresponding to the bronchopulmonary segments, and terminate in the alveolar capillary beds.

The capillary beds in the alveoli are where the gaseous exchange of oxygen and carbon dioxide from the blood to the air occurs.

The blood moves through the pulmonary capillary beds into the small venules. These unite into larger and larger channels, maintaining the same association with the bronchopulmonary segments that the arteries demonstrated. This continues until a single vein for each of the lobes of the lung is formed. The vein from the middle lobe and superior lobe of the right lung join, resulting in two pulmonary veins leaving the right lung. The veins exiting from the left lung also result in two vessels. The four pulmonary veins end in the left atrium of the heart. From here the blood is passed through to the left ventricle and out into the systemic circulation.

INDICATIONS AND CONTRAINDICATIONS

Aortography is indicated when information concerning the state of the aorta and its branches is necessary for therapeutic, surgical, or endovascular intervention. However, the procedure has been all but replaced as a screening tool for diagnosis by **magnetic resonance angiography (MRA)** and **three-dimensional computed tomography (3D CT)**. Nevertheless, catheter aortography is still used as a preoperative tool by many surgeons because it allows an accurate preoperative evaluation concerning the nature, number, and course of the great vessels of the chest and abdomen. As they become more refined, MRA and 3D CT will more than likely replace catheter aortography as the method of choice for evaluation of the aorta and its branches.

Some specific indications for the procedure include suspected aneurysms, congenital anomalies, and many acquired diseases affecting the thoracic aorta. Table 12-1 lists specific indications for angiography of the thoracic aorta, cardiac circulation, and pulmonary circulation.

Thoracic aortography and cardiac catheterization are accomplished primarily to demonstrate the coronary arteries and cardiac anatomy as well as to perform hemodynamic measurements to identify a variety of disease processes. The studies can be done to demonstrate pathophysiology of the thoracic aorta and pulmonary and peripheral vasculature. Interventions can also be accomplished as an adjunct to the diagnostic procedures or as stand-alone procedures once the pathology has been defined.

The contraindications to angiography can be divided into those that are physiologic in nature and those that are related to the toxic effects of the contrast agents. Physiologic contraindications, which are also related to the specific procedural techniques used, include femoral arteriosclerosis, which contraindicates the retrograde transfemoral approach to avoid intimal damage, and aneurysms at the injection site, which contraindicate the use of the direct puncture technique. Some other contraindications to these procedures are infection, fever, high blood pressure, acute gastrointestinal bleeding, and renal failure

Sensitivity to iodine is an example of a toxic effect of a contrast agent that contraindicates the procedure. Patients with severe hepatorenal disease should be carefully evaluated to determine the advisability of performing the study. This, however, is not an absolute contraindication to aortography.

DIAGNOSTIC PROCEDURES

Aortography

Aortography is the radiographic technique used to diagnose vascular pathology of the aorta and lower extremities. Aortography is frequently referred to by the method used to introduce the catheter into the aorta. Translumbar aortography is performed infrequently; however, this approach is still viable in patients having pathology that would preclude the use of catheterization at other access sites, such as occlusion of the suprarenal inferior vena cava and infrarenal aortic occlusion.

Aortography can be performed to visualize the thoracic or abdominal aorta. In both cases, the contrast medium is injected into the lumen of the aorta through one of the methods of vessel access. Using the percutaneous catheter approach, both flush and selective studies of the visceral vasculature can be accomplished via aortography depending on the level of catheter placement within the lumen of the aorta.

Cardiac Catheterization

Selective studies such as pulmonary angiography, left and right heart catheterization, and coronary angiography can be performed following aortography depending upon the physical examination of the anatomy, patient history, results of cardiac stress tests, electrocardiography anomalies, and findings from plain film x-rays. One of the most common selective procedures is coronary angiography. It is done to image the coronary vasculature, its branches, and collateral circulations for diagnosis and treatment planning. Right and left cardiac catheterization can also be performed to take various hemodynamic measurements and view the internal anatomy of the heart. Endomyocardial biopsies can be done as well as a variety of interventional procedures.

Coronary Arteriography

Before discussing the various procedures used for coronary arteriography, an understanding of the circulatory physiology of the coronary artery system is necessary.

Unlike other vascular filling that occurs during the systolic phase of the cardiac cycle, the coronary arteries accept blood only during diastole. This is understood easily if you recall the location of the ostia of the coronary arteries at the root of the aorta. In this location, as the systolic phase occurs, the comparatively small coronary vessels are compressed, preventing the forward flow of blood through the

TABLE 12-1   *Summary of Indications for Angiography of the Structures in the Thoracic Cavity*

Procedure	Indications
Thoracic Aortography	
Congenital anomalies	Abnormal position of specific vessels
	Abnormal number of specific vessels
	Patent ductus arteriosus
	Coarctation and pseudocoarctation of the aorta
	Aortic pulmonary window
	Aortic arch anomalies
	Pulmonary sequestration
	Truncus arteriosus
	Aortic diverticula
	Ruptured aortic sinus aneurysm
	Aortic stenosis
Acquired diseases	Preoperative mapping of aneurysms of the aorta and brachiocephalic vessels
	Aortic stenosis
	Obstructive disease of the aorta
	Aortic insufficiency
	Buckling of the aorta and brachiocephalic vessels
Coronary Arteriography	
Coronary atherosclerosis	Evaluation of collateral pathways
	Preoperative evaluation of disease
	Assessment of surgical results
	Evaluation of drug therapy
Chest pain of uncertain origin	
Valvular heart disease	
Congenital coronary abnormalities	Septal defects
	Aortic arch anomalies
	Increased cardiac size
	Anomalous left coronary artery
	Primary endocardial fibroelastosis
	Tetralogy of Fallot
	Peripheral pulmonary arterial stenosis
	Valvular pulmonary stenosis
Acquired vascular diseases	
Cardiomyopathy	
Preoperative and postoperative evaluations of patients undergoing cardiac surgery	
Pulmonary Arteriography	
Acute or chronic pulmonary embolism	
Pulmonary artery hypertension	Parenchymal lung disease
	Chronic hypoventilation
	Elevated left atrial pressure
	Elevated venous pressure
	Vasculitis
Pulmonary artery stenosis	
Pulmonary arteriovenous fistulas	
Arteriovenous malformations	
Pulmonary artery aneurysms or pseudoaneurysms	
Tumors	Chondrosarcoma
	Leiomyosarcoma
	Fibrosarcoma
	Spindle cell sarcoma
Hemoptysis	Bronchial arterial bleeding

coronary vascular system. During the diastolic phase, however, this compression is released, and the forward flow of blood in the coronary vascular system can occur. *Therefore, the optimal time for injection of contrast medium is during cardiac diastole.* This phase is relatively short, and simply attempting to inject during this phase is inadequate without improving the forward flow of the contrast medium by other means. An obvious improvement is to prolong the diastolic phase, with a corresponding increase in the inflow of the coronary vascular system.

Another factor affecting the visualization of the coronary vascular system is the cardiac output during systole. If an injection of contrast medium is made at the root of the aorta, considerable dilution occurs as a result of the high velocity of blood flow from the heart. A method by which the high concentration of contrast can be maintained is the reduction of the velocity of blood flowing from the heart, which in essence reduces cardiac output.

Successful opacification of the coronary vessels also depends on the flow of contrast agent into and through the coronary vascular system itself. Therefore, it is necessary to increase forward flow through the coronary vascular system by decreasing coronary resistance and increasing aortic diastolic pressure. This can be accomplished with the use of coronary vasodilators and occlusion of the aorta, respectively. One result of the injection of the contrast medium into the vascular system is vasodilation, which promotes an increase in flow.

The methods used to opacify the coronary vascular system can be divided into two broad categories—the nonselective, or aortic flush, methods and the selective catheterization methods.

All of the nonselective methods involve high-pressure injection of a large amount of contrast agent at the root of the aorta. Variations in the efficiency of the method occur when modifications of techniques are used. The simplest nonselective method consists of a random injection of a large amount of contrast agent at the root of the aorta. This method is grossly inefficient because of the physiologic factors discussed previously. Various modifications of the basic nonselective injection technique have been used in an attempt to create ideal physiologic conditions during the injection. Among these have been the additions of the electrocardiography-activated automatic syringe, which can phase the injection of contrast agent with the diastolic phase of the cardiac cycle. This technique results in improved coronary visualization with the use of smaller amounts of contrast agents.

Other modifications of the random nonselective injection that improve visualization of the coronary artery system include the use of acetylcholine-induced cardiac arrest, which effectively prolongs the diastolic phase and improves filling of the coronary vessels; aortic occlusion with specialized balloon catheters; and a decrease in cardiac output by using increased intrabronchial pressure or by having the patient perform a Valsalva maneuver during the injection.

All of the aortic flush methods have the limitation of superimposing the aortic root over the coronary ostia and proximal portions of the coronary arteries.

Selective coronary arteriography was first performed by Sones and coworkers. Modifications of the original catheterization technique have been used since its introduction. Of these modifications, the two most widely used today are the Amplatz and Judkins catheter techniques. The original Sones technique involves the passage of a catheter from a peripheral artery to the root of the aorta. Through various manipulations, it is placed in the orifice or in a coronary artery. The required catheter has a specially tapered tip that is unsuitable for automatic injection devices. It is important that the catheter does not occlude the coronary artery. The Sones catheter has been replaced by the multipurpose catheter that is inserted into the brachial or radial artery and advanced to the subclavian artery. This catheter is primarily a straight tapered catheter with an end hole and two side holes close to the tip. This catheter can be used for both right and left coronary arteriography as well as left ventriculography.

Both the Amplatz and the Judkins techniques involve differently shaped catheters for each coronary artery. These catheters are preshaped to allow the physician to easily access the coronary ostia. The physician can locate the arterial orifice with a minimum of catheter manipulation. The Judkins technique involves percutaneous insertion into the femoral artery and requires less manipulation than the brachial or radial approach.

Some complications that can occur during selective coronary arteriography are ventricular fibrillation, asystole, coronary spasm, and death. Because the procedure presents some risk, the patient should be monitored throughout the examination, and emergency care equipment should be available in the special procedure room in case any problems arise.

Left and Right Cardiac Catheterization

Cardiac catheterization is performed by inserting a catheter into the chambers of the heart or into the pulmonary artery. Selective cardiac catheterization is divided into right- and left-sided catheterization.

Selective **right cardiac catheterization** of the right atrium or ventricle is accomplished by inserting a catheter into a peripheral vein of the upper or lower extremity and advancing it into the chambers of the right side of the heart or pulmonary artery. Placement of the catheter should be monitored with fluoroscopy.

The Swan-Ganz balloon flotation catheter is most commonly used for right-sided heart catheterization and hemodynamic pressure measurements. The femoral approach is generally chosen. The catheter is passed into the heart across the tricuspid valve and then (because of the air in the balloon) floats in the right ventricle. Given a slight manipulation the balloon tip can be advanced into the pulmonary artery. A modification of this approach can also be used. The catheter is directed toward the lateral wall of the right atrium, allowed to loop downward, and advanced through the tricuspid valve and then into the pulmonary artery. The catheter can then be advanced and wedged in one of the smaller pulmonary vessels. The most common location for pulmonary wedge pressure is in the right lower lobe, although positioning of the balloon in any of the four lobar positions is acceptable. A variety of catheters are available for right-sided heart catheterization. Their use is governed by the physician performing the procedure and the protocol of the institution.

Selective **left cardiac catheterization** of the left ventricle and atrium can be accomplished through various methods. Generally the femoral artery approach is used.

After localization of the femoral artery and the application of anesthetic a percutaneous puncture is made. The guide wire is then inserted, and a 5 to 7 French sheath is placed over the wire and into the femoral artery. The catheter used will depend upon the ultimate goal of the procedure. For left ventriculography a pigtail catheter is usually chosen. If coronary arteriography is the objective, a Judkins or Amplatz catheter can be used as described previously. The catheter and guide wire are advanced to the level of the thoracic aorta. At this point the guide wire is removed, and pressure measurements are made at the catheter tip and the femoral artery. If normal pressures are present, the catheter is then threaded over the aortic arch, through the aortic valve, and into the left ventricle. Once catheter position has been satisfactorily confirmed, pressure measurements can be taken in the left ventricle. The left ventriculogram can then be accomplished. If the films are considered to be satisfactory the pigtail catheter can then be withdrawn into the thoracic aorta and exchanged for either the Judkins or Amplatz catheter if coronary arteriography is to be performed.

Using the images produced from two separate planes the ejection fraction (EF) can be determined. This is done by calculating the ventricular volumes at both end diastole and end systole and using the following formula to determine the volume.

$$\text{Ejection fraction} = \frac{\text{Stroke volume}}{\text{End-diastolic volume}}$$

The left side of the heart can also be accessed by the transseptal approach using a sheathed needle that is passed up the inferior vena cava to the right atrium. The needle is then exposed and used to puncture the septum between the atria. The catheter can then be advanced into the left atrium and subsequently into the left ventricle.

In cases in which a ventricular septal defect is present the catheter can be passed into the right atrium from either the radial or brachial vein to the right ventricle. It can then be moved through the septal defect into the left ventricle for the study.

Table 12-2 summarizes the normal pressures and volumes used in cardiac monitoring.

TABLE 12-2 *Normal Values of Pressures, Volumes, and Oxygen Saturation Used in Cardiac Monitoring*

NORMAL PRESSURES	
Description	**Normal Value**
Routine blood pressure	90–140/60–90 mm Hg
Brachial artery	
Peak systolic	90–140 mm Hg
End-diastolic	60–90 mm Hg
Left ventricle	
Systolic left ventricular pressure (peak systolic)	90–140 mm Hg
End-diastolic left ventricular pressure	4–12 mm Hg
Right ventricle	
Peak systolic	17–32 mm Hg
End-diastolic	1–7 mm Hg
Central venous pressure (superior vena cava)	2–14 cm H_2O
Mean pulmonary wedge pressure (arterial)	4.5–13 mm Hg
Pulmonary artery pressure	
Peak systolic	17–32 mm Hg
End-diastolic	4–13 mm Hg
Left atrium	
Mean	2–12 mm Hg
Right atrium	
Mean	1–5 mm Hg
NORMAL VOLUMES	
Description	**Normal values**
End-diastolic volume (EDV = Amount of blood in left ventricle at end of diastole)	50–90 ml/m^2
End-systolic volume (ESV = Amount of blood in left ventricle at end of systole)	25 ml/m^2
Cardiac output (CO = Amount of blood ejected by the heart in 1 minute)	36 L/min
Stroke volume (SV = Amount of blood ejected in one contraction)	45 ± 12 ml/m^2
Ejection fraction (EF = SV/EDV)	0.67 ± 0.07
NORMAL OXYGEN SATURATION VALUES	
Location	**Normal Values**
Right atrium	75%
Right ventricle	75%
Pulmonary artery	75%
Pulmonary capillary	97%
Left atrium	95%
Left ventricle	95%
Aorta	95%

Data modified from Pagana KD, Pagana TJ: *Mosby's Diagnostic and Laboratory Test Reference*, 7th ed. Philadelphia, 2005, Elsevier.

Pulmonary Arteriography

Pulmonary arteriography is accomplished using the percutaneous catheterization method either via the femoral or jugular vein. The brachial vein is sometimes used, but access to the pulmonary artery is much more difficult using this approach. Selective studies with less contrast delivery are preferred to flush angiography, yielding substantially better images with less risk to the patient. The catheter is

TABLE 12-3   *Summary of Common Catheters Used in Pulmonary Arteriography*

Catheter	Size	Advantages
Swan-Ganz	7 French	Pressure measurements can be accomplished Balloon occlusions can be performed Used with all vessel access sites
Wil 2	6 French	Used with jugular and brachial vessel access
Pigtail with a deflecting guide wire	6–8 French	Most commonly used for selective pulmonary arteriography Can be exchanged for headhunter catheter for selective catheterization of segmental arteries
Grollman	7 French	Easy manipulation because of preshaped tip
"Berman" balloon flotation catheter	4–8 French	Multiple distal side holes and no end hole or no side holes and only an end hole (wedge catheter) Introducer sheath required

advanced through the inferior vena cava into the right atrium through the tricuspid valve into the right ventricle. Once the catheter is in the right ventricle the pulmonary arteries can then be selectively accessed.

The monitoring of the pressures in the right side of the heart is commonly practiced in this procedure. Measurements are taken from the right atrium, pulmonary arteries, and right ventricle. It is important to constantly monitor the patient's pressure and electrocardiographic tracings throughout the procedure. Any abnormal rise in pressure should be noted because severe, even fatal complications can occur if the right ventricular pressure rises above 20 mm Hg.

Table 12-3 summarizes some of the catheters that can be used to accomplish pulmonary vessel access. The "J" tipped guide wire should be the catheter of choice for use within the heart. Its tip is rounded and flexible enough to be effective without causing any damage or perforation of the heart.

Vessel Access

The most common method for vessel access for all of these studies is the percutaneous route. There are several possible approaches for catheterization: translumbar (puncture at the level of L2–L3), transaxillary (puncture of the proximal brachial vein or artery), transfemoral (puncture of the common femoral vein or artery), and the transjugular approach. The transfemoral approach is the most common for aortography. Transaxillary puncture is used when pathology or aortofemoral grafts make the transfemoral approach undesirable. If the object of the procedure is to access the heart or pulmonary circulation, the transfemoral venous route is desirable. The site and location of the vessel access is established by the type of diagnostic or interventional study, as well as the projected anatomic and pathologic conditions.

Seldinger Method of Percutaneous Needle Insertion

The most common technique of catheter insertion is the *Seldinger* method of percutaneous arterial puncture. The advantage of the Seldinger technique is that smaller needles are used to effect the puncture, and a catheter approximately the same size as the needle is then inserted over a previously placed guide wire. This technique has been discussed in Chapter 8, but the following is a brief summary revisiting the basic steps of the Seldinger approach:

1. Under local anesthetic, puncture the femoral artery directly.
2. Insert a guide wire through the needle into the artery.
3. Remove the needle. Apply pressure proximal to the puncture site to control bleeding.
4. Thread a catheter over the guide wire into the artery.
5. Remove the guide wire.
6. Advance the catheter to the desired level within the lumen of the aorta.

TABLE 12-4   *Summary of Available Arterial Closure Devices*

Device	Single Wall	Double Wall	Method	Manufacturer
Angio-seal hemostasis system	X		Preloaded anchor and collagen plug. Anchor is secured on inside of artery, and collagen plug is positioned outside of the artery. A suture at the skin line maintains pressure on the collagen plug and anchor.	St Jude Medical, Minneapolis, MN
Vasoseal	X		An introducer catheter is placed in the artery. A sheath is put over the catheter, and a collagen plug is inserted. The sheath and catheter are removed, leaving the plug to assist in achieving hemostasis.	Datascope, Montvale,NJ
Prostar multiple intravascular suture device	X		Device deploys suture needles from within the vessel.	Perclose, Redwood City, CA
Duette vascular closure device		X	Balloon device provides compression for the lower wall. Sheath is removed, and collagen thrombin slurry is injected. Balloon is deflated and removed. Manual compression is applied for 5 minutes.	Vascular Solutions, Inc., Minneapolis, MN

Once catheter placement has been successfully accomplished, the catheter is flushed with heparinized saline solution, and a test injection of a small amount of contrast agent may be made to check catheter placement.

Vessel Closure

When the procedure is complete attention must be given to sealing the puncture site to prevent bleeding. In the case of venous access compression at the site of puncture is usually sufficient to attain hemostasis. Manual compression has been the primary means for providing the necessary pressure to the puncture site; however, various mechanical pressure devices have become available to accomplish this task. One such device is the FemoStop System manufactured by RADI Medical Systems, Inc. The device is available for both femoral and radial puncture sites (Fig. 12-14, *A* and *B*). Another mechanical device is the C-Clamp CompressAR System by Instromedix (see Fig. 12-14, *C*). This device is essentially a mechanical clamp that places pressure at the point of puncture. The pressure can be adjusted to suit the patient. It has primary use in femoral venous punctures.

Owing to the anatomic structure of the arteries the postcatheterization care of the puncture site is somewhat more difficult. Arterial punctures can be either single- or double-walled; that is, the technique requires the needle to pass through either one wall of the artery or both walls. Single-wall punctures are simpler to seal and achieve hemostasis.

The four approved devices that are currently being used to provide arterial closure are listed in Table 12-4.

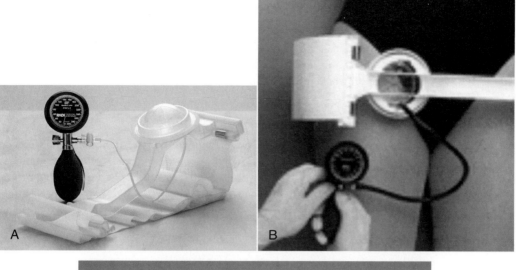

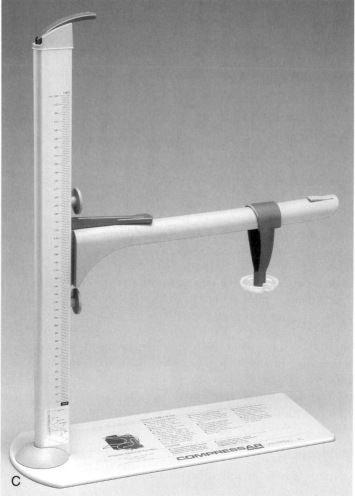

FIGURE 12-14. **A,** The RADI FemoStop closure system. **B,** The FemoStop closure system as applied to a femoral puncture site. **C,** The CompressAR C-Clamp system by Instromedix.

HEMODYNAMICS AND CALCULATIONS

Various measurements are taken during cardiac catheterization. These measurements are used to calculate cardiac functionality. The data is used to determine ventricular volume measurement, extent of stenotic valve area, shunt detections and calculations, and cardiac output. The common formulae used for these calculations are shown in the following discussions.

Calculation of Stenotic Valve Area—Gorlin Method

This method uses the difference in pressures across some type of obstruction. The difference is usually referred to as a pressure gradient. The Gorlin method uses the following formula to determine the aortic valve area. This method can be used to determine the extent of aortic valve stenosis. The pressure-flow data necessary to calculate the aortic valve area and valve resistance require the measurement of cardiac output and the pressure gradient between the left ventricle and the aorta. This can be accomplished by means of catheters placed in the left ventricle and the aorta as described earlier.

$$\text{Aortic Valvular Area} = \frac{SV/SEP}{44.3 \times (\sqrt{P})}$$

where *SV* is stroke volume (ml/beat), *SEP* is systolic ejection period (s/beat), *44.3* is a derived constant factor by Gorlin and Gorlin[1], and *P* is mean systolic pressure gradient between the left ventricle and the aorta (mm Hg).

Cardiac Output Calculation

Several methods can be used to determine the cardiac output. They are the thermodilution, dye dilution, angiographic, and Fick methods.

Thermodilution Method

The **thermodilution method** requires that a catheter (Swan-Ganz) equipped with a thermistor tip (a resistor that varies rapidly with temperature) be placed in the pulmonary artery. The indicator substance, a **cold saline solution** of a known volume and temperature (usually either iced at 4° C or at room temperature, which is approximately 20° C), is injected into the right ventricle passing into the pulmonary artery. The saline solution cools the blood, and the thermistor measures the blood temperature as it passes through the pulmonary artery. The data are fed into the thermodilution system's computer, and a thermodilution profile is computed.

Dye Dilution Method

The **dye dilution method** uses a dye, **indocyanine green** (also known as cardio green), to measure the cardiac output. The substance is nontoxic, inert, and is rapidly excreted by the liver. As the name implies, it relies on the measurement of the dilution of the dye as it passes through the circulation. The dilution is measured using a spectrophotometer equipped with a finger photosensor. The cardiac output is determined by area measurement of the dye decay curve produced by the system.

Angiographic Method

The **angiographic method** relies on measurements taken during the procedure. The formula used to calculate the cardiac output is as follows:

Cardiac output = Stroke volume × Heart rate

where stroke volume = end-diastolic volume (EDV) − end-systolic volume (ESV).

Fick Method

The **Fick method** was described in 1870 by Dr. A. Fick. His theory revolved around the principle that the amount of oxygen transferred to the blood as it passes through the lungs is equal to the amount of oxygen taken into the lungs during the act of breathing. This is expressed by the difference between the oxygen concentration in the venous and arterial blood, the arteriovenous concentration difference, times the blood flow to the lungs. The following formula is used to make this calculation:

$$\text{Cardiac output} = \frac{\text{Oxygen consumption}}{\text{Arteriovenous oxygen consumption difference}}$$

where the arteriovenous (AV) oxygen concentration difference = left ventricular oxygen concentration − pulmonary arterial oxygen content and oxygen consumption is measured using a metabolic hood.★

Shunt Detection and Calculation

Shunts are abnormal connections between the chambers of the heart. Shunts change the relationship between the pulmonary and systemic flow rates. The flow rates between these two systems are normally equal. Depending upon the type of shunt the flow rates will change the amount of blood flowing in each of the systems. For example, if there is a right-to-left shunt, more blood is sent to the left side of the heart, causing the flow to the systemic circulation to increase. The converse is true in the case of a left-to-right shunt. In this case the pulmonary circulation demonstrates an increase in flow. There will also be a corresponding increase or decrease in the oxygen content of the blood, depending upon the direction of the flow through the shunt.

A number of methods can be used to diagnose and assess the effects of a shunt. Among them are three radiographic procedures: angiography, dye dilution, and oximetry. The calculations and methodology for the Fick method and dye dilution techniques have already been discussed.

Oximetry can be used to both localize shunts and quantify the extent of the shunting. The process involves blood sampling from the left ventricle, left atrium, or pulmonary vein (arterial saturation sampling sites) and from pulmonary arteries, pulmonary vein, right ventricle, right atrium, and superior and inferior venae cavae using a balloon-tipped Swan-Ganz catheter. The process is referred to as a "saturation run" and is usually done after normal hemodynamic measurements have been accomplished.

The calculations that are performed to determine the amount of flow are accomplished by means of the Fick principle or the dye dilution curves. Using the Fick principle, the following formulae can be used to determine systemic and pulmonary flow in liters per minute.

In a left-to-right shunt situation the systemic and pulmonary flows must be calculated so that a pulmonary (**Qp**) to systemic (**Qs**) flow ratio can be generated. The calculations are accomplished using the data collected during the catheterization procedure. There are three steps to the calculation:

1.   Computation of the oxygen content for the values collected at the pulmonary artery, pulmonary vein, left ventricle and for mixed venous blood from the superior and inferior venae cavae
2.   Calculation of the pulmonary and systemic flow values
3.   Calculation of the Qp/Qs ratio

Qp/Qs ratios greater than 1.5 indicate the need for closure of the shunt. The formulae shown below for the systemic and pulmonary flow rates also include the calculations referred to in preceding Step 1.

★The Fick method is a noninvasive method of measuring the oxygen consumption. It utilizes an oxygen sensor cell (polarographic cell) to measure the oxygen content of exhaled air. This is referred to as a rebreathing technique. The two variations of this technique are partial and total rebreathing. The patient is required to rebreathe into a bag containing a mixture of oxygen and carbon dioxide while data on the venous carbon dioxide level are measured. The data are then used to calculate the cardiac output.

Left-to-Right Shunt Calculations

Systemic Flow

$$\text{Systemic flow (Qs)} = \frac{\text{Oxygen consumption}}{\text{Arterial oxygen content} - \text{Mixed venous oxygen content}}$$

where arterial oxygen content is calculated as follows:

$$\text{Arterial oxygen content} = 1.36 \times \text{Hemoglobin value} \times \text{LV oxygen content} \times 10$$

and mixed venous oxygen content is calculated as follows:

$$\text{Mixed venous oxygen content} =$$
$$\frac{(3)\ (SVC) + (1)\ (IVC) \times 1.36 \times \text{Hemoglobin value} \times \text{PA oxygen sat.} \times 10}{4}$$

Pulmonary Flow

$$\text{Pulmonary flow (Qp)} = \frac{\text{Oxygen consumption}}{\text{Pulmonary vein oxygen content} - \text{Pulmonary artery oxygen content}}$$

where pulmonary vein oxygen content is calculated as pulmonary vein oxygen saturation $\times$ 1.36 $\times$ hemoglobin value $\times$ 10 and pulmonary artery oxygen content is calculated as pulmonary artery oxygen saturation $\times$ 1.36 $\times$ hemoglobin value $\times$ 10.

Pulmonary to Systemic Flow Ratio

$$\text{Pulmonary to systemic flow rate} = Qp/Qs$$

where Q is flow, P is pulmonary, and S is systemic.

The calculation of the Qp/Qs ratio can also be accomplished using only the saturation values collected during the catheterization. The formula would be represented as follows:

$$\frac{Qp}{Qs} = \frac{\text{Arterial oxygen saturation} - \text{Mixed venous oxygen saturation}}{\text{Pulmonary vein oxygen saturation} - \text{Pulmonary artery oxygen saturation}}$$

where

$$\text{Mixed venous oxygen saturation} = \frac{(3)\ SVC + (1)\ IVC}{4}$$

Right-to-Left Shunt Calculations

The steps are similar for right-to-left shunts. The oxygen content must be calculated; however, it is only necessary to compute oxygen content values for the, pulmonary artery, pulmonary vein, and systemic artery saturation. Once this is accomplished, then the systemic and pulmonary blood flows can be calculated and the results used to create the Qp/Qs ratio. The formula for the systemic flow varies slightly from the one used in a left-to-right shunt situation. The formula utilizes the pulmonary artery oxygen content for both of the calculations as shown below:

Systemic Flow

$$\text{Systemic flow (Qs)} = \frac{\text{Oxygen consumption}}{\text{Arterial oxygen content} - \text{pulmonary artery oxygen content}}$$

where arterial oxygen content is calculated as 1.36 $\times$ hemoglobin value $\times$ LV oxygen content $\times$ 10 and the pulmonary artery oxygen content is calculated as the pulmonary artery oxygen saturation $\times$ 1.36 $\times$ hemoglobin value $\times$ 10.

Pulmonary Flow

$$\text{Pulmonary flow (Qp)} = \frac{\text{Oxygen consumption}}{\text{Pulmonary vein oxygen content} - \text{Pulmonary artery oxygen content}}$$

where the pulmonary vein oxygen content is equal to the pulmonary vein oxygen saturation $\times 1.36 \times$ hemoglobin value $\times 10$ and the pulmonary artery oxygen content equals the pulmonary artery oxygen saturation $\times 1.36 \times$ hemoglobin value $\times 10$.

CONTRAST AGENTS

Water-soluble organic iodine contrast agents are used for angiography of the aorta, heart, and pulmonary vessels. The iodine content, concentration, and amount of the substance vary with the area to be opacified, the type of pathology, and the imaging system used. Both nonionic and the ionic contrast agents are suitable for this study; however, the ultimate choice of contrast agent rests with the physician performing the procedure.

The amount of contrast agent delivered to the patient during catheter aortography varies with the area of the aorta or the specific vessel(s) under investigation. The flow rate of the injection should approximate the flow rate within the vessel(s) being investigated. Some general guidelines can be summarized as follows:

Aortic Arch and Thoracic Aortography★

Transfemoral or transaxillary approach	20 ml/s × 2–3 s
Cardiac catheterization	
Left ventriculography	13–15 ml/s × 3 s
Coronary arteriography	
Left coronary artery	7–10 ml per injection
Right coronary artery	3–5 ml per injection
Pulmonary arteriography	
Main pulmonary artery	30–35 ml/s × 2 s
Right pulmonary artery	25–30 ml/s × 2 s
Left pulmonary artery	22–26 ml/s × 2 s
Lobar and segmental arteries	5–15/s × 2 s

★The amount of contrast is dependent upon weight. The value listed is for a normal adult patient.

These general guidelines may be adjusted by the physician performing the procedure to compensate for vessel diameter (e.g., dilated aortic aneurysms), decreased cardiac output, or severe atherosclerotic disease.

EQUIPMENT

The cardiovascular laboratory differs from the normal angiography/interventional suite in that additional equipment is necessary for the monitoring of the patient and the acquisition of the hemodynamic data required by the studies. Box 12-1 summarizes the specialized equipment required, although the list is not inclusive by any means and will vary depending upon the institution.

PATIENT POSITIONING

The radiographic positioning for aortography depends on the injection procedure chosen and the information desired. Preliminary films should be taken so that proper positioning, technique, and coverage of area of interest can be determined before the injection is made, thereby minimizing the possibility of subjecting the patient to another injection.

BOX 12-1   *Summary of Special Equipment for Cardiac Catheterization*

Blood gas and oxygen content and saturation analyzer
Pacemakers
   Temporary
   External
   Transvenous pacing catheters
   Ancillary cables and devices
Intra-aortic balloon pump
Pressure transducers
Electrocardiograph
   Pressure recorder
   Analyzer
Cardiac output thermodilution device and computer

Percutaneous catheter aortography begins with the patient in the supine position for the introduction of the catheter. After successful placement, the patient may be rotated into the right posterior oblique position for demonstration of the brachiocephalic vessels during thoracic aortography. This is usually the position of choice for the delineation of any type of aneurysm. If a biplane study is done, the patient is maintained in the supine position, and anteroposterior and lateral projections can be taken with one injection. With catheter aortography, the selective injection of any of the major branches may be done easily, if necessary. Table 12-5 summarizes the positioning used in the various procedures for cardiac angiography.

COMPLICATIONS

Complications can arise during the procedures discussed in this chapter. The complications caused by the administration of contrast agents have already been discussed in Chapter 6. The complications related to the mechanics of the catheterization procedure have also been discussed previously in Chapter 8. The complications specific to the various procedures are listed in the box at the bottom of the page.

This is by no means a complete catalog of potential complications that can arise during the angiographic procedures. Many of these will also apply to the interventional procedures associated with the diagnostic procedures. Although the risk for any major complications in a low-risk patient is minimal, the possibility of an occurrence should be expected. Careful patient monitoring before, during, and after the procedure is critical to an event-free procedure. Many of the complications can be identified at the early stages of their occurrence, and treatment can be administered.

Aortography (thoracic)
   Aortic dissection
   Compression of adjacent anatomic structures
   Infection
   Rupture of aneurysm
Cardiac catheterization /coronary arteriography and pulmonary arteriography
   Acute pulmonary edema
   Air embolism
   Angina
   Aortic dissection
   Arteriovenous fistula

Continued

Continued	Hypotension
Atrial fibrillation	Infection
Bradycardia	Myocardial infarction
Cardiac perforation	Pseudoaneurysm
Cardiogenic shock	Pulmonary congestion
Cerebrovascular event	Renal dysfunction and renal failure
Congestive heart failure	Respiratory distress
Death	Thrombosis
Heart block	Ventricular tachycardia
Hemorrhage	

SUMMARY

The thoracic aorta and heart are frequently imaged for the diagnosis and treatment of vascular disease. Malfunctions in the body's vascular system are divided into two primary categories: those that increase the blood flow and those that decrease it. Angiography is performed to assess the aorta, pulmonary circulation, heart function, and pulmonary circulation. Indications for the studies span a wide range of pathologic conditions that are specific to the area being studied.

The common procedures include aortography, cardiac catheterization (left- and right-sided), coronary arteriography, and pulmonary arteriography. Various pressure measurements are taken during cardiac catheterization and pulmonary arteriography which help the radiologist make an accurate diagnosis of the pathology and determine the proper intervention that should be accomplished.

Percutaneous catheter placement is the primary route for vessel access. A number of entry sites are available for use. These include transfemoral, transaxillary, translumbar, and the transjugular approach. The choice of approach is determined by the type of study and is dictated by the radiologist performing the procedure. The most common method used is the Seldinger technique for percutaneous catheter insertion. Vessel closure is an important facet of the studies performed in this area. Various systems are available for compression and vessel closure in order to achieve hemostasis.

The various measurements taken during the studies of the heart and pulmonary circulation are used to determine cardiac function. Among these is the Gorlin method for calculation of stenotic valve area, cardiac output calculations either by the dye dilution, thermodilution, or Fick methods, pulmonary flow, pulmonary-to-systemic flow ratio, and right-to-left shunt calculations. Normal values for the various measurements are given in the chapter.

The nonionic water-soluble organic iodine contrast agents are used for these studies. The amount used varies with the area under investigation and is dictated by the radiologist in charge of the study. These studies also require specialized equipment for patient monitoring and to facilitate the necessary measurements to assess cardiac function.

The complications that can arise from the performance of these studies are procedure dependent. Attention to detail and patient monitoring will reduce the probability of a major reaction; the radiographer should always expect the possibility that a complication can occur.

REFERENCE

1. Gorlin R, Gorlin SG: Hydraulic formula for calculation of stenotic mitral valve, other cardiac valves, and central circulatory shunts. *Am Heart J* 41:1–29, 1951.

TABLE 12-5 *Positions for Aortography and Cardiac Angiography*

Procedure	Projection	Patient Position	Central Ray	Anatomy
Translumbar aortography	Posteroanterior	Patient prone, centered to table, arms next to body, lower legs supported	Vertical beam to center of image receptor, area of interest over image receptor	Aorta and major branches
Percutaneous catheter midstream aortography	Anteroposterior	Patient supine, arms next to body (single plane), arms above head (biplane)	Vertical beam to center of image receptor, area of interest centered to image receptor	Aorta and major branches in area of interest demonstrated in frontal view
	Lateral	Patient in true lateral position, arms above head (single plane)	Vertical beam to center of image receptor	Aorta and major branches in area of interest demonstrated in lateral view
		Patient supine, centered to table (biplane)	Horizontal beam to center of image receptor	
	Posterior oblique	Patient in supine oblique position	Vertical beam to center of imager receptor	Anatomy best demonstrated by posterior oblique projections
Cardiac catheterization		Supine with arms above head or by side (femoral approach)	Various positions when using "C-arm" equipment. "C-arm" should be capable of filming from the inguinal area to the upper thorax	Intracardiac anatomy including the LV, LA, RV, RA, PA, and PV
		Supine with arm on arm board (brachial or radial approach)		
	Right anterior oblique (30 degrees) for left ventriculography			Left ventricular contour in profile. The anterior wall, apex, inferior wall and mitral valve are well demonstrated
	Left anterior oblique (60 degrees) with 25 – 30 degree cephalic angle for left ventriculography			Outflow portion of the LV, posterior wall, and mitral valve

TABLE 12-5   *Positions for Aortography and Cardiac Angiography (cont'd)*

Procedure	Projection	Patient Position	Central Ray	Anatomy
Coronary arteriography (left coronary artery)	Anteroposterior A 5–10 degree RAO can also be employed.	Supine with arms above head or by side (femoral approach)	Various positions when using "C-arm" equipment. "C-arm" should be capable of filming from the inguinal area to the upper thorax	Left main coronary artery
	Left anterior oblique (30–45 degrees) with a 20–30 degree cephalic angle)			Left anterior descending branch/ circumflex bifurcation
	30–40 degree RAO with 20–30 degree caudal angle			Circumflex and marginal branches
	5–30 degree RAO with 20–45 degree cephalic angle			Left anterior descending
	50–60 degree LAO with 10–20 degree caudal angulation			Left anterior descending branch/ circumflex bifurcation
Coronary arteriography (right coronary artery)	30–45 degree LAO with 15–20 degree cephalic angle 30–45 degree RAO			Posterior descending artery and posterior and midportion of the right coronary artery
Pulmonary angiography	Anteroposterior	Supine with arms above head or by side (femoral approach)	Various positions when using "C-arm" equipment. "C-arm" should be capable of filming from the inguinal area to the upper thorax	Main pulmonary artery Selective branch catheterization (specific to branch)
	15–20 degree LAO with 35–40 degree cephalic angle			Pulmonary artery bifurcation
	45–60 degree oblique of the suspected side			Demonstrates pulmonary vasculature of the side in question

LA, left atrium; LAO, left anterior oblique; LV, left ventricle; PA, pulmonary artery; PV, pulmonary vein; RA, right atrium; RAO, right anterior oblique; RV, right ventricle.

SUGGESTED READINGS

Cardiac Catheterization

Andrews RE, Tulloh RM: Interventional cardiac catheterization in congenital heart disease. *Arch Dis Child* 89(12):1168–1173, 2004.

Campbell RM, Strieper MJ, Frias PA, et al: Quantifying and minimizing radiation exposure during pediatric cardiac catheterization. *Pediatr Cardiol* 26(1):29–33, 2005.

Giles ER, Murphy PH: Measuring skin dose with radiochromic dosimetry film in the cardiac catheterization laboratory. *Health Phys* 82(6):875–880, 2002.

Nishikawa T, Dohi S: Errors in the measurement of cardiac output by thermodilution. *Can J Anaesth* 40:142–153, 1993.

Razavi R, Hill DL, Keevil SF, et al: Cardiac catheterization guided by MRI in children and adults with congenital heart disease. *Lancet* 362(9399):1877–1882, 2003.

Segal AZ, Abernethy WB, Palacios IF, et al: Stroke as a complication of cardiac catheterization: risk factors and clinical features. *Neurology* 56(7):975–977, 2001.

Vincent RN, Diehl HJ: Interventions in pediatric cardiac catheterization. *Crit Care Nurs* Q 25(3):37–47, 2002.

Coronary Arteriography

Baglini R, Sesana M, Capuano C, et al: Left ventricular diastolic impairment during coronary arteriography with a non-ionic contrast medium. *Minerva Cardioangiol* 52(4):323–328, 2004.

Bell PD, Hudson S: Equity in the diagnosis of chest pain: race and gender. *Am J Health Behav* 25(1):60–71, 2001.

Carlisle DM, Leape LL, Bickel S, Bell R, Kamberg C, Genovese B, French WJ, Kaushik VS, Mahrer PR, Ellestad MH, Brook RH, Shapiro MF: Underuse and overuse of diagnostic testing for coronary artery disease in patients presenting with new-onset chest pain. *Am J Med* 106(4):391–398, 1999.

Ferguson JA, Adams TA, Weinberger M: Racial differences in cardiac catheterization use and appropriateness. *Am J Med Sci* 315(5):302–306, 1998.

Frances CD, Go AS, Dauterman KW, Deosaransingh K, Jung DL, Gettner S, Newman JM, Massies BM, Browner WS: Outcome following acute myocardial infarction: are differences among physician specialties the result of quality of care or case mix? *Arch Intern Med* 159(13):1429–1436, 1999.

Hemingway H, Crook AM, Feder G, Banerjee S, Dawson JR, Magee P, Philpott S, Sanders J, Wood A, Timmis AD: Underuse of coronary revascularization procedures in patients considered appropriate candidates for revascularization. *N Engl J Med* 344(9):645–654, 2001.

Hofmann R, Kypta A, Steinwender C, Kerschner K, Grund M, Leisch F: Coronary angiography in patients undergoing carotid artery stenting reveals a high incidence of significant coronary artery disease. *Heart* 91(11):1438-1441, 2005.

Khairy P, Triedman JK, Juraszek A, Cecchin F: Inability to cannulate the coronary sinus in patients with supraventricular arrhythmias: congenital and acquired coronary sinus atresia. *J Intervent Card Electrophysiol* 12(2):123–127, 2005.

Mahla E, Vicenzi M, Schrottner B, Maier R, Tiesenhausen K, Watzinger N, Rienmuller R, Moser RL, Metzler H: Coronary artery plaque burden and perioperative cardiac function. *Anesthesiology* 95:1133–1140, 2001.

Pohle K, Maffert R, Ropers D, Moshage W, Stilianakis N, Daniel WG, Achenbach S: Progression of aortic valve calcification: association with coronary atherosclerosis and cardiovascular risk factors. *Circulation* 104(16):1927–1932, 2001.

Sablayrolles JL, Al Attar N, Nataf P: New trends in non-invasive coronary angiography with multislice CT. *Surg Technol Int* 13:205–213, 2004.

Vaseghi M, Cesario DA, Ji S, Shannon KM, Wiener I, Boyle NG, Fonarow GC, Valderrabano M, Shivkumar K: Beyond coronary sinus angiography: the value of coronary arteriography and identification of the pericardiophrenic vein during left ventricular lead placement. *Pacing Clin Electrophysiol* 28(3):185–190, 2005.

Yang EH, Lerman A: Angina pectoris with a normal coronary angiogram. *Herz.* 30(1):17–25, 2005.

Percutaneous Catheter Aortography

Chessa M, Dindar A, Vettukattil JJ, et al: Balloon angioplasty in infants with aortic obstruction after the modified stage I Norwood procedure. *Am Heart J* 140(2):227–231, 2000.

Fedson S, Jolly N, Lang RM, et al: Percutaneous closure of a ruptured sinus of Valsalva aneurysm using the Amplatzer duct occluder. *Catheter Cardiovasc Intervent* 58(3):406–411, 2003.

Godart F, Haulon S, Houmany M, et al: Transcatheter closure of aortocaval fistula with the amplatzer duct occluder. *J Endovasc Ther* 12(1):134–137, 2005.

Lim JS, Desai T, Stumper O: Dual-catheter balloon occlusion aortography in pulmonary atresia with ventricular septal defect and major aorto-pulmonary collaterals. *Pediatr Cardiol* 25(5):500–502, 2004.

Parker MV, O'Donnell SD, Chang AS, et al: What imaging studies are necessary for abdominal aortic endograft sizing? A prospective blinded study using conventional computed tomography, aortography, and three-dimensional computed tomography. *J Vasc Surg* 41(2):199–205, 2005.

Stavropoulos SW, Baum RA: Catheter-based treatments of endoleaks. *Semin Vasc Surg* 17(4):279–283, 2004.

Pulmonary Angiography

Anorbe E, Alvarez S: CT pulmonary angiography. *AJR Am J Roentgenol* 184(4):1360, 2005.

Gruden JF, Tigges S, Baron MG, Pearlman H: MDCT pulmonary angiography: image processing tools. *Semin Roentgenol* 40(1):48–63, 2005.

Loud PA, Katz DS, Bruce DA, et al: Deep venous thrombosis with suspected pulmonary embolism: detection with combined CT venography and pulmonary angiography. *Radiology* 219(2):498–502, 2001.

McRae SJ, Ginsberg JS: The diagnostic evaluation of pulmonary embolism. *Am Heart Hosp J* 3(1):14–20, 2005.

Quiroz R, Schoepf UJ: CT pulmonary angiography for acute pulmonary embolism: cost-effectiveness analysis and review of the literature. *Semin Roentgenol* 40(1):20–24, 2005.

STUDY QUESTIONS

1. The structural layer in the arteries that separates the blood from the blood vessels proper is called the:
   a. tunica intima
   b. tunica media
   c. tunica externa
   d. tunica adventitia

2. The anatomic structure that supplies the pulmonary circulation with blood is called the:
   a. aorta
   b. pulmonary artery
   c. pulmonary vein
   d. left ventricle

3. The aortic arch directly gives off three major branches, which are the _____ arteries.
   i. left subclavian
   ii. brachiocephalic
   iii. right subclavian
   iv. left common carotid
   a. i, ii, and iii
   b. i, ii, and iv
   c. i, iii, and iv
   d. ii, iii, and iv

4. Vieussens' ring is considered to be a(n):
   a. means of collateral circulation between the right and left coronary arteries
   b. fibrous structure around the mitral valve
   c. pseudonym for the pulmonary circulation
   d. abnormal opening between the right and left ventricles

5. All of the following are catheter types used for pulmonary angiography except:
   a. Berman balloon flotation
   b. Swan-Ganz
   c. Grollman
   d. Miller-Levine

STUDY QUESTIONS (*cont'd*)

6. Which of the following are considered to be congenital abnormalities?
    i. tetrology of Fallot
    ii. septal defect
    iii. aortic insufficiency
    a. i only
    b. iii only
    c. i and ii only
    d. i, ii, and iii

7. The optimal time for the injection of contrast agent into the coronary arteries is usually:
    a. cardiac systole
    b. cardiac diastole
    c. cardiac asystole
    d. cardiac tamponade

8. Complications of selective coronary arteriography include which of the following?
    i. death
    ii. valvular regurgitation
    iii. coronary spasm
    iv. ventricular fibrillation
    a. i and iii only   c. ii, iii, and iv only
    b. i, iii, and iv only   d. i, ii, iii, and iv

9. Which of the following formulas represents the calculation necessary for the determination of the ejection fraction?
    a. stroke volume/end-diastolic volume
    b. cardiac output/end-diastolic volume
    c. end-diastolic volume/stroke volume
    d. stroke volume/cardiac output

10. The principle that the amount of oxygen transferred to the blood as it passes through the lungs is equal to the amount of oxygen taken into the lungs during the act of breathing is the basis for the:
    a. Gorlin theory of stenotic valve dissection
    b. Berman theory of pulmonary flotation
    c. Fick principle for cardiac output calculations
    d. Swan-Ganz method of stroke volume calculation

13 Abdominal Aortography and Genitourinary System Procedures

CHAPTER OBJECTIVES

After completing this chapter, the reader will be able to perform the following:

▪ Identify the anatomy of the abdominal aorta

▪ Identify the vascular anatomy of the urinary system and celiac and mesenteric circulation

▪ Describe the vascular anatomy of the reproductive system

▪ List the various procedures that can be performed in these areas

▪ List the indications and contraindications for angiography in these areas

▪ Identify vessel access for these procedures

▪ Describe the contrast agents used in angiography of the genitourinary system

▪ Identify common complications of these procedures

CHAPTER OUTLINE

The abdominal portion of the descending aorta begins as it passes through the diaphragm and enters the abdominal cavity at approximately the level of the twelfth thoracic vertebra. Several vessels branch off the abdominal aorta to service the kidneys, intestines, and reproductive organs and to supply the diaphragm with nutrients. Conventional abdominal aortography can be performed as a "flush" study to visualize the vasculature of the vessel and to determine the presence or absence of relevant pathology. This is usually done by positioning the catheter in the lumen of the aorta at the level of T12–L1. Pelvic aortography can also be performed by placing the catheter tip approximately 2 to 3 cm (1 inch) above the aortic bifurcation. Depending on the area of interest and the suspected pathology, the catheter can be placed selectively into any of the branches to demonstrate specific vasculature.

ANATOMIC CONSIDERATIONS

Abdominal Aorta

The abdominal aorta courses toward the midline anterior to the vertebral column. At the level of the fourth lumbar vertebra, the abdominal aorta bifurcates (splits) into the right and left common iliac arteries (Fig. 13-1, *A* and *B*). The bifurcation can be topographically located slightly inferior and to the left of the navel. This point is considered the termination of the aorta. The common iliac arteries are the major arteries of the pelvis. Each common iliac artery divides into an internal and an external iliac artery. The external iliac arteries then form the femoral arteries of the lower extremities.

Some of the branches of the abdominal aorta are paired and others are unpaired. All of the parietal vessels are paired with the exception of the median sacral artery, which branches off at the level of the aortic bifurcation and courses toward the sacrum and coccyx. The branches of the descending abdominal aorta can be classified as either parietal or visceral and may be summarized as follows:

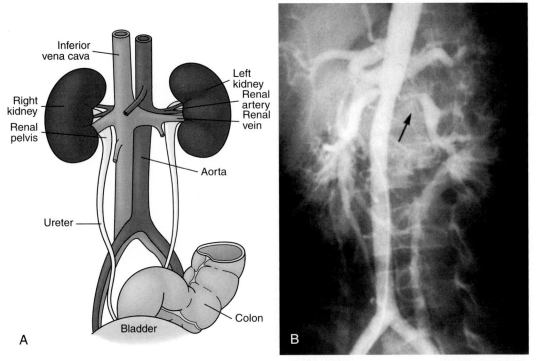

FIGURE 13-1. **A,** Location of the abdominal portion of the descending aorta and its bifurcation and their relationships with the inferior vena cava and abdominal viscera. **B,** Radiograph of an aortogram showing the filling of the renal vessels.

Descending abdominal aorta

Parietal branches
- Inferior phrenic arteries
- Lumbar arteries
- Common iliac arteries
- Median sacral artery

Visceral branches
- Middle suprarenal (adrenal) arteries
- Renal arteries
- Gonadal arteries
- Celiac trunk
- Superior mesenteric artery
- Inferior mesenteric artery

During aortography, it is not uncommon for some of the branches to visualize. Frequently, the circulatory supply of the kidneys will be well demonstrated. The middle adrenal arteries can occasionally be seen on an abdominal aortogram, especially in cases of renal or adrenal pathology. These are paired vessels arising from the lateral wall of the aorta at a level between the celiac trunk and the superior mesenteric arteries.

Celiac Trunk and Mesenteric Circulation

The first main branch originating on the ventral aorta is the **celiac trunk**. The main areas supplied by this vessel are the esophagus, stomach, liver, spleen, and pancreas (Fig. 13-2). The celiac trunk bifurcates and gives

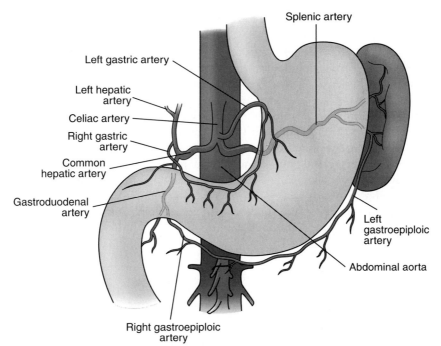

FIGURE 13-2. Illustration of the origin of the celiac artery and its major branches.

off the left gastric, splenic, and the common hepatic arteries. The left gastric artery, as its name implies, runs off to the left to supply the stomach coursing along the lesser curvature and connects with the right gastric artery. The splenic artery also runs off to the left and gives off numerous branches to supply the pancreas.

The common hepatic artery courses to the right. It subsequently divides into the right gastric, gastroduodenal, and hepatic arteries. The hepatic artery runs superiorly to divide into the right and left hepatic arteries. As stated earlier the right gastric artery follows the lesser curvature of the stomach to join with the left gastric artery. The gastroduodenal artery courses posteriorly and divides into the pancreaticoduodenal artery and the right gastric epiploic, which continues along the greater curvature of the stomach to become the left gastric epiploic artery.

The superior and inferior mesenteric arteries are unpaired vessels. They are considered visceral branches of the aorta and primarily supply the small and large intestines. The superior mesenteric arises ventrally just below the origin of the celiac trunk. The inferior mesenteric artery is also ventrally located and originates just above the bifurcation of the aorta.

The capillaries of the stomach, intestine, spleen, and pancreas bring the blood into the portal vein which carries it to the capillary-like liver sinusoids. The portal vein, the large collecting vein, collects all of the venous blood from the gastrointestinal system, spleen, and pancreas. It is formed by the superior mesenteric vein and the splenic vein. Although the inferior mesenteric vein empties into one of the two other major veins in the portal system, it is considered to be one of the veins that make up the portal vein. The portal vein then courses superiorly and divides into right and left branches. These vessels then break up into interlobular and then smaller intralobular veins, which form the sinusoids. These sinusoids drain into the central vein of each liver lobule, which merges into the hepatic veins, which drain into the inferior vena cava.

Urinary System

The kidneys are bean-shaped organs that lie in the abdomen next to the vertebral column at the level of the twelfth thoracic vertebra to the second or third lumbar vertebra. The renal hilum, an indented area on the medial border of the kidneys, can usually be found at the level of the interspace of the first and second lumbar vertebrae. This level can vary by as much as one vertebral body in either direction. It is here that the major vessels and ureters enter and leave the kidney.

The internal structure of the kidney is divided into two areas—the *cortex*, or outer area, and the *medulla*, or inner portion. The cortex contains the glomeruli, which are capsules that enclose a convoluted group of capillaries. The *glomeruli* are portions of the nephrons, the functional units of the kidney (Fig. 13-3). The cortex also comprises other portions of the nephron, the convoluted tubules, and portions of the origins of the collecting ducts.

The medulla comprises straight tubules, continuations of the convoluted tubules called Henle's loop, and collecting ducts. The medulla has the appearance of many pyramids, the apex of which terminates in the cuplike indentation of the minor renal calyx (Fig. 13-4).

The *nephrons* filter blood plasma and permit selective reabsorption of water and dissolved materials necessary for maintaining the ionic balance of the blood back into the circulation. There are 1 million or more of these nephrons in each kidney. During renal arteriography, the interlobular arteries are not outlined as separate channels but instead appear as a diffuse accumulation over the entire kidney. This is usually called the *nephrogram phase* of the arteriogram.

Adrenal Gland Vasculature

The adrenal glands sit on top of each kidney. They are embedded in the adipose tissue that surrounds the kidney and consists of a cortex (outer portion) and the medulla (inner portion). Both of these areas are well supplied with blood vessels.

The medullary portion of the adrenal glands is responsible for the secretion of epinephrine (adrenaline) and norepinephrine (noradrenalin). Tumors in the adrenal glands can affect the amount of

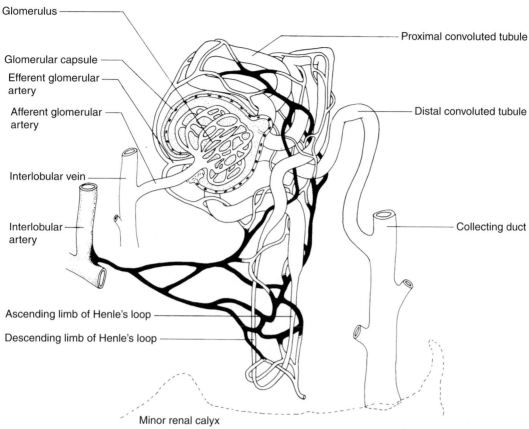

Glomerulus

Glomerular capsule

Efferent glomerular artery

Afferent glomerular artery

Interlobular vein

Interlobular artery

Ascending limb of Henle's loop

Descending limb of Henle's loop

Proximal convoluted tubule

Distal convoluted tubule

Collecting duct

Minor renal calyx

FIGURE 13-3. Microscopic anatomy of the kidney showing the nephron, the functional unit of the organ.

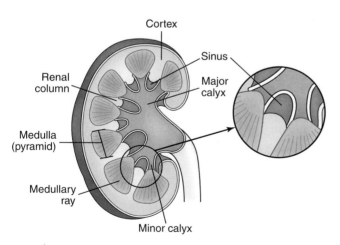

Cortex

Sinus

Major calyx

Renal column

Medulla (pyramid)

Medullary ray

Minor calyx

FIGURE 13-4. Gross internal structure of the kidney showing the renal pyramids and their termination in the renal calyx.

hormone that is secreted. Norepinephrine is usually increased, causing a variety of different bodily responses such as high blood pressure and increased heart rate.

The adrenal cortex also gives off a number of steroids and hormones. Three of these secretions are important for the proper maintenance of electrolyte balance and glucose metabolism: (1) the adrenal sex hormones—adrenal androgen in the male and its converted form, estrogen, in the female; (2)

aldosterone; and (3) cortisol (hydrocortisone). Unlike the secretions from the medulla of adrenal medulla, if the cortical secretions are interrupted for even a week, survival of the patient is questionable.

The adrenal glands are supplied with blood via three arteries to each gland: the superior, middle, and inferior adrenal arteries. The superior adrenal artery is a branch of the inferior phrenic artery. The middle adrenal is a direct branch from the aorta, arising at some point between the celiac and the renal arteries. The inferior adrenal artery branches off each of the renal arteries. These vessels break into many smaller branches that infuse both the cortical and medullary portions of the gland. As the vessels pass through the medulla they become smaller capillaries that begin to take on the characteristics of venules.

When they approach the center of the medullary area they join into a central vein. The venous vasculature differs between the left and right adrenal gland. In the right adrenal gland there are generally three major branches coming from the posterior, superior, and inferior portions of the gland. These join into a larger branch which communicates with the inferior vena cava.

The left adrenal gland has a single central vein that joins the left phrenic vein just before emptying into the left renal vein.

Renal Circulation

The renal arteries originate as branches of the abdominal aorta at about the level of the interspace of the first and second lumbar vertebrae (Fig. 13-5). They run transversely toward each kidney, with the right renal artery passing posterior to the inferior vena cava. The superior mesenteric artery is just above the origin of the renal arteries.

The renal artery gives off an extrarenal branch called the inferior suprarenal artery, which supplies the largest portion of the adrenal gland. Other portions are supplied by the superior and middle suprarenal arteries, which are branches originating directly from the aorta. The adrenal glands are usually demonstrated during renal angiography.

Before the renal arteries enter the hilum of the kidney, each divides into five branches corresponding to the five renal segments. These enter the renal sinus and course both anteriorly and posteriorly to the renal pelvis (Fig. 13-6). The renal sinus is a recess containing the renal vessels and the renal pelvis, the upper expanded portion of the ureter.

In the renal sinus, the larger branches of the renal artery subdivide to form smaller interlobar branches. These vessels course between the lobes, in the renal columns, toward the periphery of the kidney. At the level of the renal cortex, the interlobar branches become the arcuate arteries. These arteries course along the line between the cortex and medulla and give off branches called the interlobular arteries.

The interlobular arteries subdivide into the afferent arterioles that course into the glomerulus. In the glomerulus, the afferent arteriole becomes an efferent arteriole and then forms a capillary plexus surrounding the straight and convoluted tubules.

The efferent arteriole plexus is continuous with small venules that unite to form interlobular and medullary veins. These drain into the arcuate veins, which course along the boundary of the cortex and medulla. Interlobar veins are formed by the arcuate veins and converge to form the renal vein, which ultimately drains into the inferior vena cava.

Table 13-1 summarizes, in order of filling, the vessels seen during the various phases of renal arteriography. It should be noted that when renal masses are evaluated with intravenous digital subtraction angiography (DSA), the catheter is placed in the inferior vena cava via the femoral approach. This technique demonstrates the patency of the inferior vena cava during the initial phase of the study. The later phases appear as stated in Table 13-1.

Reproductive System Vasculature

The arteries that supply the testes and ovaries, the **gonadal** arteries, originate as another set of paired arteries originating from the abdominal aorta. Depending on the sex of the patient they can be referred

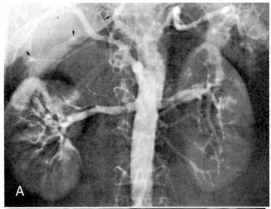

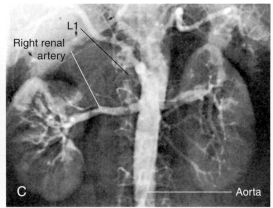

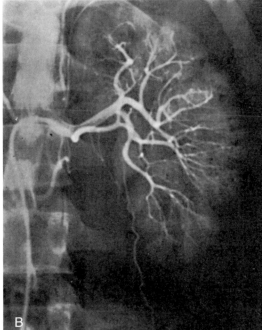

FIGURE 13-5. **A,** Radiograph of a renal arteriogram made by the flush method. Note that the catheter is placed at the level of the renal vessels. Both kidneys are visualized in this manner. **B,** Selective angiogram (arterial phase) showing wrapping of normal vessels around upper pole mass. Note the location of the catheter in the orifice in the renal artery. **C,** Tracing of radiograph showing location of renal arteries in relationship to the lumbar spine.

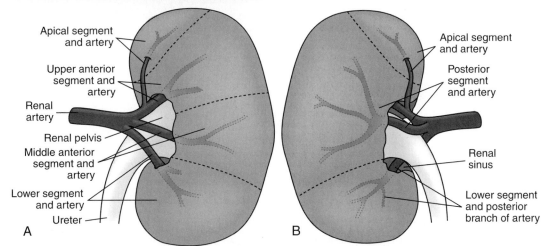

FIGURE 13-6. Segmental branches of the renal arteries shown in the anterior (**A**) and posterior (**B**) aspects. Note that the renal artery gives branches both anteriorly and posteriorly to the renal pelvis.

TABLE 13-1 *Summary of Renal Circulatory Pattern*

Phase	Vessels Observed
Arterial	Abdominal aorta (nonselective studies only)
	Renal artery with extrarenal branches
	Segmental branches
	Interlobular arteries
Nephrogram	Arcuate arteries
	Interlobular arteries
	Afferent arterioles
	Efferent arterioles
	Venules
	Interlobular and medullary veins
	Arcuate veins
	Interlobular veins
Venous	Main renal veins

to as the **testicular** or **ovarian** arteries. The testicular arteries course inferolaterally, on the psoas muscle, to enter the testicular canal and supply the spermatic cord and testis. The ovarian arteries, as their name implies, follows a similar path entering the suspensor ligament of the ovary providing its blood supply.

Venous return from the gonads is accomplished through the left and right gonadal veins. In the male each of the gonadal veins drains its respective testicle while in the female they drain the ovaries. The right gonadal vein travels upward and drains directly into the inferior vena cava, while the left gonadal vein empties into the left renal vein close to its junction with the inferior vena cava.

In the male the **spermatic** veins from the testes and epididymis drain into the **pampiniform plexus**, a group of 8 to 10 anastomosing veins. These vessels join to form three to four vessels ascending through the inguinal ring, converging once again into two vessels, which rise along the psoas muscle to unite into a single vein that empties into the inferior vena cava on the right side and on the left side enters the left renal vein. In the female the ovarian veins become the uterine plexus following a similar path as in the male.

One of the major pathologic processes that can be identified through venography is the presence of a varicocele. A **varicocele** is a dilation and tortuosity of the pampiniform venous plexus and the internal spermatic vein. They are primarily found on the left side because of the anatomic structure of the veins. The absence of venous valves combined with the acute angle of anastomosis with the renal vein and the higher blood pressures associated with the renal vein create ideal conditions for this abnormality. Varicoceles can usually be identified through venography or ultrasonography.

DIAGNOSTIC PROCEDURES

The vasculature of the genitourinary system is supplied by the abdominal aorta. The studies that can be used to diagnose various pathologic conditions in this system begin with **aortography**. Either a percutaneous or translumbar approach can be used to visualize the aorta and its branches. Once the flush study has been accomplished, selective catheterization of specific vessels can then be done. **Renal angiography** is one of the more commonly performed procedures both for diagnoses and for interventional procedures. **Adrenal angiography** is utilized in the diagnoses of various hormonal pathologies. The reproductive system in both males and females can also be carried out using **uterine angiography** in the female and **testicular angiography** in the male.

The patient positioning for aortography will be dependent upon the type of vessel access, either translumbar or via the percutaneous femoral artery puncture, both summarized in Table 13-2. Once a flush study has been completed, selective and superselective catheterization of the various organ systems

TABLE 13-2 *Positions for Aortography*

Procedure	Projection	Patient Position	Anatomy
Translumbar aortography	Posteroanterior	Patient prone, centered to table, arms next to body, lower legs supported	Aorta and major branches
Percutaneous catheter midstream aortography	Anteroposterior	Patient supine, arms next to body (single plane), arms above head (biplane)	Aorta and major branches in area of interest demonstrated in frontal view
	Lateral	Patient in true lateral position, arms above head (single plane)	Aorta and major branches in area of interest demonstrated in lateral view
		Patient supine, centered to table (biplane)	Aorta and major branches in area of interest demonstrated in anteroposterior and lateral views
	Posterior oblique	Patient in supine oblique position	Aorta and major branches in oblique projections; primarily used to circumvent overlying vessels when digital subtraction angiography is not used

can be carried out. The patient positioning for each of these studies also is variable depending upon the architecture of the vasculature, the pathology, and the physician and institution protocols. The use of bilateral "C-arm" equipped x-ray systems and digital subtraction will limit the requirements for patient positioning during the examination. When using conventional equipment it may be necessary to reposition the patient during the procedure.

INDICATIONS AND CONTRAINDICATIONS

Aortography

Abdominal aortography is indicated for evaluating a variety of pathologic conditions. Arteriosclerosis at various sites in the abdominal aorta causing aortic occlusions either complete or incomplete can be well demonstrated using this procedure. Despite the fact that arteriosclerosis is a progressive disease that develops over many years, the morphologic changes can demonstrate the severity, location, and extent of the disease.

Localized abdominal aortic aneurysm (AAA) is another indication for this procedure. Identification and preoperative assessment of the suspected aneurysm as well as postoperative evaluation of treatment can be accomplished by angiography in this area. Abdominal aortography can reveal the following in cases of suspected aneurysm: evidence of rupture, assessment of renal arteries, patency of mesenteric arteries, inflammation, and any potential inferior vena caval or renal vein anomalies.

The contraindications for abdominal aortography are similar to those that have already been discussed for thoracic aortography, including physiologic and mechanical (inability to perform the catheterization procedure) contraindications and the toxic effect of the contrast agent.

Renal Angiography

Renal angiography is indicated for the diagnosis of various vascular lesions and as an adjunct to surgery or interventional therapy. Renovascular hypertension is the greatest indication for the use of this procedure. The following is a list of some of the renovascular problems that cause renal hypertension and that can be diagnosed with this procedure:

- Atherosclerosis
- Stenosis
- Fibromuscular disease
- Medial fibroplasia with mural aneurysm
- Perimedial fibroplasia
- Intimal fibroplasia
- Periarterial fibroplasia
- Selective venous sampling for renin

In addition, this procedure is indicated for the presurgical mapping of renal neoplasms and for renal transplantation.

Renal angiography is also indicated for evaluating certain aspects of renal trauma. Although computed tomography and excretory urography are used extensively to diagnose renal contusions, tears, and infarctions, these studies are not as sensitive as renal angiography in determining renal arterial involvement. Angiography is usually indicated when arterial involvement such as laceration or occlusion is suspected.

Renal hypertension can result from stenosis of one or more renal arteries. In these cases it is the initiation of the renin/angiotensinogen/aldosterone system. Renin is a proteolytic enzyme that aids in the control of the glomerular filtration rate in the kidney and ultimately the blood pressure. Renin is released by the kidney in response to the following stimuli:

- A drop in blood pressure detected by special cells in the afferent arterioles
- Sympathetic (autonomic nervous system) stimulation
- A decrease in the amounts of chlorine, potassium, and sodium ions reaching the distal tubule
- Renal vascular occlusion or renal disease

Renin is released into the renal veins, resulting in the activation of the renin–angiotensin system. In the blood renin reacts with angiotensinogen (a plasma protein released by the liver). The interaction produces a substance called angiotensin I. Another enzyme (angiotensin-converting enzyme) is released into the blood stream by the lungs and converts the angiotensin I into angiotensin II. This substance is a powerful vasoconstrictor that narrows the efferent arterioles, causing a backup of blood into the glomerulus.

Angiotensin II also stimulates the adrenal cortex to release aldosterone. The aldosterone stimulates the kidney tubules to reabsorb more sodium, causing a reduction in water lost to urine. The result is an increase in blood volume causing a rise in blood pressure. The posterior pituitary releases antidiuretic hormones as a result of stimulation from the hypothalamus's reaction to the reduction in blood pressure.

Although the renal veins can usually be seen during the venous phase of the angiogram (Fig. 13-7), renal venography via selective catheterization is the procedure of choice when the diagnosis of renal vein thrombosis is warranted.

Renal venography is also performed in order to achieve renin sampling to diagnose renal vascular hypertension. Once the catheter is in place in the inferior vena cava and the renal veins have been localized, blood samples are taken. These samples are usually collected at each of the renal veins and in the inferior vena cava. Approximately 7 ml of blood is taken at each site. These specimens are labeled, packed in ice, and sent to the laboratory for assay. Indication of renal vascular hypertension is diagnosed if the ratio of renal venous renin is equal to or greater than 1.5:1. The normal values for plasma renin activity are listed on the opposite page.

The contraindications for renal angiography are few. Because the excretory pathway of most angiographic contrast agents is through glomerular filtration, severe renal disease should be a major contraindication. However; severe renal disease is not a definite contraindication for renal angiography because complications are rare. Renal angiography has been performed on patients with severe renal

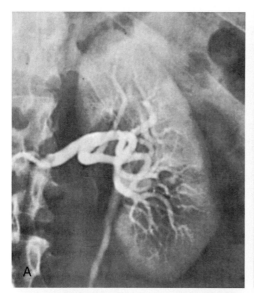

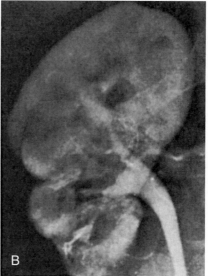

FIGURE 13-7. Radiographs of the phases of renal arteriography: **A**, arterial phase; **B**, early nephrogram phase; **C**, venous phase.

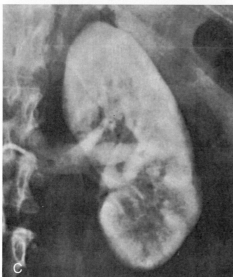

Patient Type	Conditions	Age	Normal Values (ng/ml/hr)
Adult/elderly	Upright position, sodium-restricted diet	20–39	2.9–24
		>40	2.9–10.8
Adult/elderly	Upright position, normal sodium diet	20–39	0.1–4.3
		>40	0.1–3.0
Child		0–3	<17
		3–6	<7
		6–9	<4.4
		9–12	<6
		12–15	<4.2
		15–18	<4.2

Data modified from Pagana KD, Pagana TJ: *Mosby's Diagnostic and Laboratory Test Reference*, 7th ed. Phildelphia, 2005, Elsevier.

disease without resulting in any major reactions. Catheter techniques may be contraindicated in the presence of certain vascular disease states. In these cases, other routes or methods of demonstrating the renal vascular anatomy may be used.

Adrenal Angiography

The primary and probably the sole indication for adrenal angiography is the treatment of tumors through percutaneous ablation. Venous sampling to evaluate hormonally active tumors of the adrenal glands can also be an indication for adrenal angiography. The following is a summary of some of the other indications for adrenal angiography:

- Pheochromocytoma
- Large masses of the adrenal glands
- Malignant adrenal carcinoma
- Cushing syndrome
- Adrenal adenoma
- Adrenal hyperplasia

Adrenal venography is generally required to determine the location of catheter placement in adrenal vein sampling.

Reproductive System Angiography and Venography

Arteriography is performed more commonly in the female patient than in the male. The primary indications in the woman would be to identify and treat symptomatic fibroids or uterine myomas (leiomyoma). The diagnosis of these pathologic conditions can be accomplished by means of either hysteroscopy or arteriography. Fibroids may require treatment if they are showing rapid growth, causing pressure on other organs, or causing abnormal bleeding between periods (menorrhagia) or if the patient is experiencing fertility problems. Angiography is generally performed unless contraindicated by pregnancy, malignancy, endometritis, connective tissue disease, and severe renal insufficiency.

In the male venography is indicated in cases of suspected varicocele. The indications for this procedure are infertility, scrotal pain, testicular atrophy, scrotal edema, and as a result of recurrence after surgical intervention. Although varicoceles are prevalent in the left internal spermatic vein, they do often appear in the right internal spermatic vein also. The contraindications are coagulation abnormalities and potential adverse reaction to contrast agents.

Vessel Access

The vessel access for these studies is generally through percutaneous puncture of the femoral vasculature. If the procedure is arterial, the femoral artery is used. The femoral vein is the choice of vessel access for venography. The transaxillary approach is also used, especially if the use of femoral vein or artery puncture is contraindicated. The Seldinger technique is usually employed when percutaneous access is used.

In rare cases the translumbar approach can be used (Fig. 13-8). The specific technique of direct puncture of the aorta differs according to the physician performing the procedure. There are two basic variations—high and low—and the approach chosen depends on the anatomic information desired. The procedure is accomplished with a specially designed 18-gauge catheter with a 6F sheath 18 to 24 cm in length. The patient is placed into the prone position. The insertion point can be at the level of the twelfth thoracic vertebra (high approach) or at the third lumbar vertebra (low approach), and it is always made from the left flank approximately one hand's width from the spinous process.

In the low approach, the needle is directed in the axial plane at an angle of approximately 40 degrees. This approach provides opacification of the vessels of the lower extremity without superimposition of the vessels of the abdominal viscera.

The high approach is used when there is a suspected aortic aneurysm or occlusion. The needle is directed cranially to avoid accidental injury to the renal artery. The angle is similar to that of the low approach, but there is the added risk of inducing a pneumothorax through accidental puncture of the lung. This approach is less desirable than the low approach because of the opacification of the vessels of the abdominal viscera.

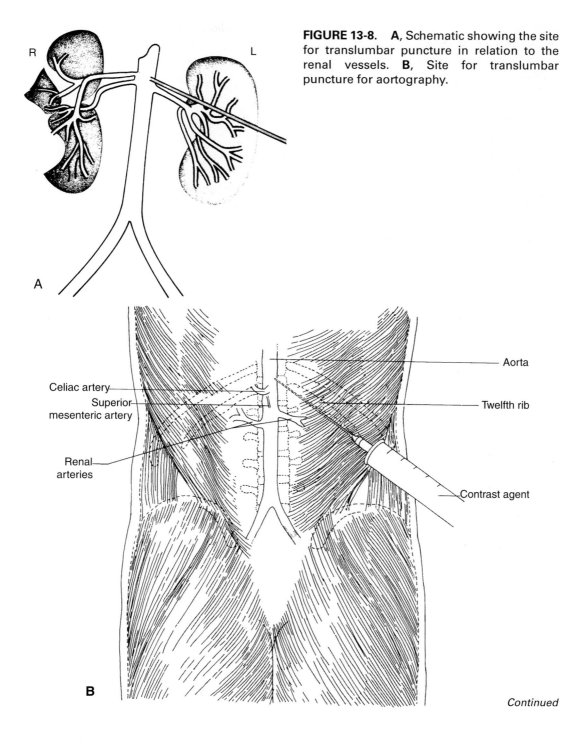

FIGURE 13-8. **A,** Schematic showing the site for translumbar puncture in relation to the renal vessels. **B,** Site for translumbar puncture for aortography.

Continued

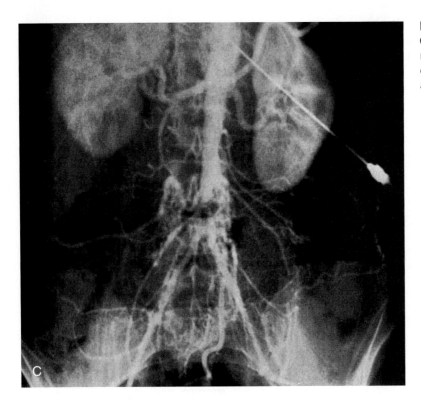

FIGURE 13-8, *cont'd.* **C,** Radiograph showing needle placement during translumbar aortography.

Once aortic puncture has been accomplished, a guide wire is inserted and advanced through the needle into the aorta. The sheath is then placed in the vessel over the guide wire. The injection of contrast agent is made through the sheath. In many cases a flush aortogram will yield useful diagnostic information; however, in many cases selective catheterization of the specific arteries can be performed for a more detailed study.

Venous studies require that the femoral vein access be used and the catheter passed into the inferior vena cava. As with the arterial studies, selective catheterization can be accomplished after a flush study assessment of the inferior vena cava has been completed.

CONTRAST AGENTS

The following flow rates and total volumes of contrast agents will vary with the disease process and the physician's preference. Although the technologist is often responsible for setting the flow rate and total contrast volume on the automatic injector, the radiologist is ultimately responsible for dictating both parameters.

Abdominal Aortography

Translumbar approach:
Flow rate   8–12 ml/s
Total volume   25–30 ml
Transfemoral or transaxillary approach:
Flow rate   20 ml/s
Total volume   40 ml

Adrenal Arteriography

Femoral artery approach:

Flow rate	1–3 ml/s
Total volume	4–6 ml

Adrenal Venography

Femoral vein approach:

Flow rate	2 ml/s
Total volume	3–4 ml

Renal Arteriography

Nonselective DSA:

Flow rate	20 ml/s
Total volume	30–40 ml

Selective DSA:

Flow rate	5 ml/s
Total volume	8–10 ml

TABLE 13-3 *Summary of Complications for Abdominal Angiographic Studies*

Procedure	Complications
Aortography	Mechanical complications resulting from the catheterization procedure
	Abdominal aortic aneurysm rupture
Adrenal angiography	Acute hypertension in cases of unsuspected pheochromocytoma
	Intra-adrenal extravasation of contrast agent
	Mechanical complications resulting from the catheterization procedure
Renal angiography	Local thrombus formation
	Arterial damage
	Rupture
	Dissection
	Renal infarction
	Embolus
	Renal
	Peripheral
	Renal failure
	Acute
	Chronic
	Myocardial infarction
	Perinephric hematoma
Testicular angiography	Venous perforation
	Phlebitis of pampiniform plexus
	Testicular atrophy
	Mechanical complications associated with intervention
	Balloon migration
	Misplaced coils
	Infection
	Hematoma at puncture site
Uterine angiography	Severe pelvic cramping
	Uterine infection

Renal Venography

Renal veins and intrarenal vasculature:
Flow rate   15 ml/s
Total volume   30 ml

COMPLICATIONS

Table 13-3 summarizes the potential complications for each of the procedures listed here. In all procedures that utilize a contrast agent there is a risk of complication from the administration of the substance. Contrast agent reactions can be reduced by the use of nonionic water-soluble compounds. Infections are also general complications that can be either systemic or localized to the puncture site. Also, as with any of the angiographic procedures, there is a risk of complications at the site of puncture and intravascular damage. These complications have been enumerated in previous chapters.

SUMMARY

Aortography is a valuable source of diagnostic information about the abdominal aorta, the urinary tract, and reproductive system. Other visceral structures such as the liver, spleen, pancreas, and gastrointestinal system can also be visualized using aortography. Vessel access techniques include the percutaneous catheter and the translumbar approach. The translumbar approach is rarely performed, but it remains viable when access to the vessel by the percutaneous approach is restricted.

The vasculature of the urinary system is easily demonstrated using selective catheterization techniques. Renal angiography specifically focuses on the kidneys and is used to demonstrate renovascular hypertension. The adrenal glands can also be studied, and interventions can be applied in the treatment of tumors.

Selective catheterization as an adjunct to aortography is also a useful tool in the diagnosis and treatment of disease processes associated with the male and female reproductive system. The study is used in the female to diagnose and treat fibroids, and in the male the primary indication is a suspected varicocele.

The water-soluble organic iodine compounds are used to provide the necessary contrast for the visualization of the anatomy. Indications for aortography vary; however, the major pathologic processes include arteriosclerosis and localized abdominal aortic aneurysm. The primary contraindications are the inability to perform the procedure and the potential for contrast agent reactions. Other contraindications are specific to the type of procedure being performed.

SUGGESTED READINGS

Renal Angiography

Bokhari SW, Faxon DP: Current advances in the diagnosis and treatment of renal artery stenosis. *Rev Cardiovasc Med* 5(4):204–215, 2004.

Dunnick NR: Renal lesions: great strides in imaging. *Radiology* 182:305–306, 1992.

Liss P, Eklof H, Hellberg O, Hagg A, Bostrom-Ardin A, Lofberg AM, Olsson U, Orndahl P, Nilsson H, Hansell P, Eriksson LG, Bergqvist D, Nyman R: Renal effects of CO_2 and iodinated contrast media in patients undergoing renovascular intervention: a prospective, randomized study. *J Vasc Interv Radiol* 16(1):57–65, 2005.

Michaely HJ, Schoenberg SO, Rieger JR, Reiser MF: MR Angiography in patients with renal disease. *Magn Reson Imaging Clin North Am* 13(1):131–151, 2005.

Textor SC: Pitfalls in imaging for renal artery stenosis. *Ann Intern Med* 141(9):730–731, 2004.

Pelvic Angiography

Bierdrager E, Van Rooij WJ, Sluzewski M: Emergency stenting to control massive bleeding of injured iliac artery following lumbar disk surgery. *Neuroradiology* 46(5):404–406, 2004.

Blattler W, Blattler IK: Relief of obstructive pelvic venous symptoms with endoluminal stenting. *J Vasc Surg* 29(3):484–488, 1999.

Gulsun M, Balkanci F, Cekirge S, Deger A: Pelvic kidney with an unusual blood supply: angiographic findings. *Surg Radiol Anat* 22(1):59–61, 2000.

Hak DJ: The role of pelvic angiography in evaluation and management of pelvic trauma. *Orthop Clin North Am* 35(4):439–443, 2004.

Ley EJ, Hood DB, Leke MA, Rao RK, Rowe VL, Weaver FA: Endovascular management of iliac vein occlusive disease. *Ann Vasc Surg* 18(2):228–233, 2004.

Metz CM, Hak DJ, Goulet JA, Williams D: Pelvic fracture patterns and their corresponding angiographic sources of hemorrhage. *Orthop Clin North Am* 35(4):431–437, 2004.

Pelage JP, Walker WJ, Le Dref O, Rymer R: Ovarian artery: angiographic appearance, embolization and relevance to uterine fibroid embolization. *Cardiovasc Intervent Radiol* 26(3):227–233, 2003.

Shapiro M, McDonald AA, Knight D, Johannigman JA, Cuschieri J: The role of repeat angiography in the management of pelvic fractures. *J Trauma* 58(2):227–231, 2005.

Strouse PJ: Magnetic resonance angiography of the pediatric abdomen and pelvis. *Magn Reson Imaging Clin North Am* 10(2):345–361, 2002.

Translumbar Aortography

Biswal R, Nosher JL, Siegel RL, et al: Translumbar placement of paired hemodialysis catheters (Tesio catheters) and follow-up in 10 patients. *Cardiovasc Intervent Radiol* 23(1):75–78, 2000.

Bove PG, Long GW, Shanley CJ, et al: Transrenal fixation of endovascular stent-grafts for infrarenal aortic aneurysm repair: mid-term results. *J Vasc Surg* 37(5):938–942, 2003.

Chan TY, Brown I, Sathanathan N, Punnyadasa HD: Position of skin puncture in translumbar aortography. *Acta Radiol* 34(6):631–632, 1993.

Henry GA, Williams B, Pollak J, Pfau S: Placement of an intracoronary stent via translumbar puncture. *Catheter Cardiovasc Interv* 46(3):340–342, 1999.

Kinney TB: Translumbar high inferior vena cava access placement in patients with thrombosed inferior vena cava filters. *J Vasc Interv Radiol* 14(12):1563–1568, 2003.

Patel NH: Percutaneous translumbar placement of a Hickman catheter into the azygous vein. *AJR Am J Roentgenol* 175(5):1302–1304, 2000.

Rial R, Serrano FF, Vega M, et al: Treatment of type II endoleaks after endovascular repair of abdominal aortic aneurysms: translumbar puncture and injection of thrombin into the aneurysm sac. *Eur J Vasc Endovasc Surg* 27(3):333–335, 2004.

Stavropoulos SW, Carpenter JP, Fairman RM, et al: Inferior vena cava traversal for translumbar endoleak embolization after endovascular abdominal aortic aneurysm repair. *J Vasc Interv Radiol* 14(9 Pt 1):1191–1194, 2003.

STUDY QUESTIONS

1. Which of the following parietal vessels is not paired?
   a. inferior phrenic
   b. median sacral
   c. lumbar
   d. common iliac

2. Which of the following organs is not supplied by the celiac trunk?
   a. esophagus
   b. liver
   c. kidney
   d. pancreas

3. The nephrogram phase of the renal angiogram demonstrates all of the following except:
   a. segmental branches of the renal artery
   b. venules
   c. arcuate arteries
   d. afferent arterioles

STUDY QUESTIONS (*cont'd*)

4. The pampiniform plexus can be found in the:
   a. male reproductive system
   b. female reproductive system
   c. renal vasculature
   d. splenic vasculature

5. A dilatation accompanied by tortuosity of the veins of the male reproductive system is referred to as a:
   a. fistula
   b. volvulus
   c. dissection
   d. varicocele

6. All of the following are indications for the performance of adrenal angiography except:
   a. leiomyoma
   b. malignant carcinoma
   c. pheochromocytoma
   d. Cushing's syndrome

7. The total volume of contrast agent recommended for a nonselective DSA examination of the renal vasculature is:
   a. 1–8 ml
   b. 10–15 ml
   c. 20–30 ml
   d. 30–40 ml

8. Which of the following would be considered a contraindication for uterine angiography?
   i. pregnancy
   ii. malignancy
   iii. endometritis
   a. i only
   b. i and ii only
   c. ii and iii only
   d. i, ii, and iii

9. Aldosterone is a compound that is secreted by the:
   a. liver
   b. adrenal medulla
   c. adrenal cortex
   d. pancreas

10. The renal arteries normally branch off from the aorta at the level of the _____ interspace.
   a. T11–T12
   b. L1–L2
   c. 2–L3
   d. L4–L5

14 *Visceral Angiography*

CHAPTER OBJECTIVES

After completing this chapter, the reader will be able to perform the following:

- Describe the vascular anatomy of the abdominal viscera
- List the various procedures that can be performed in these areas
- List the indications and contraindications for angiography in these areas
- Explain vessel access for these procedures
- Describe the contrast agents used in visceral angiography
- List suggested patient positions for various visceral angiography studies
- Identify common complications of these procedures

CHAPTER OUTLINE

The descending abdominal aorta provides the blood supply for the abdominal viscera. We have seen in Chapter 13 some of the major branches of the aorta. In this chapter we will discuss the vasculature of the gastrointestinal system, liver, spleen, and pancreas and the studies that relate to each of the respective organ systems.

ANATOMIC CONSIDERATIONS

The blood supply for the abdominal viscera comes from the branches of the descending aorta (Fig. 14–1). These branches include the paired **inferior phrenic**, unpaired **celiac trunk**, **superior mesenteric**, paired **middle adrenal**, paired **renal**, paired **gonadal**, **inferior mesenteric,** and **median sacral** arteries in order of their origins from superior to inferior. Also between the levels of the paired renal arteries

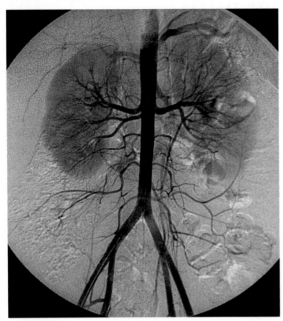

FIGURE 14-1. Radiograph of a flush aortogram showing how the major vessels from the aorta supply the various abdominal viscera with their blood supply.

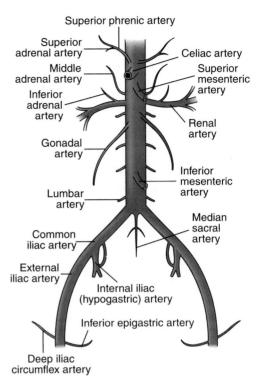

FIGURE 14-2. Schematic drawing showing the major branches of the descending abdominal aorta. Note the locations of both the superior and inferior mesenteric arteries in relationship to the other major arteries of the aorta.

and the aortic bifurcation there are four paired **lumbar arteries**. We will confine our discussion of the vasculature to the following branches: celiac trunk and its branches and the superior and inferior mesenteric arteries (Fig. 14-2).

Celiac Trunk

This is the first major branch arising from the abdominal aorta. It is located between the twelfth thoracic and first lumbar vertebral disk space. It gives rise to three major branches: the left gastric, hepatic, and splenic arteries. These three arteries are responsible for providing the blood supply to the organ systems in the superior portion of the abdomen, the liver, spleen, stomach, and pancreas.

In order of their origin the **left gastric artery** is the first to branch from the celiac trunk. This vessel runs along the lesser curvature of the stomach to supply the fundus and the gastroesophageal junction. It courses back toward the aorta and finally joins with the **right gastric artery,** which is a branch of the common hepatic artery.

The celiac trunk then bifurcates into two vessels, the **common hepatic** and the **splenic** arteries. The **splenic artery** is considered to be the largest branch of the celiac trunk. As its name implies, it runs toward the spleen, providing a supply of blood to various organs along the way. It is a tortuous vessel that gives off several branches including the **pancreatic** vessels, **left gastroepiploic** artery, **short gastric** arteries, and finally the splenic branches at its terminus.

The first branch of the common hepatic artery is the **gastroduodenal** artery. This vessel gives off the **superior pancreaticoduodenal** artery, which supplies the head of the pancreas with blood.

TABLE 14-1   *Summary of the Vasculature of the Celiac Trunk*

Major Branch	Primary Branch	Secondary Branch	Organ(s) Supplied
Left gastric artery	None	None	Fundus of the stomach Gastroesophageal junction
Splenic artery	Pancreatic arteries Left gastroepiploic Short gastric Splenic branches	None	Pancreas Greater curvature of stomach Fundus of stomach Spleen
Hepatic artery	Right gastric artery Gastroduodenal artery	Superior pancreaticoduodenal artery	Lesser curvature of the stomach Pancreatic head Duodenum
	Right hepatic artery	Cystic artery	Stomach Right lobe of liver Gallbladder
	Left hepatic artery		Left lobe of liver

Another branch continues as the **right gastric epiploic** artery to join with the left gastric epiploic artery. The common hepatic artery also gives rise to the **right gastric** artery, which runs toward the lesser curvature of the stomach and joins with the left gastric artery. At this point the hepatic artery is referred to as the **hepatic artery proper**. It courses upward to the liver and divides into the **left and right hepatic** arteries. The right hepatic artery usually gives off the **cystic** artery, which supplies the gallbladder with blood. The right and left hepatic arteries give off many branches and run in close proximity with branches from the hepatic portal vein. They empty into the hepatic sinusoids, which carry the blood to the central veins and out of the liver. Table 14–1 summarizes the various branches of the celiac trunk and the organ systems that are supplied by these vessels.

Superior Mesenteric Artery

The superior mesenteric artery (Fig. 14–3) arises from the aorta approximately 1.5 cm below the celiac trunk. It lies at about the level of the first and second lumbar intervertebral space. It is responsible for providing the blood supply for the viscera from the middle portion of the duodenum to the transverse colon.

The first major branch of the superior mesenteric artery is the **inferior pancreaticoduodenal**. It generally travels caudally, giving off approximately 10 to 14 branches to the small intestine. These intestinal arteries are referred to as the **jejunal** and **ileal** arteries. These branches usually join with branches above and below to form arches. As the arches approach the intestine they get smaller and smaller, finally giving rise to small straight vessels called the **vasa recta** that run to both sides of the small intestine.

The **middle colic artery** also arises in the same vicinity as the inferior pancreaticoduodenal artery. This artery divides into a right and left branch. The right branch of the middle colic artery joins with the right colic artery, and the left branch joins with the left colic branch of the inferior mesenteric artery. These form the **marginal artery**, which runs along the mesenteric border of the colon.

The **right colic** artery is the next vessel to arise from the superior mesenteric artery. It runs toward the ascending colon where it divides into an ascending and descending branch. There is an anastomosis between the descending branch of the right colic artery and the ascending branch of the ileocolic artery. The ascending branch of the right colic artery joins with the middle colic artery.

The **ileocolic** branch of the superior mesenteric artery is the most inferior of the major branches. It courses toward the cecum and gives off an ascending branch, which joins with the descending branch of the right colic artery. The ileocolic branch terminates at the level of the ileocecal junction

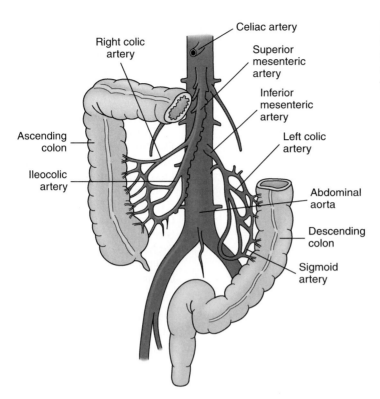

FIGURE 14-3. Drawing of the descending abdominal aorta showing the origin of the superior and inferior mesenteric artery and their branches.

and divides into a number of smaller branches (Table 14–2). One of these branches, the **appendicular** artery, supplies the appendix with blood.

Inferior Mesenteric Artery

The third major branch arising from the abdominal aorta is the **inferior mesenteric** artery (see Fig. 14–3). This vessel also provides a portion of the blood supply to the gastrointestinal system from the midtransverse colon to the rectum. It can be found on the ventral surface of the aorta at about the level of the third lumbar vertebra. The main trunk is longer than the superior mesenteric and is usually about 3 to 5 cm in length before it divides. The major branches from the vessel are the **left colic** artery, **sigmoid** arteries, and the **superior rectal (hemorrhoidal)** artery.

The left colic artery divides into an **ascending** and a **descending** branch. The ascending branch joins with the left branch of the middle colic artery and services the upper portion of the descending colon and a portion of the transverse colon. The descending branch supplies the midportion of the descending colon. It joins with the ascending branch of the sigmoid artery to supply the lower portion of the descending and sigmoid portions of the colon. There are usually two to three **sigmoid** arteries which give off both ascending and descending branches that form arcades or loops from which vasa recta are given off to supply the sigmoid colon with blood.

The inferior mesenteric artery continues into the **superior rectal (hemorrhoidal)** arteries, which divide to form **middle** and **inferior rectal** branches. These vessels supply the rectum and the anal canal. Table 14–3 summarizes the vasculature of the inferior mesenteric artery.

Venous Circulation

The major vein in the abdominal cavity that is responsible for bringing the blood back to the heart is the inferior vena cava. It collects the venous blood from the lower extremities, the back, and the viscera located in the abdomen and the pelvis (Fig. 14–4).

TABLE 14-2　*Summary of Vasculature of the Superior Mesenteric Artery*

Major Branch	Primary Branch	Secondary Branch	Organ(s) Supplied
Inferior pancreaticoduodenal	Anterior inferior pancreaticoduodenal Posterior inferior pancreaticoduodenal	Anterior duodenal arcades Posterior duodenal arcades	Pancreatic head and duodenum
Jejunal and ileal arteries	Intestinal arcades	Vasa recta	Small intestine
Middle colic artery	Right middle colic joins with the right colic artery Left middle colic joins with the left colic branch of the inferior mesenteric artery	Marginal artery	Transverse colon and ascending colon
Right colic artery	Ascending branch Descending branch	Joins with middle colic artery and gives off secondary branches Joins with ascending branch of ileocolic artery and gives off secondary branches	Ascending colon and the beginning portion of the transverse colon
Ileocolic artery	Ascending branch	Colic branch Anterior cecal branch Posterior cecal branch Appendicular artery Ileal branch	Cecum, terminal ileum, and appendix

TABLE 14-3　*Summary of Vasculature of the Inferior Mesenteric Branch of the Aorta*

Major Branch	Primary Branch	Secondary Branch	Organ(s) Supplied
Left colic artery	Ascending branch Descending branch	Joins with the left branch of the middle colic artery Joins with ascending branch of sigmoid artery	Left portion of the transverse colon and upper descending colon Lower portion of descending colon and sigmoid colon
Sigmoid arteries	Ascending branch Descending branch	Both branches join to form loops or arcades giving off vasa recta	Sigmoid colon
Superior rectal (hemorrhoidal)	Middle rectal arteries Inferior rectal arteries	Smaller branches	Rectum and anal canal

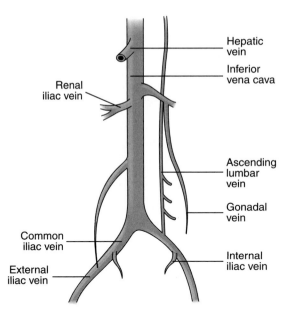

FIGURE 14-4. The vena cava and its major branches.

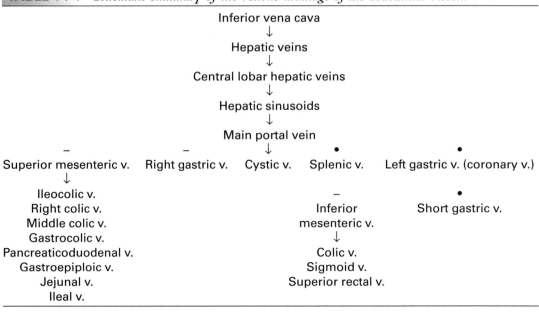

TABLE 14-4 *Schematic summary of the venous drainage of the abdominal viscera*

The blood from the stomach and intestine, pancreas, and spleen is received by the portal vein and transported to the sinusoids of the liver. There are many branches that contribute venous blood to the portal vein. These vessels are summarized in Table 14-4.

In the schematic in Table 14-4 it can be seen that the superior mesenteric vein collects the venous blood from the small bowel, right side of the colon, specifically from the cecum to the midtransverse portion, pancreas, and the duodenum. The balance of the colon from the rectum to the midtransverse colon delivers the venous blood to the inferior mesenteric vein before emptying into the splenic vein. The splenic vein primarily carries the blood from the spleen but also receives a venous flow from the stomach via the short gastric veins as well as the pancreas. The right and left gastric veins take the venous blood from the stomach and lower esophagus before emptying into the main portal vein.

The portal vein enters the liver, and branches are given off in a similar manner to the arterial blood supply. The capillaries of the portal vein and its branches join with their corresponding arterial capillaries in the hepatic sinusoids. From the sinusoids the venous blood enters the hepatic veins. These are distributed throughout the liver in the intersegmental planes draining their respective segments. There are three major hepatic veins: the left, middle, and right. These vessels usually enter the inferior vena cava individually; however, a union of the left and middle hepatic veins can occur shortly before the inferior vena cava, emptying into it as one vessel.

DIAGNOSTIC PROCEDURES

Aortography of the abdominal aorta has already been discussed in Chapter 13, along with procedures specific to the genitourinary system. It can be seen from the description of the anatomy of the abdominal viscera that there are a number of major vessels that would lend themselves to study via angiography. Collectively these procedures are grouped under the heading of visceral angiography. Specifically, the following vessels are usually studied selectively: celiac, splenic, hepatic, left gastric, gastroduodenal, inferior mesenteric, and superior mesenteric arteries. It should also be noted that there is quite a lot of variation in the normal visceral vasculature, making the studies both interesting and challenging. Most visceral studies are done primarily for interventional reasons.

Hepatic Angiography

Angiographic studies of the hepatic vasculature include hepatic arteriography, portal venography, and transhepatic portography. Selective catheterization of the portal vein and its branches cannot be accomplished. A direct hepatic or splenic puncture technique must be used if direct opacification of the portal vasculature is required. This technique is considered to be highly invasive, and practitioners have resorted to indirect portal studies by selectively catheterizing the mesenteric and splenic vessels.

Another approach is the catheterization of the celiac trunk, injecting the contrast agent and imaging through the arterial, capillary, and venous phases. The hepatic artery can also be superselectively catheterized directly. This technique yields excellent information of the intrahepatic branches in the arterial phase. It has the disadvantage of not providing a good visualization of the venous phase.

Pancreatic Angiography

The procedure is accomplished by means of an antegrade approach using the axillary artery as the means of vessel access or through catheterization of the femoral artery in a retrograde approach. The pancreas is fed by the celiac and superior mesenteric arteries, and a complete study of the vasculature of this organ should include opacification of both vessels. This can be accomplished by a single injection using a "Y" connector between the catheters or two separate injections, one in each of the vessels. Visualization of the vessels can be enhanced if the stomach is distended with air prior to the injection(s).

The projections required for a complete study include an anteroposterior and a slight right posterior oblique to demonstrate the venous system. The injection of a vasodilator can increase the blood flow, enabling the bolus of contrast agent to provide excellent vessel opacification. Digital subtraction techniques can provide a better study with the use of less contrast agent. It is important in pancreatic angiography to demonstrate all phases of blood flow through the organ.

Splenic Angiography

Most of the diagnostic splenic studies are being done using either computed tomography or magnetic resonance imaging. Splenic arteriography is generally done in conjunction with an interventional

TABLE 14-5 *Summary of Indications for Visceral Angiography*

Indication	Location / Structure / Vessel	Etiology
Acute ischemia	Mesenteric artery Superior Inferior	Embolus Vasculitis Vessel dissection Venous thrombosis
Chronic ischemia	Mesenteric artery Superior Inferior	Abdominal aortic coarctation Aneurysm Atherosclerosis Fibromuscular dysplasia Vasculitis Vessel dissection
Neoplasm	Pancreatic Hepatic	Assess presurgical anatomy Cholangiocarcinoma Hepatoma Metastatic adenocarcinoma Metastatic sarcoma
Benign lesions	Hepatic	Abscess Adenoma Cysts Hemangioma
Trauma	Gastrointestinal Hepatic Splenic	Blunt Penetrating
Gastrointestinal bleeding	Gastrointestinal tract	Arteriovenous malformations Bowel inflammation Diverticulosis Infection Ischemia Meckel's diverticulum Portal hypertension Tumors Ulcers Vasculitis
Aneurysms	Celiac Hepatic Splenic	Celiac artery stenosis Fibromuscular dysplasia Pancreatitis Superior mesenteric artery stenosis Vascular inflammation

procedure. It can be accomplished through a selective catheterization of the splenic artery following investigation of the anatomy by injection into the celiac trunk.

INDICATIONS AND CONTRAINDICATIONS

The indications for visceral angiography and endovascular intervention are varied. The general indications are ischemia, acute gastrointestinal bleeding (both upper and lower tracts), aneurysm, neoplasms (pancreatic and hepatic), benign masses, pre- and post-surgical assessment of liver transplantation, trauma, vascular hemorrhage or infarction (splenic), fibromuscular dysplasia, vessel dissection, vascular malformations, vasculitis, enlarged spleen, and cirrhosis. Table 14-5 summarizes the indications for visceral angiography.

The contraindications for the procedure are similar to those already discussed in previous chapters. The primary contraindication would be contrast agent reaction.

VESSEL ACCESS

The vessel access is similar to that discussed for aortography in Chapter 13. Selective catheterization of the various visceral vessels requires different guide wires and catheter shapes. Flush aortography can be performed prior to selective catheterization and can give the physician information about the vessels to make an accurate assessment of catheter and guide wire selection. This information can also be gleaned from the results of previous computed tomographic angiography or magnetic resonance angiography studies, if available. Some of the abdominal viscera are difficult to selectively catheterize and will require opacification by means of injections in the vicinity of the major vessels that supply more than one organ.

TABLE 14-6 *Suggested Contrast Agent Amounts for Various Visceral Angiographic Studies*

Study	Vessel Access	Flow Rate (ml/s)	Total Volume (ml)
Aortography	Percutaneous transfemoral approach	20	40
	Translumbar puncture	8–12	25–30
Celiac trunk angiography	Retrograde percutaneous femoral artery with selective catheterization of the celiac trunk	4–8	30–60
Common hepatic angiography	Retrograde percutaneous femoral artery with superselective catheterization of the common hepatic artery	5–6	40
Superior mesenteric angiography	Retrograde percutaneous femoral artery with selective catheterization of superior mesenteric artery	5–7	30–60
Inferior mesenteric angiography	Retrograde percutaneous femoral artery with selective catheterization of the inferior mesenteric artery	3–6	10–20
	Flush study from antegrade approach	16	35
Pancreatic angiography*	Bilateral femoral artery approach with simultaneous injection	10	60 (30 ml per vessel)
Splenoportography	Percutaneous transsplenic puncture	5–14	30–50
Splenic angiography	Percutaneous femoral approach with selective catheterization of the splenic artery	5–6	30–50
Arterial portography	Percutaneous femoral approach with selective catheterization of the superior mesenteric artery	6–8	30–60
Hepatic wedge venography	Percutaneous transfemoral vein puncture with selective wedge catheterization of a hepatic vein	2	6
Hepatic flush venography	Percutaneous transfemoral vein puncture with selective catheterization of the main hepatic vein	8–10	24

*Survey of vasculature uses selective celiac and superior mesenteric arteriography.

TABLE 14-7 *Summary of Suggested Patient Positioning for Various Visceral Angiography Studies*

Study	Anatomy Visualized	Recommended Projections
Aortography	Upper abdominal aorta and its branches	Anteroposterior Lateral Posteroanterior
Celiac trunk angiography	Intrahepatic branches, pancreas, spleen, and portions of the stomach and gastroesophageal junction	Anteroposterior Left anterior oblique
Common hepatic angiography	Hepatic arterial system	Anteroposterior
Superior mesenteric angiography	Duodenum, small bowel, large bowel to the splenic flexure	Anteroposterior Left anterior oblique
Inferior mesenteric angiography (retrograde percutaneous femoral artery approach)	Left side of large bowel, sigmoid and portion of the rectum	Anteroposterior
Inferior mesenteric angiography (flush study from antegrade approach)	Vasculature of the inferior mesenteric artery	Anteroposterior
Pancreatic angiography	Vasculature of the pancreas*	Anteroposterior Left anterior oblique
Splenoportography	Splenic vasculature and portal veins	Anteroposterior
Splenic angiography	Splenic vasculature and the main splenic and portal veins	Anteroposterior Right posterior oblique
Arterial portography	Extra- and intrahepatic portal veins	Conventional angiography use a 15-degree right posterior oblique Digital subtraction angiography uses anteroposterior
Hepatic wedge venography	Hepatic veins, portal vein branches	Anteroposterior
Hepatic flush venography	Visualization of the hepatic vein branches	Anteroposterior

*Selective pancreatic angiography requires selective catheterization of various arteries to visualize the different portions of the pancreatic vasculature.

CONTRAST AGENTS

The contrast agents that are used to image the visceral vasculature are also of the water–soluble iodine category. They can be ionic, low osmolar, or nonionic. The choice is made by the physician performing the study or determined by the protocol of the institution. The diagnostic procedures discussed are imaged using either the antegrade approach through percutaneous puncture of upper extremity vessel and catheter advancement into the abdominal aorta or via the transfemoral retrograde approach. The catheter is placed in the lumen of the aorta or is manipulated to selectively or superselectively catheterize specific vessels.

Table 14–6 lists some suggested flow rates and total volumes for the procedures discussed here.

PATIENT POSITIONING

Table 14-7 summarizes suggested patient positioning for the various procedures used for visceral angiography. Additional projections may be required depending upon the reason for the study and the need to demonstrate specific vasculature. Most projections can be achieved with a minimum of patient movement when using bilateral "C-arm" equipped angiography suites.

COMPLICATIONS.

The complications that can result from these procedures follow the same pattern as those discussed in previous chapters. They fall into several major categories: contrast agent reactions; systemic complications; mechanical complications resulting from the puncture technique, catheter insertion, and manipulation; and death. The factors mitigating the appearance of complications are related to the age and condition of the patient, the length and complexity of the procedure, and the severity of the disease. These factors should be considered when assessing the patient for the procedure. The successful management of these complications depends upon the preparedness of the staff and the presence of proper medical protocols. These should be established by the institution and reviewed prior to the procedure.

The contrast agent reactions have already been discussed in Chapter 6. The complications resulting from systemic disturbances are divided into cardiovascular, neurologic, and renal system failure. Cardiac events can result in complete cardiovascular collapse and death. Seizures can result from the procedure, and a danger of renal complications always exists with the injection of contrast agents.

The complications resulting from vessel access have also been addressed in previous chapters and include pseudoaneurysms, thrombosis, hemorrhage, arteriovenous fistula, mechanical failure of guide wires, catheters, and accessory items, vessel perforation, and emboli.

SUMMARY

The descending abdominal aorta provides the blood supply for the major organ systems in the abdomen. The celiac trunk is the first major vessel that originates from the aorta. Several major branches come from the celiac trunk, providing nutrients for much of the gastrointestinal system and the liver. The superior mesenteric artery arises from the aorta slightly below the level of the celiac trunk, providing the large intestine with a supply of blood. The third major branch is the inferior mesenteric artery, which also feeds the gastrointestinal system.

The major vessel responsible for bringing the blood back to the heart is the inferior vena cava. The hepatic venous system collects the blood from the abdominal viscera and delivers the blood to the inferior vena cava.

A variety of studies are performed in this area including hepatic, pancreatic, and splenic angiography. The techniques for vessel access are similar in all of these studies varying with the location of catheter placement and delivery of a satisfactory flow rate and total volume of contrast medium. Indications for these examinations include acute or chronic ischemia, neoplasm, benign lesions, trauma, gastrointestinal bleeding, and suspected aneurysms.

The water-soluble contrast agents are used for standard catheter studies. Flow rates and total volumes are dictated by the radiologist responsible for the case. Complications are similar to those discussed in previous chapters and are grouped into several categories: contrast agent reactions, systemic complications, and mechanical complications. These can be mild to severe and occasionally result in death. Attending to detail and establishing accurate baseline vital signs as well as taking a comprehensive patient history can reduce the number and severity of complications from the studies.

Fundamentals of Special Radiographic Procedures

SUGGESTED READINGS

Hepatic Angiography

Corazziari E: Biliary tract imaging. *Curr Gastroenterol Rep* 1(2):123–131, 1999.

Holland-Fischer P, Gronbaek H, Astrup L, Keiding S, Nielsen DT, Vilstrup H: Budd-Chiari and inferior caval vein syndromes due to membranous obstruction of the liver veins: successful treatment with angioplasty and transcaval transjugular intrahepatic porto-systemic shunt. *Scand J Gastroenterol* 39(10):1025–1028, 2004.

Kojima H, Tanigawa N, Komemushi A, Kariya S, Sawada S: Computed tomography perfusion of the liver: assessment of pure portal blood flow studied with CT perfusion during superior mesenteric arterial portography. *Acta Radiol* 45(7):709–715, 2004.

Martinez-Cuesta A, Elduayen B, Vivas I: CO(2) wedged hepatic venography: technical considerations and comparison with direct and indirect portography with iodinated contrast. *Abdom Imaging* 25(6):576–582, 2000.

Pilleul F, Beuf O: Diagnosis of splanchnic artery aneurysms and pseudoaneurysms, with special reference to contrast enhanced 3D magnetic resonance angiography: a review. *Acta Radiol* 45(7):702–708, 2004.

Uflacker R, Pariente DM: Angiographic findings in biliary atresia. *Cardiovasc Intervent Radiol* 27(5):486–490, 2004.

Weimann A, Ringe B, Klempnauer J: Benign liver tumors: differential diagnosis and indications for surgery. *World J Surg* 21(9):983–990; discussion 990–991, 1997.

Yamamoto K, Shiraki K, Nakanishi S, Fuke H, Hashimoto A, Shimizu A, Nakano T: Usefulness of digital subtraction imaging with Levovist in the diagnosis of hepatocellular carcinomas. *Oncol Rep* 13(1):95–99, 2005.

Pancreatic Angiography

ASGE guidelines for clinical application. The role of ERCP in diseases of the biliary tract and pancreas. American Society for Gastrointestinal Endoscopy. *Gastrointest Endosc* 50(6):915–920, 1999.

.Coakley FV, Schwartz LH: Magnetic resonance cholangiopancreatography. *J Magn Reson Imaging* 9(2):157–162, 1999.

Jackson JE: Angiography and arterial stimulation venous sampling in the localization of pancreatic neuroendocrine tumours. *Best Pract Res Clin Endocrinol Metab* 19(2):229–239, 2005.

Weber CH, Pfeifer KJ, Tato F, Reiser M, Rieger J: Transcatheter coil embolization of an aneurysm of the pancreatico-duodenal artery with occluded celiac trunk. *Cardiovasc Interv Radiol* 28(2):259-261, 2005.

Splenic Angiography

Bilbao JI, Vivas I, Elduayen B: Limitations of percutaneous techniques in the treatment of portal vein thrombosis. *Cardiovasc Interv Radiol* 22(5):417–422, 1999.

Pilleul F, Beuf O: Diagnosis of splanchnic artery aneurysms and pseudoaneurysms, with special reference to contrast enhanced 3D magnetic resonance angiography: a review. *Acta Radiol* 45(7):702–708, 2004.

Shanmuganathan K, Mirvis SE, Boyd-Kranis R, Takada T, Scalea TM: Nonsurgical management of blunt splenic injury: use of CT criteria to select patients for splenic arteriography and potential endovascular therapy. *Radiology* 217(1):75–82, 2000.

Vlachogiannakos J, Patch D, Watkinson A, et al: Carbon-dioxide portography: an expanding role? *Lancet* 355(9208):987–988, 2000.

STUDY QUESTIONS

1. The first major branch of the abdominal aorta is the:
   a. middle phrenic
   b. celiac trunk
   c. renal artery
   d. inferior mesenteric

2. The right gastric artery, which runs toward the lesser curvature of the stomach and joins with the left gastric artery, arises as a branch of the _____ artery.
   a. gastroepiploic
   b. short gastric
   c. pancreaticoduodenal
   d. common hepatic

3. The splenic artery supplies all of the organs listed here except the:
   a. right lobe of the liver
   b. spleen
   c. pancreas
   d. fundus of the stomach

STUDY QUESTIONS (*cont'd*)

4. The ascending colon and the beginning portion of the transverse colon receive their supply of blood from the _____ artery.
    a. vasa recta
    c. appendicular
    b. right colic
    d. pancreaticoduodenal

5. Which of the following major vessels supplies the rectum with blood?
    a. celiac trunk
    c. renal artery
    b. inferior mesenteric
    d. superior mesenteric

6. Which of the following studies will demonstrate the arterial, capillary, and venous phases of the hepatic vasculature?
    a. transhepatic portography
    b. selective catheterization of the portal vein
    c. direct splenic puncture
    d. superselective catheterization of the hepatic artery

7. Which of the following viscera would be candidates for the performance of angiography to evaluate the result of either blunt or penetrating trauma?
    i. gastrointestinal tract
    ii. liver
    iii. spleen
    a. i only
    c. i and iii only
    b. ii and iii only
    d. i, ii, and iii

8. The superior mesenteric artery arises from the aorta _____ in relationship to the celiac trunk.
    a. superiorly
    c. medially
    b. inferiorly
    d. laterally

9. The liver contains _____ major hepatic vein(s).
    a. 1
    c. 5
    b. 3
    d. 12

10. The suggested flow rate for celiac trunk angiography is _____ ml/s:
    a. 2–4
    c. 6–8
    b. 4–8
    d. 8–10

15 *Peripheral Vascular Procedures*

CHAPTER OBJECTIVES

After completing this chapter, the reader will be able to perform the following:

- Discuss the vascular anatomy of the upper and lower extremities and the pelvis
- List the various procedures that can be performed in these areas
- List the indications and contraindications for angiography in these areas
- Discuss vessel access for these procedures
- List the contrast agents that are suggested for peripheral angiography
- Discuss the patient positioning for peripheral angiography
- Identify common complications of these procedures

CHAPTER OUTLINE

Peripheral angiography involves demonstration of the circulation of the upper and lower extremities. Arteriography of the extremities has gained importance in the identification of many vascular abnormalities, including embolism, aneurysm, and arterial injury, and many bone and soft tissue lesions.

Femoral arteriography involves the entire lower extremity and can be accomplished with a single-film technique, digital subtraction angiography (DSA), single-plane serial radiography, or biplane serial radiography. Femoral arteriography is a commonly performed procedure primarily used to diagnose a variety of vascular diseases and is a common site for percutaneous intervention.

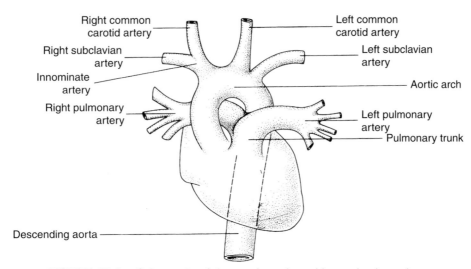

FIGURE 15-1. Schematic of the aortic arch and its major branches.

Arteriography on the upper extremity is performed less frequently for arterial disease than for venous pathophysiology. It is also not as frequent an examination as arteriography of the lower extremity.

ANATOMIC CONSIDERATIONS

Arterial Supply

Upper Extremity

The aortic arch gives off three major vessels: the brachiocephalic, left common carotid, and left subclavian arteries (Fig. 15-1). The brachiocephalic artery is the first major branch coming off the aorta. It splits into the right subclavian and the right common carotid arteries.

The subclavian arteries course over the apex of the lungs and give off several branches. These branches are the vertebral artery, thyrocervical trunk, dorsal scapular artery, costocervical trunk, and internal mammary artery (also known as the internal thoracic artery).

The vertebral artery courses up to enter the skull. This vessel supplies the deep structures in the neck. It also gives off branches referred to as the spinal arteries to supply the spinal cord and the meninges. It then courses into the skull where it joins the basilar artery. The anatomy of the vertebral artery will be discussed in depth in Chapter 16.

Another branch of the subclavian artery that supplies the deep neck structures is the costocervical artery, which, as its name implies, provides the supply for the upper two intercostal spaces. The thyrocervical vessels supply the thyroid gland, superficial neck structures, and upper scapula. Branches to the upper six intercostal spaces, the pleura, pericardium, and the breast are given off by the internal mammary (internal thoracic) artery. The final branch emanating from the subclavian artery is the dorsal or descending scapular artery, which sends branches to the scapular musculature and both surfaces of the scapula.

When the subclavian artery enters the axilla, at approximately the level of the first rib, it becomes the axillary artery. The axillary artery and its branches supply the axilla, shoulder joint, upper humerus, and structures of the chest wall. There are six major branches that arise from the axillary artery: superior thoracic, lateral thoracic, thoracoacromial trunk, subscapular artery, and anterior and posterior humeral circumflex arteries.

Upon leaving the axilla, the axillary artery becomes the brachial artery. Initially, this vessel courses adjacent to the humerus, and as it descends it runs anterior to the humerus until it crosses the humeral epicondyles at the elbow. It gives off several branches, among them the deep brachial artery, the nutrient humeral artery, the superior and inferior ulnar collateral arteries, and its terminal branches are radial and ulnar arteries. The deep brachial artery courses around the posterior of the humerus and provides the blood supply to the triceps muscle. The nutrient artery enters the nutrient canal on the humerus. The ulnar collateral arteries provide an anastomosis with the recurrent ulnar and radial arteries in the forearm.

The terminal branches of the brachial artery are the radial and the ulnar arteries. The ulnar artery is the larger vessel beginning at the cubital fossa (the triangular space at the bend of the elbow) and coursing toward the medial side of the forearm. A branch of the ulnar artery, the common interosseous artery, usually divides into an anterior and posterior branch, which follows the interosseous membrane. Some other branches of the ulnar artery are the anterior and posterior recurrent arteries, the palmar carpal branch, the dorsal carpal branch, and several muscular branches that supply the medial side of the forearm.

The smaller radial artery arises at the level of the radial head and runs down the lateral side of the forearm toward the hand. It gives off the following branches: the radial recurrent artery, the palmar carpal branch, the superficial palmar branch, and several muscular branches.

The radial and ulnar arteries supply the hand with blood. As it passes the wrist, the radial artery moves from the palmar surface to the posterior side of the hand. The ulnar artery passes through the wrist to the palmar side of the hand. These two arteries form the superficial and deep palmar arches. The superficial palmar arch gives off branches, the common palmar digital arteries, which provide the blood supply to the fingers. The deep and superficial arches along with the radial and ulnar arteries supply the thumb and forefinger with blood.

Lower Extremity

At about the level of the fourth lumbar vertebra, the abdominal aorta terminates in a bifurcation. At this point, the aorta becomes the common iliac arteries. These arteries travel for a short distance (about 5 cm), and at about the upper level of the sacrum, they divide into the external and internal iliac arteries.

The internal iliac arteries supply blood to the pelvic region, whereas the external iliac arteries are the origin of the blood supply to the lower extremities (Fig. 15-2, *A* and *B*). The external iliac artery courses for about 10 cm before becoming the femoral artery at a point midway between the anterior superior iliac spine and the symphysis pubis. This is also the level at which the femoral artery enters the lower extremity. The branches of the femoral artery are divided into superficial and deep branches, as summarized in Box 15-1.

As the femoral artery passes into the popliteal space, it becomes the popliteal artery. It courses in a lateral oblique direction to its termination, where it divides into the anterior and posterior tibial arteries. The popliteal artery usually has six major branches—lateral superior genicular, medial superior genicular, middle genicular, lateral inferior genicular, medial inferior genicular, and sural arteries.

The anterior tibial artery courses forward from its origin to descend into the interosseous membrane of the lower leg to the level of the anterior aspect of the ankle joint, where it becomes the dorsalis pedis artery. The major branches of the anterior tibial artery are located around the knee and

BOX 15-1	*Major Branches of the Femoral Artery*
Superficial	**Deep**
Epigastric	Muscular branches
Circumflex iliac	Deep external pudendal
External pudendal	Deep femoral
	Lateral circumflex
	Medial circumflex
	Descending genicular

ankle joints, and many smaller muscular branches are given off along its descending route. The anterior tibial artery is the smaller of the two branches of the popliteal artery.

The posterior tibial artery is a direct continuation of the popliteal artery. Coursing downward toward the ankle, it passes between the medial malleolus of the tibia and the calcaneus and terminates in the foot. As in the anatomy of the anterior tibial artery, the major branches of the posterior tibial artery—the peroneal, nutrient, communicating, posterior medial malleolar, and medial calcaneal arteries—are concentrated around the knee and ankle joints. A summary of the circulation from the level of the anterior and posterior tibial arteries is given in Figure 15-3.

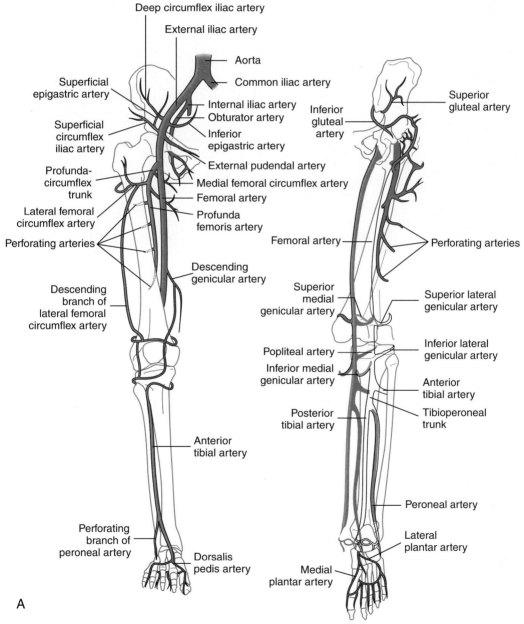

FIGURE 15-2.   A, Arteries on the lower limb shown from the anterior and posterior aspects.
Continued

Fundamentals of Special Radiographic Procedures

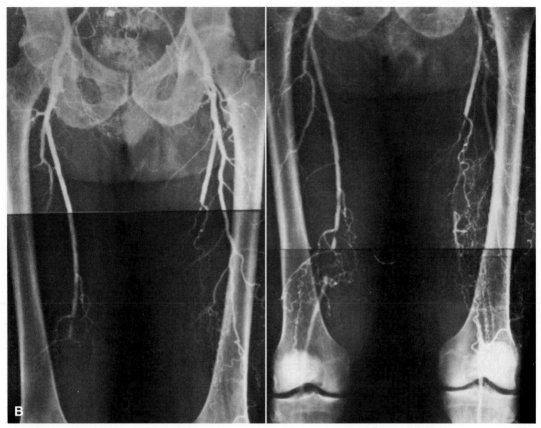

FIGURE 15-2, *cont'd*. B, Selected films from a femoral arteriogram depicting the contrast agent in the lower extremity.

Veins
Upper Extremity

The veins of the body collect the blood from the systemic circulation and return it to the heart and lungs for reoxygenation. The venous system of the body is extensive, and consideration is given here only to major veins with significance in venous angiography. The venous system of the body ultimately empties into two major veins—the inferior and superior venae cavae—which direct the venous blood into the right atrium of the heart (Fig. 15-4). All of the major veins are tributaries of these vessels and compose the venous circulation. The superior vena cava receives blood from the upper portion of the body, and the inferior vena cava serves the lower portion.

The venous system of the upper extremity consists of both superficial and deep veins. The deep veins are usually small and paired; they accompany the arteries and ultimately drain into the axillary vein. The veins of the upper extremity contain valves that prevent backflow of the blood and aid in movement of the blood to the heart.

There are two major superficial veins of the upper extremity—the cephalic vein and the basilic vein of the forearm (Fig. 15-5). These vessels are the primary means of drainage in the upper extremity. The cephalic vein starts in the distal forearm, receives the drainage from the dorsal aspect of the hand, runs along the lateral aspect of the arm, and ends just below the clavicle. At this point, the vein courses medially and joins the axillary vein. The median cubital vein forms a connection between the cephalic and the basilic veins of the upper extremity and is located on the anterior aspect of the arm at the level of the elbow. This vein is the usual location for blood

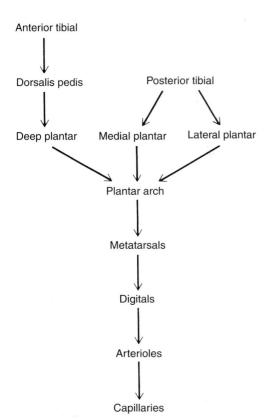

Anterior tibial

Dorsalis pedis

Posterior tibial

Deep plantar   Medial plantar   Lateral plantar

Plantar arch

Metatarsals

Digitals

Arterioles

Capillaries

FIGURE 15-3. Flowchart summarizing the arterial circulation of the lower extremity.

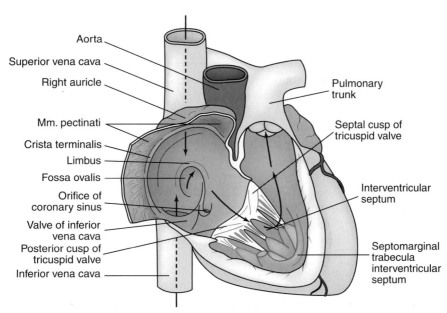

Aorta

Superior vena cava

Right auricle

Pulmonary trunk

Mm. pectinati

Septal cusp of tricuspid valve

Crista terminalis

Limbus

Fossa ovalis

Orifice of coronary sinus

Interventricular septum

Valve of inferior vena cava

Posterior cusp of tricuspid valve

Septomarginal trabecula interventricular septum

Inferior vena cava

FIGURE 15-4. External and internal anatomy of the right atrium, right ventricle, and the tricuspid orifice. Blood circulation is identified by the arrows.

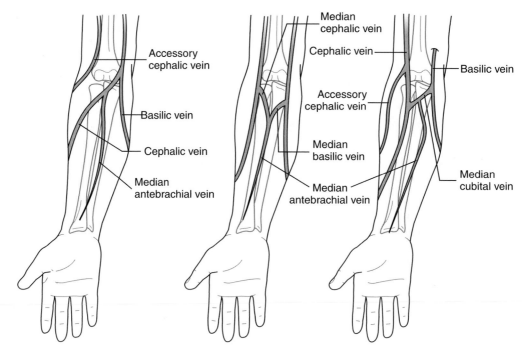

FIGURE 15-5. The superficial branches of the upper limb.

sampling, intravenous injection, blood transfusion, and introducing catheters for contrast radiography. The basilic vein runs up from the distal forearm toward the medial side of the arm, where it ultimately becomes the axillary vein. The median vein collects the venous return from the palmar aspect of the hand. It then courses over the anterior of the arm until it joins the basilic vein. In another variant of the normal anatomy, the median vein can also join the median cubital vein. The axillary vein continues a short distance and becomes the subclavian vein at approximately the level of the first rib. The subclavian vein is then joined by the internal jugular vein to form the brachiocephalic vein. The brachiocephalic vein also collects blood from the vertebral, internal mammary, intercostal, and thyroid veins.

The left and right brachiocephalic veins, which are formed by the union of the internal jugular and subclavian veins, join to form the superior vena cava. The superior vena cava then courses down on the right side of the ascending aorta, where it receives the azygos vein before entering the right atrium of the heart.

The azygos and hemiazygos system comprises unpaired vessels that lie on each side of the spine (Fig. 15-6). There are several normal variants of the anatomic presentation of this system of veins.

The azygos vein arises at about the level of the right renal vein and courses up to the right of midline. It collects venous blood from a variety of vessels, including the intercostal, subcostal, mediastinal, esophageal, right ascending lumbar, pericardial, bronchial, accessory hemiazygos, and hemiazygos veins. The hemiazygos and accessory hemiazygos veins are located to the left of midline and are considered to correspond to the azygos vein. These vessels collect blood from a variety of vessels on the left side of the body and ultimately empty into the azygos vein for transport to the heart.

Lower Extremity

The venous system of the lower extremity comprises both deep and superficial veins. Unlike in the upper extremity, here the deep veins provide the primary drainage. There is some communication throughout the venous system of the lower extremity; however, this is limited to one-way flow from the superficial system to the deep veins.

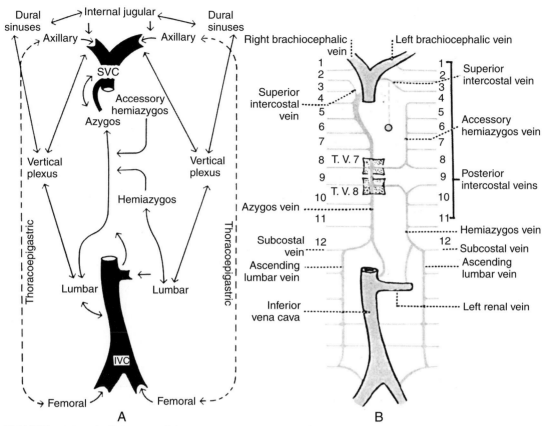

FIGURE 15-6. **A,** Scheme of the main connections of the azygos, caval, and vertebral systems of veins. Connections of the azygos and hemiazygos veins with the posterior intercostal veins also occur. **B,** The main veins of the thorax. A dashed line indicates the course of a left superior vena cava (a rare anomaly) on its way to the coronary sinus.

The superficial veins are represented primarily by the great and small saphenous veins. The accessory saphenous vein also contributes to the return of blood from the lower extremity, when it is present. It is usually located over the posteromedial aspect of the thigh and communicates with both the great and small saphenous veins. The great saphenous vein originates at the medial side of the foot at the level of the median marginal vein. It continues in front of the medial malleolus, ascends along the anteromedial aspect of the lower leg and thigh, and ends in the common femoral vein. The location of this vessel at the medial malleolus provides an excellent avenue for intravenous administration of medications, if necessary. The small saphenous vein, also called the lesser saphenous vein, originates on the lateral side of the foot at the level of the lateral marginal vein. It then courses toward the posterior of the lower leg and ascends to above the knee joint. Several normal variants may be present at this level, and the small saphenous vein joins the popliteal, greater saphenous, or deep muscular calf veins (Fig. 15-7).

The deep veins of the lower extremity consist primarily of the femoral and popliteal. These are usually paired and accompany the arteries. These normally originate with the vessels in the plantar surface of the foot and follow the course of the anterior tibial, posterior tibial, and peroneal arteries. The anterior and posterior tibial veins ascend to just below the level of the knee, where they anastomose to form the popliteal vein (Fig. 15-8). At approximately the level of midthigh, the popliteal veins become the superficial femoral vein. This vein ascends until it is joined by the deep femoral vein. This occurs about 5 to 10 cm below the inguinal ligament; the resultant vessel is called the common

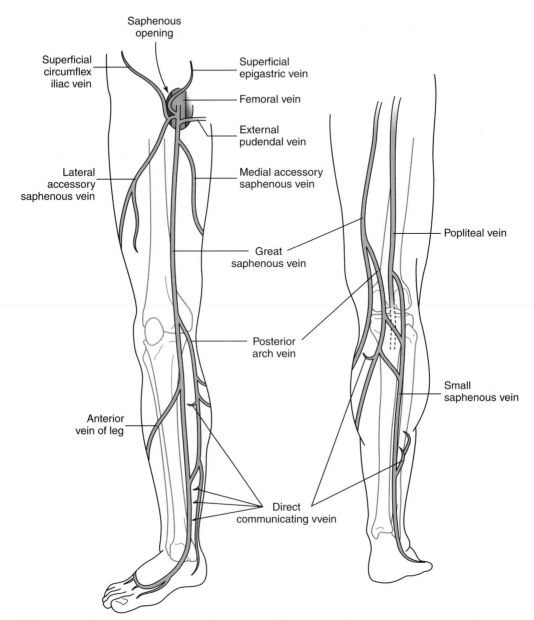

FIGURE 15-7. Schematic drawing of the superficial veins of the lower extremity. For ease of visualization only the major vessels are included.

femoral vein. The common femoral vein becomes the external iliac vein above the inguinal ligament. It connects with the internal iliac vein to become the common iliac vein. At about the level of the fifth lumbar vertebra, the left and right iliac veins join to become the inferior vena cava.

As in all veins, those of the lower extremity have thinner walls than the arteries and are equipped with valves to prevent the backflow of blood. The veins of the lower extremity begin as small channels; they are both superficial and deep in the foot. There are more valves in the deep-set veins; the veins become progressively larger along their ascending courses. These veins run with the arteries and are named similarly. The veins of the superficial group collect in the great and small saphenous veins.

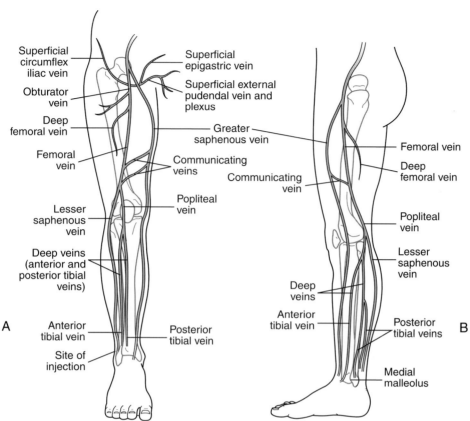

FIGURE 15-8. The major veins of the lower leg as they would appear in a normal venogram. **A,** Anteroposterior projection. **B,** Lateral projection.

The veins of the deep-set group and those of the small saphenous vein empty into the popliteal vein, whereas the great saphenous vein drains into the femoral vein. From this point, the blood flows up through the external and common iliac veins and ultimately into the inferior vena cava to the heart.

A summary of the venous circulation of the lower extremity is given in Figure 15-9.

Pelvic Circulation

The abdominal aorta bifurcates at the level of the fourth lumbar vertebra forming the left and right common iliac arteries. As the common iliac arteries approach the level of the sacrum, they once again divide into the external and internal iliac arteries. These are the only normal branches off the common iliac arteries.

Table 15-1 summarizes the branches that arise from the external and internal iliac arteries.

DIAGNOSTIC PROCEDURES
Upper Extremity and Superior Vena Cava

In the upper extremity, the site of puncture is dependent on the area of investigation. If the entire arm is to be imaged, a distal forearm vein is punctured. The physician may use either a 19-gauge butterfly needle or a small angiocatheter. The median cubital vein is usually the site of choice for evaluation of the axillary vein or central structures. This route is the same as that for the evaluation of the superior vena cava and can be done by direct injection or catheterization. The patient is prepared with the palm

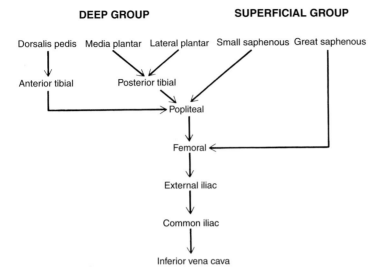

DEEP GROUP   **SUPERFICIAL GROUP**

FIGURE 15-9. Flowchart summarizing the venous circulation of the lower extremity.

TABLE 15-1 *Summary of Branches from the External and Internal Iliac Arteries*

Artery	Branch	Sub Branches
External iliac	Inferior epigastric artery	
	Deep iliac circumflex	
Internal iliac	Anterior trunk	Superior vesical
		Inferior vesical
		Middle hemorrhoidal
		Obturator
		Internal pudendal
		Uterine
		Prostatic
		Inferior gluteal
	Posterior trunk	Iliolumbar
		Lateral sacral superior gluteal

facing up and the arm abducted 90 degrees from the body. A tourniquet is applied proximal to the puncture site for manual injection methods. The contrast agent is then injected. During the last 5 ml of the injection, the tourniquet is released, and filming can proceed.

If the study is for diagnosis in the superior vena cava, the injection can be performed using a simultaneous bilateral direct injection of contrast agent into the median cubital vein. Catheter angiography in this area can be accomplished through catheterization of the median cubital vein, the jugular vein, or the femoral vein; the usual routes are the cubital and femoral approaches. An automatic injection device is used, and visualization of the contrast can be accomplished with fluoroscopy; filming can be accomplished in a single plane or biplane mode.

Azygos and Hemiazygos System

To visualize the vessels in the azygos and hemiazygos system, selective catheter venography is used. A catheter is maneuvered from the median cubital or femoral vein and selectively positioned in the azygos vein. An automatic injector is used to deliver the contrast agent at a rate of 15 ml/s for a total volume of 30 ml. Filming is usually accomplished in the biplane mode.

Inferior Vena Cava and Pelvis

The inferior vena cava is imaged with the median cubital or femoral approach. The technique involves the introduction of a catheter into the inferior vena cava. The type and size of the catheter depend on the approach and physician's preference. The cubital vein approach is contraindicated if thrombosis is suspected. Contrast agent is delivered by automatic injection at a rate of 20 ml/s for a total volume of 40 ml.

The veins of the pelvis, including the iliac veins, are usually imaged using a catheter sheath technique from a femoral vein approach. The external iliac vein can also be studied by catheter insertion at the median cubital vein. The rate and total volume of contrast agent vary with the site to be examined.

Lower Extremity

A number of techniques are used for contrast venography of the lower extremity. In general, the patient is positioned supine on a tilting radiographic table. The opposite leg is placed on a support that allows the leg of interest to be suspended or non–weight bearing. Tourniquets can be used to slow the progress of venous return; they can also help compress the superficial veins, allowing the contrast easier access to the deep veins. When this method is used, one tourniquet is placed above the ankle and the other is affixed slightly above the knee. Other variants of this procedure do not require the use of the second tourniquet or, as in the Greitz technique, require no tourniquets at all. When **ascending** venography is performed on the lower extremity a superficial vein on the dorsum of the foot is chosen for the puncture site, and a butterfly needle is used for the cannulation. The ankle tourniquet will prevent the contrast agent from filling the superficial veins and direct it into the deep venous system. Depending upon the preference of the physician, the table can be placed in an upright position between 45 and 90 degrees. This technique makes use of gravity to slow the progression of the contrast agent through the venous system. The contrast agent can then be introduced into the vein by means of manual or automatic injection with a slow flow rate. Continuous monitoring for extravasation is imperative. If extravasation is noted, the procedure should be aborted, and recannulation should be accomplished before the injection continues.

Descending venography is performed with the catheter approach using a femoral vein puncture. In the case of a unilateral study; the catheter is placed in the ipsilateral vein. When bilateral studies are done, a single femoral puncture will produce satisfactory images while reducing patient discomfort. The patient is placed in a 60-degree semierect position with the contralateral leg supported to provide non–weight-bearing status for the leg under study. From 30 to 100 ml of contrast agent is slowly injected into the catheter at a rate of 50 to 75 ml/min. Contrast flow can be followed by fluoroscopy, and filming is accomplished by spot film or cine camera.

If the equipment does not permit placement of the patient in the angled position, supine venography can be performed. The puncture site is the same, and tourniquets are used to slow the venous blood flow. The contrast agent is injected manually. After 50% of the contrast agent has been injected, the lower tourniquet is removed, and filming can proceed. As the contrast agent moves up the leg, the upper tourniquet is removed, and overhead films can be made of the upper leg and pelvis. The study should include imaging of the iliac vein and the inferior vena cava.

In both descending and ascending venography, filming can be accomplished with cine camera or large-format film radiography. The use of a stepping table is an advantage for this type of study.

Figure 15-10 shows examples of some venous angiograms of the upper and lower extremities and azygos systems.

INDICATIONS AND CONTRAINDICATIONS

Peripheral angiography is indicated in a number of instances. The primary focus in most cases is occlusive vascular disease. The procedure also has usefulness in mapping the vasculature as a presurgical tool and identification of complications from surgical procedures as well as being widely used in interventional radiology. Specific indications for the procedure are listed in Table 15-2 (p. 279).

The indications for arteriography include many vascular disorders of the upper and lower extremities and pelvis. Trauma to the lower extremity with clinical evidence of vascular involvement requires arteriography for injury assessment. The primary indication for femoral arteriography is in the diagnosis of vascular lesions. The procedure is also useful in the diagnosis of bone and soft tissue tumors, especially when interventional embolization is being considered.

Venography is performed primarily in the assessment of superficial and deep vein thrombosis. It also has use in the mapping of the vasculature for the placement of dialysis access sites, transvenous pacemakers, central venous catheter placement and external compression syndrome caused by trauma or neoplastic processes.

The contraindications for the procedure are minimal. They are limited to patients having previous history of contrast agent reaction, pregnancy and compromised physical condition resulting from renal insufficiency or reduced cardiopulmonary function.

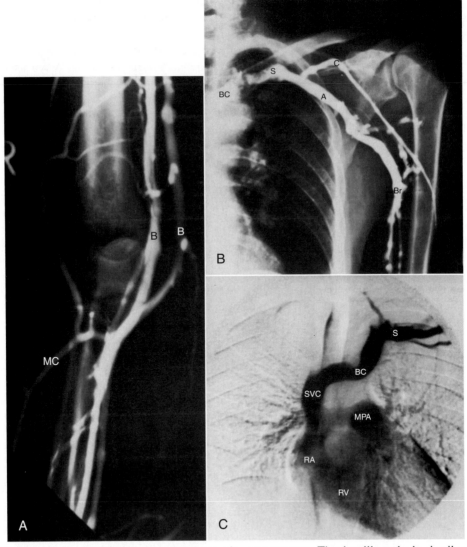

FIGURE 15-10. **A** to **C,** Normal upper extremity venograms. The basilic vein is duplicated. *A,* axillary; *B,* basilic; *BC,* brachiocephalic; *Br,* brachial; *C,* cephalic; *MC,* median cubital; *MPA,* main pulmonary artery; *RA,* right atrium; *RV,* right ventricle; *S,* subclavian vein; *SVC,* superior vena cava. *Continued*

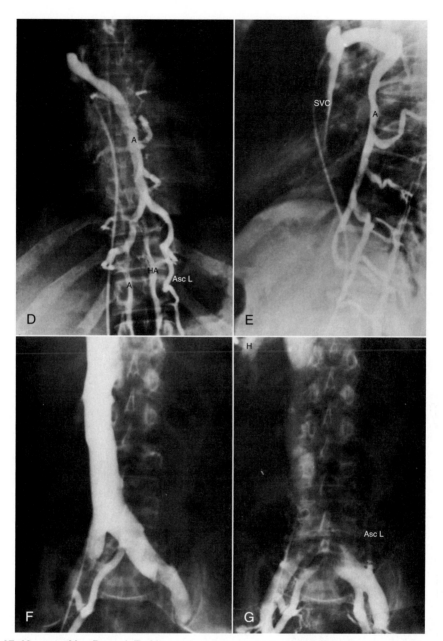

FIGURE 15-10, *cont'd.*   **D** and **E,** Normal anteroposterior and lateral azygos venograms. *A,* azygos; *Asc L,* ascending lumbar; *HA,* hemiazygos veins; *SVC,* superior vena cava. Normal inferior vena cavagram. **F,** Early phase. **G,** Later film shows reflux of contrast medium into pelvic and hepatic *(H)* veins.   *Continued*

VESSEL ACCESS

Arterial Access

The most common method of introducing the contrast agent into the aorta and lower extremity arteries is by the percutaneous transfemoral route. Retrograde percutaneous arterial puncture with catheterization via the femoral artery is the method of choice; however, antegrade percutaneous

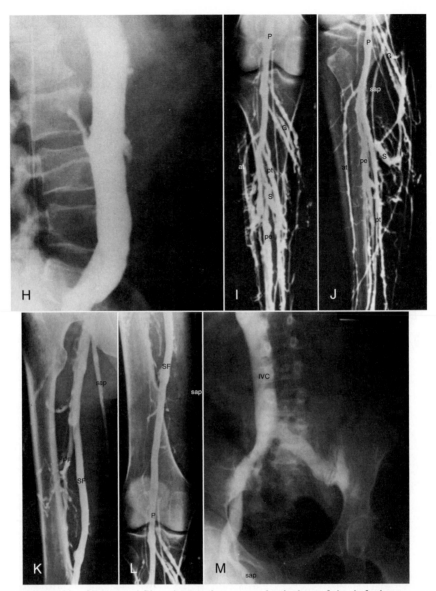

FIGURE 15-10, *cont'd*.   H, Lateral film shows the normal relation of the inferior vena cava to the spine. *ASC L,* ascending lumbar vein. Normal leg venogram. **I,** Anteroposterior and **J,** lateral distal leg. **K** and **L,** Proximal and distal thigh. **M,** Iliac vein and inferior vena cava. *at,* anterior tibial; *G,* gastrocnemius; *IVC,* inferior vena cava; *P,* popliteal; *pe,* peroneal; *PF,* profunda femoris; *pt,* posterior tibial; *S,* soleal; *sap,* saphenous; *SF,* superficial femoral veins.

puncture is an acceptable route for vessel access. If the transfemoral approach is not possible, left axillary artery or brachial artery puncture can be used, although there appears to be a greater incidence of complications with these approaches. An infrequently used technique is the translumbar aortic puncture with or without catheterization. This approach is used when both the transfemoral and the transaxillary approaches are compromised or contraindicated. The techniques of percutaneous catheter insertion as well as translumbar puncture have been discussed previously. The ultimate choice of injection technique is determined by institutional protocol and physician preference.

TABLE 15-2   *Summary of Indications for Arteriography and Venography of the Upper and Lower Extremity and Pelvis*

Procedure	General Pathology	Specific Conditions
Arteriography	Vascular lesions	Aneurysms
		Arterial spasm
		Arterial trauma
		Arteriosclerosis obliterans
		Arteriovenous fistula
		Arteriovenous malformation
		Embolism
		Grafts
		Occlusive disease
		Thromboangiitis obliterans
	Bone tumors	Angioma
		Chondroma
		Chondrosarcoma
		Ewing's tumor
		Giant cell tumor
		Intraosseous sarcoma
		Osteoid osteoma
		Osteoma
		Osteosarcoma
		Reticulum cell sarcoma
	Soft tissue tumors	Differentiated (blastic) sarcoma
		Fibroma
		Fibrosarcoma
		Lipoma
		Myxoma
		Neurofibroma
		Undifferentiated (ablastic) sarcoma
	Surgical/interventional planning	Presurgical mapping
		Postsurgical treatment /interventions
Pelvic angiography	Planning and intervention	Assessment of male impotence
		Atherosclerosis
		Iliac artery occlusions
		Localization of neoplastic lesions
		Localization of traumatic lesions
Venography	Venous disease of the upper, lower extremities and pelvis	Acute deep venous thrombosis
		Aneurysms
		Chronic deep vein thrombosis
		Congenital venous malformations
		Evaluation of tumors
		External compression syndrome
		Superficial vein thrombosis
		Trauma
		Upper extremity vein mapping for transvenous pacemaker placement or dialysis access

In many cases the lower extremity vessels are not adequately imaged due to delayed or decreased blood flow. Obstructive disease processes, diminished cardiac output, vasoconstriction, and poor collateral circulation are some of the causes. Two major techniques have been used to compensate for this factor: reactive hyperemia and vasodilatation. **Reactive hyperemia** refers to the mechanical increase in blood flow as a result of some action. Ischemia (decreased blood supply) is produced in the lower extremity with a blood pressure cuff inflated to 150 mm Hg for 5 to 7 minutes. The ischemia can be increased if exercise is added. The patient may be asked to flex or extend the foot during the period of time that the blood pressure cuff is inflated. Upon release of the pressure, the blood flow is increased to the lower extremity. **Vasodilatation** is induced by means of pharmacologic agents (vasodilators) or by the use of calcium-channel blockers.

Venous Access

Venous angiography can be performed with the percutaneous catheter technique or by direct injection. The choice of method is dictated by area of interest, physician preference, and type of pathology present.

CONTRAST AGENTS

Arteriography

The contrast agents used for peripheral arteriography are the water-soluble organic iodine compounds. Each institution will have its own protocol as to which type of contrast agent to use. In many cases the nonionic water-soluble contrast agents are used exclusively, and at other institutions these agents are reserved specifically for use in high-risk patients.

If the ionic contrast agents are used, either sodium or meglumine may be the choice; however, the N-methylglucamine salts are better tolerated for intravascular injection. Highly concentrated compounds, in the range of 50% to 76%, are recommended.

The amount of contrast agent injected depends on the vessel access, equipment, and procedure (see Table 15-3 for suggested contrast agent rates and volumes). If the injection is made into the distal aorta through percutaneous catheter insertion or translumbar aortography, a total of 40 to 60 ml is introduced at a rate of 10 to 15 ml/s over 3 to 4 s. Direct puncture of the femoral artery requires 20 to 30 ml injected at a rate of 10 to 15 ml/s for 2 to 3 s. If a specialized large-field cassette changer or cineradiography is used, the amount injected can be reduced because the entire system can then be recorded with a single injection. DSA allows the use of less concentrated contrast agents. Dilutions of 1:1 or 1:3 with saline are common utilizing this methodology. The lower concentrations have a tendency to reduce the reactions to the contrast material as well as the pain experienced with the intravascular injection of ionic iodine compounds. When DSA is performed, the total amount of contrast agent required for adequate arterial opacification is 20 to 25 ml.

Venography

It is recommended that a 60% concentration be used for upper extremity and superior vena cavography and a 76% concentration be used for all other types of studies. If DSA is being performed, the concentration of the contrast agent can be reduced to 20%. The amount suggested for a selective study of the common femoral vein is 25 ml introduced at 8 ml/s for 3 s and inferior vena cavography, 50 ml total injected at 20 ml/s for 2 to 2.5 s. The amount of material used varies with physician's preference, the area being examined, and hospital protocol. In venography the contrast agent should be mixed with the blood rather than administered as a bolus that replaces the blood. The diluted contrast agent will allow the visualization of smaller clots.

PATIENT POSITIONING

The positioning of the patient is dependent upon the type of procedure being performed. The upper limb can be imaged in its entirety or the procedure may be directed at a specific portion of the arm. If the study is limited to the hand, the patient is generally supine with the extremity extended and the

TABLE 15-3 *Summary of Contrast Agent Rates and Volumes for Peripheral Angiographic Procedures*

Anatomic Area	Puncture Site	Injection		Rate (ml/s)	Volume (ml)
		Manual	Automatic		
Upper extremity	Site dependent on area to be investigated	X		2–4	8–20*
	Digital subtraction	X		Bolus	20–40
	Screen film imaging				
Superior vena cava	Bilateral cubital vein injection	X		Bolus	25 each arm
	Catheter angiography				
	Cubital		X	15	30
	Femoral		X	15	30
Azygos and hemiazygos system	Catheter angiography				
	Cubital		X	5	12
	Femoral		X	5	12
Inferior vena cava	Catheter angiography				
	Cubital		X	20	40
	Femoral		X	20	40
Pelvis	Catheter sheath angiography, bilateral femoral		X	20	40
	Catheter angiography, aortic bifurcation		X	8–10	16–30
Lower extremity	Superficial dorsal pedis vein	X		Bolus	50–100†
Ascending Descending	Common femoral vein	X		Bolus	15
Iliac veins					
External	Femoral vein		X	10	20
Internal	Ipsilateral		X	10	20
	Contralateral		X	10	20
	Cubital vein		X	8	15
	Femoral vein				

* Contrast: saline ratio = 1:2.
† Low iodine content contrast agent < 200 mg/ml.

hand in either a prone or supine position. If the entire limb is the subject of the study, the anteroposterior projection is also used. Both venography and arteriography utilize the same patient position. If the entire limb is the subject of the examination, it should be imaged from the hand to the thoracic area.

Lower extremity angiography is also performed with the patient in the supine position because vessel access is generally accomplished via a transfemoral vessel approach or through a superficial dorsal pedal vessel. For single extremity studies the side of interest should be centered to the image receptor. Bilateral procedures require that the midline of the patient be centered to the image receptor, being sure to include both extremities. The same principle applies as in routine positioning of the lower extremity. The lower limbs should be internally rotated 30 degrees to achieve a true anteroposterior projection. Single limb studies may require lateral projections as well as those in the anteroposterior planes. When the entire limb is the subject of the study imaging should include from the foot to the aortic bifurcation for arteriography and to the common iliac vein in lower limb venography.

Table 15-4 provides a summary of the patient positions for peripheral angiography.

TABLE 15-4 *Summary of Patient Positioning for Peripheral Angiography*

Type of Angiography	Anatomic Location	Position	Projection
Arteriography	Upper limb	Patient supine, upper extremity extended with the hand in the supine or prone position	Anteroposterior
	Lower limb Femoral approach Femoral approach Translumbar approach	Patient supine, toes pointed up Patient supine, legs internally rotated 30 degrees. Improved visualization of popliteal arterial region Patient prone, legs internally rotated 30 degrees to place legs in true posteroanterior position	Anteroposterior Posteroanterior
	Pelvis (flush)	Patient supine, imaging to include from distal aorta to common femoral artery bifurcation Patient angled in posterior oblique positions	Anteroposterior Right and left posterior oblique
Venography	Upper limb Hand or forearm vein	The hand is placed in the anatomic position, the arm is abducted	Anteroposterior
	Lower limb (ascending) Superficial dorsal pedis vein	Patient supine in a reverse Trendelenburg position Imaging should include foot through the iliac veins	Anteroposterior
	Lower limb (descending) Femoral vein Femoral vein	Patient supine with head elevated 60 degrees Patient supine with no elevation of the head, patient required to perform a Valsalva maneuver upon injection of contrast agent	Anteroposterior Anteroposterior

COMPLICATIONS

The complications for peripheral angiography are similar to those already discussed in previous chapters. The complications associated with these procedures can primarily be associated with the establishment of vessel access or catheter manipulation. The patient's condition can influence the probability of adverse reactions. Higher risk patients exhibit a greater probability of sustaining complications as a result of the procedure. The skill of the physician performing the procedure also influences the potential for complications. Many of the problems can be linked to the vessel puncture. Situations such as hemorrhage, pseudoaneurysms, and thrombosis can be avoided by

BOX 15-2	*Summary of Some Major Complications Resulting from Peripheral Angiography*
Complication	**Treatment**
Aneurysm	Vessel reconstruction
Death	None
Distal embolization	Thrombolysis
	Surgical intervention
	Percutaneous intervention
Hemorrhage	Proper compression techniques
	Surgical intervention
Pseudoaneurysm	Percutaneous intervention with thrombin injection
	Percutaneous intravascular compression
Thrombosis	Preprocedure heparinization reduces risk
	Thrombolysis
Vessel dissection (false lumen or intimal flap)	Percutaneous catheter intervention
Vessel occlusion	Percutaneous angioplasty
Vessel spasm	Heparin bolus, 3000–5000 units
	Vasodilator injection
	Reserpine (0.5–1.0 mg)
	Tolazoline (25 mg)

carefully assessing the proper location for and the angle of the percutaneous puncture. Adequate compression at the conclusion of the study is important to avoid the possibility of hemorrhage at the puncture site.

Box 15-2 summarizes some of the major complications that have been reported as a result of peripheral angiography.

SUMMARY

The peripheral vasculature system is a commonly performed procedure used to both demonstrate and treat pathologic conditions of the upper and lower extremity and the pelvis. The upper extremity, head, and neck are fed via the major vessels arising from the aortic arch. On the right side of the body the brachiocephalic artery gives off the subclavian artery, which ultimately becomes the axillary artery, which services the shoulder, upper humerus, and some of the structures of the chest wall. At the level of the elbow the axillary artery branches into the brachial artery, which terminates in the radial and ulnar arteries. These two vessels supply the lower arm, wrist, and hand with a supply of blood. The left subclavian artery, which arises directly from the aortic arch, follows a similar path to feed the upper extremity.

The lower extremity is supplied from the abdominal aorta. This vessel terminates in a bifurcation at about the level of the fourth lumbar vertebra into the left and right common iliac arteries. At about the level of the sacrum these become the external iliac arteries, which give off several major branches to supply the pelvic structures and lower extremities.

The veins of both the upper and lower extremities begin distally and ultimately terminate in the inferior and superior venae cavae, which empty into the right atrium of the heart.

Imaging of either the lower or upper extremities can be accomplished using the techniques for vessel access and contrast media as described in previous chapters. The indications for the procedure include vascular lesions, bone tumors, surgical planning and intervention, and venous diseases of the upper and lower extremity and pelvis.

Water-soluble contrast agents are used in the procedures; the flow rates and total volumes will vary with the procedure being performed.

Complications of these procedures are related to vessel access, contrast agent reactions, and unacceptable patient care practices at the conclusion of the study.

SUGGESTED READINGS

Adriaensen ME, Kock MC, Stijnen T, et al: Peripheral arterial disease: therapeutic confidence of CT versus digital subtraction angiography and effects on additional imaging recommendations. *Radiology* 233(2):385–391, 2004.

Becker, GJ, McClenny TE, Kovacs ME, Raabe RD, Katzen BT: The importance of increasing public and physician awareness of peripheral arterial disease. *J Vasc Interv Radiol* 13:7–11, 2002.

Donnelly R, Hinwood D, London NJM: Non-invasive methods of arterial and venous assessment. *Br Med J* 320:698–701, 2000.

Higgins D: Peripheral venous cannulation. *Nurs Times* 100(41):32–33, 2004.

Hirsch AT, Criqui MH, Treat-Jacobson D, et al: Peripheral arterial disease detection, awareness and treatment in primary care. *JAMA* 286:1317–1324, 2001.

Meaney JF, Sheehy N: MR angiography of the peripheral arteries. *Magn Reson Imaging Clin N Am* 13(1):91–111, 2005.

Patel H: Peripheral magnetic resonance angiography. *J Ark Med Soc* 101(4):114–116, 2004.

Shearman CP: Management of intermittent claudication. *Br J Surg* 89:529–531, 2002.

Vorwerk D, Gunther RW: Percutaneous interventions for treatment of iliac artery stenoses and occlusions. *World J Surg* 25:319–327, 2001.

Wahlgren CM, Pekkari K: Elevated thioredoxin after angioplasty in peripheral arterial disease. *Eur J Vasc Endovasc Surg* 29(3):281–286, 2005.

STUDY QUESTIONS

1. Which of the following is not a branch of the subclavian artery?
   a. thyrocervical
   b. brachiocephalic
   c. vertebral
   d. internal mammary

2. The terminal branch(es) of the brachial artery include the:
   i. radial artery
   ii. nutrient artery
   iii. ulnar artery
   a. i only
   b. i and iii only
   c. ii and iii only
   d. i, ii, and iii

3. The abdominal aorta terminates in a bifurcation at the level of _____.
   a. T11
   b. L2
   c. L4
   d. the sacrum

4. Which of the following is not considered to be a deep branch of the femoral artery?
   a. lateral circumflex
   b. circumflex iliac
   c. medial circumflex
   d. descending genicular

5. The vein that is the usual location for blood sampling, intravenous injection, blood transfusion, and introducing catheters for contrast radiography is the _____.
   a. median cubital
   b. brachial
   c. anterior popliteal
   d. subclavian

STUDY QUESTIONS (*cont'd*)

6. The internal gluteal artery arises from which of the following vessels?
   a. external iliac
   b. internal iliac
   c. internal epigastric
   d. external pudendal

7. The primary indication for the use of venography as a diagnostic procedure is:
   a. confirmation of the presence of fibrosarcoma
   b. identification of Ewing's syndrome
   c. localization of vascular tumors
   d. identification of deep vein thrombosis

8. When imaging the azygos and hemiazygos vasculature the total amount of contrast agent recommended is:
   a. 8 ml   c. 40 ml
   b. 12 ml   d. 100 ml

9. The mechanical increase in blood flow as a result of some action is referred to as:
   a. ischemia
   b. interactive hypoxemia
   c. reactive hyperemia
   d. orthostatic hypotension

10. When ascending venography is performed the vessel chosen to provide access for the contrast agent is the:
    a. popliteal vein
    b. superficial vein on the dorsum of the foot
    c. common femoral vein
    d. brachial vein

16 *Neurologic Vascular Procedures*

CHAPTER OBJECTIVES

After completing this chapter, the reader will be able to perform the following:

- Describe the extracranial and intracranial vascular anatomy
- List the various procedures that can be performed in these areas
- List the indications and contraindications for angiography in these areas
- Describe vessel access for these procedures
- Identify the contrast agent used for these procedures
- List the equipment required for cerebral angiography
- List the patient positions used during diagnostic cerebral angiography
- Identify common complications of these procedures

CHAPTER OUTLINE

The demonstration of the cerebrovascular system by means of catheter placement with the administration of contrast medium is called **cerebral angiography**. This procedure had its official beginnings in 1927 when it was presented to the Neurologic Society of Paris by Egas Moniz, a Portuguese neurologist. There have been many improvements in technique, contrast media, and equipment since the origin of the procedure. Computed tomography (CT) angiography and magnetic resonance (MR) angiography are taking center stage in the diagnosis of neurologic pathology. The percutaneous catheter method is still viable in the practice of neurologic interventional radiography and as part of the diagnostic protocol.

ANATOMIC CONSIDERATIONS

Cerebral angiography provides the physician with a wealth of information regarding the anatomy of the cerebrovascular system as well as indirect information regarding the superficial and deep-lying structures of the brain. A great deal of knowledge has been compiled concerning the anatomy of the cerebrovascular system, most of which is beyond the scope of this text. However, a general summary of the major vessels of the cerebrovascular system is presented. The variations in arteries and veins are not considered to avoid the possibility of confusion.

Arterial Supply

A discussion of the cerebrovascular system must begin with the aortic arch, which is where the major vessels originate. In Chapter 15, we saw that the aortic arch has three major branches—the **brachiocephalic trunk**, the **left common carotid artery**, and the **left subclavian artery** (see Fig. 15-1). The brachiocephalic trunk is about 4 to 5 cm long at the upper border of the right sternoclavicular articulation and bifurcates into the right subclavian and right common carotid arteries. The left common carotid artery originates at the highest point of the aortic arch. It ascends to the left sternoclavicular joint, where it enters the neck. The common carotid arteries are **unequal** in length, with the left being 4 to 5 cm longer than the right. The carotid line, which begins at the sternoclavicular joint and terminates midway between the angle of the mandible and the mastoid process of the temporal bone, defines the course of the carotid artery. At the cranial edge of the thyroid cartilage, the common carotid arteries divide terminally into two main branches—the **internal** and **external carotid arteries**. At its bifurcation, there is a dilation of the terminal portion of the common carotid artery and the base of the internal carotid artery; this dilated portion is called the **carotid sinus**. The carotid sinus is similar to the aortic sinus in that it contains certain receptors that help to control blood pressure.

Internal Carotid Artery

The internal carotid artery has no named branches in the cervical segment. It supplies chiefly the frontal, parietal, and temporal lobes of the brain and orbital structures. It accompanies the internal jugular vein to the base of the skull and enters the carotid canal in the petrous portion of the temporal bone.

　　The course of the internal carotid is illustrated in Figure 16-1. The path of the internal carotid artery ascends from the underside of the petrous bone to the peak of the petrous pyramid. This path resembles an inverted "L." It then curves forward and medially, running laterally to the sphenoidal structures (**S5**). The artery then enters the cavernous sinus and passes next to the sella turcica (**S4**). It ascends, passes through the dural roof of the sinus under the base of the anterior clinoid process (**S3**), and then courses backward, passing under the optic nerve. At this point, the artery lies in the subarachnoid space (**S2**). It then ascends, dividing into the **anterior** and **middle cerebral** arteries (**S1**). The curving portions of the internal carotid artery, designated S2, S3, and S4, were called the **carotid siphon** by Moniz. The ophthalmic artery originates at point S3 of the carotid siphon. Two other arteries arise as branches of the carotid siphon—the **anterior choroidal** and **posterior communicating** arteries.

　　The two main terminal branches of the internal carotid artery are the **anterior cerebral** and **middle cerebral** arteries. The anterior cerebral artery is the smaller of the two main branches. It continues from the bifurcation of the internal carotid as the medial branch, entering the longitudinal fissure of the cerebrum. (The longitudinal fissure separates the right and left cerebral hemispheres.) At this point, the two anterior cerebral arteries are near one another and are joined by the **anterior**

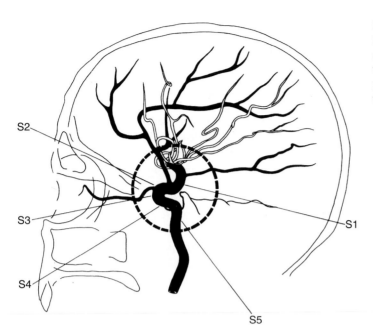

FIGURE 16-1. Schematic of the lateral view of the skull with arteries showing the course of the internal carotid artery. The portion in the circle is termed the "carotid siphon."

communicating artery. This is the shortest of the cerebral arteries and connects the arterial systems of both hemispheres. It is generally thought that the anterior cerebral artery runs to the origin of the **callosomarginal** artery. From this point, it is called the **pericallosal** artery.

The largest branch of the internal carotid artery is the middle cerebral artery. It courses laterally and is considered a direct continuation of the internal carotid artery. The middle cerebral artery appears to have many coils and loops as a result of the fetal growth of the cerebral hemisphere. During fetal development, the middle cerebral artery and its branches course smoothly over the **insula,** the central lobe of a cerebral hemisphere, also called the **isle of Reil**. With further fetal evolution, the insula sinks deeply into the cerebral hemisphere, giving the middle cerebral artery and its branches a coiled appearance in this area. This occurs when the branches of the middle cerebral artery course superiorly in the sylvian fissure until they rise to the top of the isle of Reil. From this point, they course laterally and inferiorly to the opening of the sylvian fissure and become dispersed in the cerebral hemispheres.

The isle of Reil is a triangular structure that can be delineated by the middle cerebral artery and its branches, which form the **sylvian triangle** (Fig. 16-2). This is a very important anatomic landmark; it is usually affected by most mass lesions, and any shift will probably be demonstrated.

The middle cerebral artery gives off many branches that are usually named for the areas they supply. They have a fan-shaped appearance and can be best seen in the lateral projection. The last branch leaving the sylvian triangle denotes the sylvian point and is called the angular branch. The middle cerebral artery and its branches supply the sensory, auditory, and motor areas of the brain.

Vertebrobasilar System

Another important arterial system that supplies the posteroinferior portion of the brain, brain stem, and cerebellum is the **vertebrobasilar** system (Fig. 16-3). The vertebral arteries originate as branches of the subclavian arteries. The left is longer than the right, because the right subclavian artery originates as a branch of the brachiocephalic artery. The **vertebral arteries** run through the cervical region and then pass through the foramen magnum to enter the skull. Running parallel to each other for a short distance, the vertebral arteries begin to converge and then unite to form the **basilar artery**.

The basilar artery begins at the lower border of the pons and terminally divides into the paired **posterior cerebral arteries**. In general, the basilar artery can be found traveling in the longitudinal

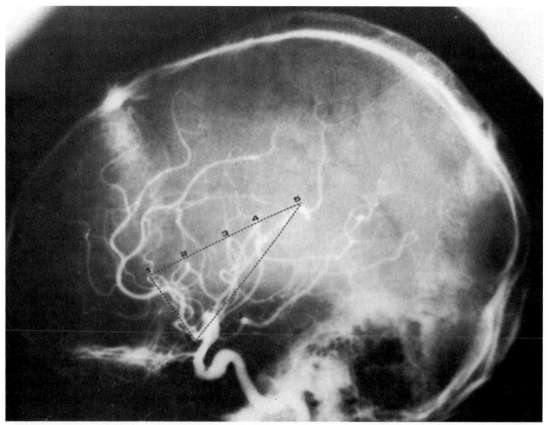

FIGURE 16-2. Lateral projection of the skull showing the middle cerebral artery and its branches. The triangular dotted line illustrates the sylvian triangle. The upper border or roof can be formed by drawing a line across the loops of the branches of the middle cerebral artery (numbered from 1 to 5 as they rise to the top of the sylvian fissure). Number 5 denotes the angular branch and the sylvian point. The floor of the sylvian triangle is shown by a dotted line drawn from the sylvian point to the genu (the area in which the middle cerebral artery bifurcates at its most lateral point). The anterior part of the sylvian triangle is demonstrated by connecting the anterior loop of the middle cerebral artery with the genu.

groove at the front of the pons (Fig. 16-4). A short distance after the union of the vertebral arteries, the paired **anteroinferior cerebellar** arteries arise as branches of the basilar artery. There are numerous **pontine** branches (paramedian arteries) coursing perpendicularly into the pons. As their name implies, these branches provide the blood supply to the pons. The paired **superior cerebellar** arteries can be found just before the terminal bifurcation of the basilar artery. These arteries supply the upper surface of the cerebellum. The posterior cerebral arteries supply the inferior and medial surfaces of the temporal and occipital lobes.

Circle of Willis

Many cerebral arteries anastomose with each other on the surface of the brain. One major anastomosis, the **circle of Willis (circulus arteriosus)**, is a union of the four major arteries supplying the brain (Fig. 16-5). This is not a direct union of the internal carotid and vertebral arteries but rather is formed by the major branches of these arteries. Through this anastomosis, an important means of collateral circulation is formed. In the event of obstruction of one of the arteries, circulation to the area may be

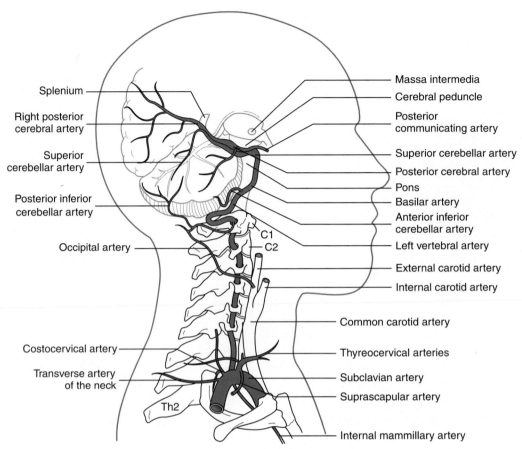

Splenium

Right posterior
cerebral artery

Superior
cerebellar artery

Posterior inferior
cerebellar artery

Occipital artery

Costocervical artery

Transverse artery
of the neck

Th2

C1
C2

Massa intermedia

Cerebral peduncle

Posterior
communicating artery

Superior cerebellar artery

Posterior cerebral artery

Pons

Basilar artery

Anterior inferior
cerebellar artery

Left vertebral artery

External carotid artery

Internal carotid artery

Common carotid artery

Thyreocervical arteries

Subclavian artery

Suprascapular artery

Internal mammillary artery

FIGURE 16-3. Schematic of the course of the arteries in the vertebrobasilar system.

continued through the circle of Willis. Each branch of the anastomosis has minute branches to the brain.

Venous Drainage

The venous drainage of the intracranial area can be considered in three segments—the **cerebral veins**, the **dural sinuses**, and the **internal jugular vein**.

Cerebral veins can be either superficial or deep-lying, inner veins. The superficial veins drain directly into the sinuses from the cortical region of the hemispheres and cerebellum. The inner, or deep, veins also empty into the sinuses, but they do so through a more circuitous route. The veins of the brain are thin-walled and do not contain valves. A summary of the cortical and deep veins of the brain is given in Table 16-1.

The **dural sinuses** receive blood from the cerebral veins. These sinuses are simply dilated areas lined with endothelium continuous with that of the veins formed by a separation of the layers of the dura mater. The dural sinuses include the **superior sagittal, inferior sagittal, occipital, right and left transverse, right and left sigmoid, straight,** and **cavernous sinuses** (Fig. 16-6). The superior and inferior sagittal sinuses lie on the borders of the falx cerebri, the fold of the dura mater that separates the cerebral hemispheres. The straight sinus is located at the junction of the falx cerebri and the tentorium cerebelli, which forms a partition between the cerebrum and the cerebellum.

The **confluence of sinuses** (torcular Herophili) is the junction of the superior, sagittal, and occipital sinuses with the right and left transverse sinuses. It is near the internal occipital protuberance.

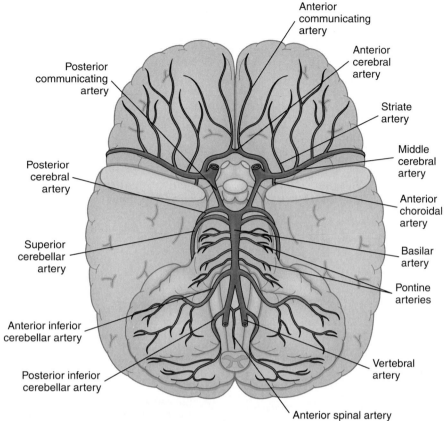

FIGURE 16-4.   The inferior aspect of the brain showing the location of the basilar artery.

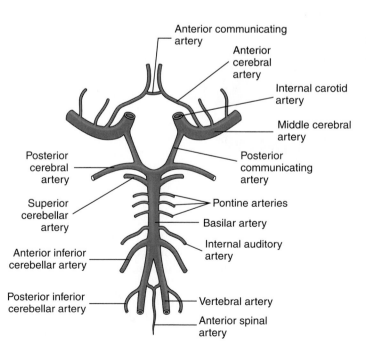

FIGURE 16-5. Schematic of the vessels that make up the circle of Willis.

TABLE 16-1 *Major Cerebral and Cerebellar Veins*

Type	Veins	Number	Termination
Superficial or external cerebral veins	Superior cerebral	8–10	Superior sagittal sinus
	Middle cerebral	1	Cavernous sinus
	Inferior cerebral	Numerous	Cavernous, petrosal, and transverse sinuses
	Basal	1	Great cerebral vein to straight sinus
Deep or internal veins	Internal cerebral	2	Join to form the great cerebral vein that terminates in the straight sinus
Cerebellar veins	Superior cerebellar	Numerous	Internal cerebral veins and straight sinus
	Inferior cerebellar	Numerous	Inferior petrosal, occipital, and sigmoid sinuses

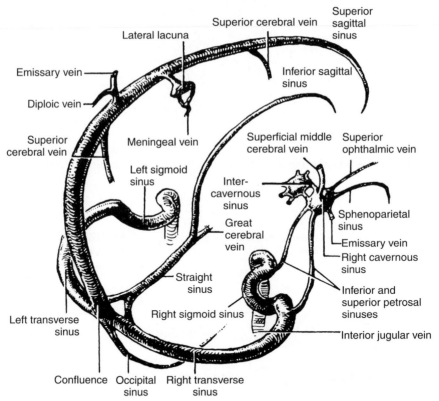

FIGURE 16-6. Schematic of the venous sinuses of the brain in the right lateral aspect.

The sigmoid sinuses are extensions of the transverse sinuses. They are located in a deep groove on the mastoid portion of the temporal bone and are contiguous with the internal jugular vein in the jugular foramen (Fig. 16-7).

The **internal jugular** segment begins with the sigmoid sinus in the jugular foramen. Its course can be represented on the surface of the body by a line from the lobe of the ear to the sternal end of the clavicle. The paired internal jugular veins join with the subclavian vein to form the **innominate** or

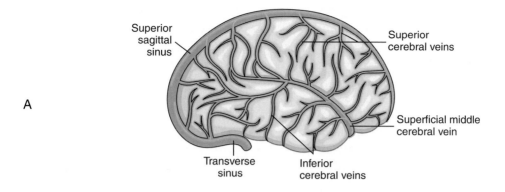

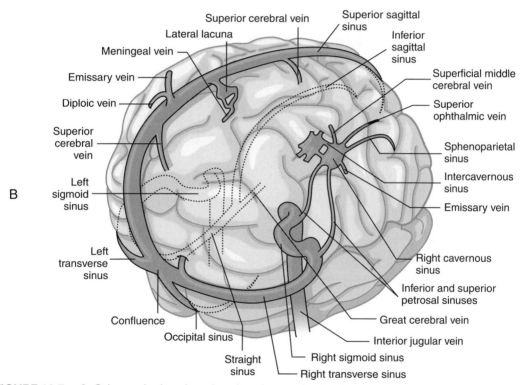

FIGURE 16-7.   **A,** Schematic drawing showing the cerebral veins as seen through the arachnoid after removal of the dura mater. **B,** The venous sinus of the dura mater.

brachiocephalic vein, which terminates in the superior vena cava. This segment receives blood from the dural sinuses and veins of the cranial cavity and the superficial veins of the face and the neck.

DIAGNOSTIC PROCEDURES

Cerebral arteriography and venography are the procedures that are usually performed both diagnostically and for the purpose of intervention. In the past these procedures were performed for a wide variety of indications; however, the improvements and use of noninvasive procedures such as magnetic resonance angiography (MRA) and magnetic resonance venography (MRV) have limited the use of these procedures. The basic cerebral angiogram can be used to investigate different areas of the cerebral vasculature, depending upon the catheter chosen and the vessel(s) selected to opacify. If the

BOX 16-1	*Summary of Indications for Cerebral Angiography*
Indication	**Pathology**
Diagnosis	Extracranial vessels
	Traumatized vessels
	Blunt trauma
	Penetrating trauma
	Atherosclerotic disease
	Aneurysmal dissections
	Facial fractures with oral or nasal bleeding
	Mapping of tumor vascularization
	Inferior petrosal venous sampling for ACTH levels
	Intracranial vessels
	Arteriovenous malformation
	Vessel spasm
	Arteritis
	Atherosclerotic disease
	Aneurysms
	Pseudoaneurysms
Intervention	Extracranial lesions prior to embolization
	Tumors
	Angiofibromas
	Extracranial blood supply to meningiomas
Evaluation	Intracranial lesions
	Hemodynamic significance of lesions
	Gliomas
	Presurgical mapping
	Postsurgical assessment
	Postintervention assessment
	Trauma to the neck
	Penetrating intracranial injury

vertebral arterial system is the desired target, the procedure is referred to as vertebral angiography. If the carotid artery is the target, then the study can be referred to as a carotid angiogram. Both extracranial and intracranial vasculature can be easily demonstrated using the basic technique. The major areas that are investigated using this procedure are internal carotid arteries, external carotid arteries, internal maxillary arteries, and the facial arteries.

INDICATIONS AND CONTRAINDICATIONS

Much of the diagnostic investigation of pathology of the brain is being relegated to computed tomography and magnetic resonance imaging, especially in identifying intracranial saccular aneurysms and carotid artery disease in the neck. The proportion of cerebral angiograms performed has declined, and it is no longer considered a primary diagnostic tool for cerebral pathology. However, the study will remain important in interventional neuroradiology and presurgical mapping. Box 16-1 summarizes the indications for cerebral angiography, which fall into three broad categories—diagnosis, intervention, and evaluation.

Cerebral angiography can be used in the differential diagnosis of cerebrovascular disease for the differentiation of various intracerebral hematomas and vascular lesions and in the diagnosis and localization of intracranial tumors. These pathologic conditions can also be demonstrated by magnetic

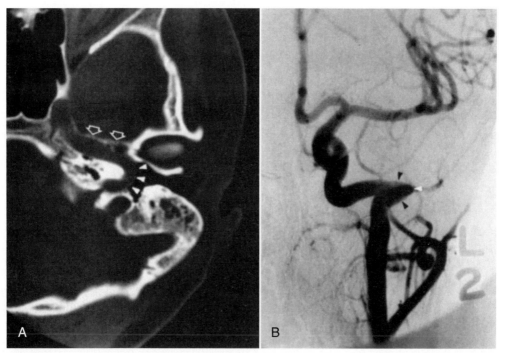

FIGURE 16-8.   An aberrant left internal carotid artery. **A,** An axial CT scan shows what appears to be a vascular structure coursing through the middle ear cavity (*arrowheads*) and then entering the carotid canal (*arrows*). **B,** An anteroposterior view of a left common carotid angiogram confirms that this is an aberrant loop (*arrowheads*) of the internal carotid artery.

resonance imaging and computed tomography; however, correlation with conventional or digital subtraction angiography cerebral studies should be made to confirm diagnosis (Fig. 16-8).

It can also be indicated as an evaluative procedure after intracranial surgery or for diagnosis of postsurgical complications.

Contraindications for cerebral angiography include contrast media sensitivity, advanced arteriosclerosis, extremely ill or comatose patients, severe hypertension, or severe subarachnoid or intracerebral hemorrhaging. The examination can be hazardous and is generally contraindicated in very old patients.

VESSEL ACCESS

The most common method of vessel access for neuroangiography is via the transfemoral artery approach. Figure 16-9 illustrates the various entrance sites that can be used for percutaneous catheter insertion. The access site used will depend upon the information desired and the personal preference of the physician performing the procedure. A brief discussion of the direct puncture technique is provided.

Percutaneous catheterization has already been discussed in Chapter 8. The basic puncture technique is the same and will not be discussed here. The most common approach for cerebrovascular studies is through the femoral artery. Because of a greater threat of thrombosis, the brachial artery is the second choice, followed by the axillary artery.

Various catheters are available for use in cerebral angiography. These catheters differ in the configuration of the catheter tip, although they all contain only one end hole; the choice is dependent upon the physician and the patient's anatomy.

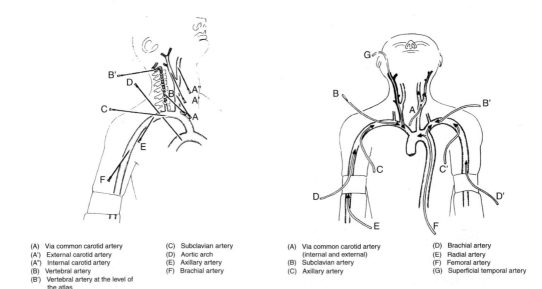

(A) Via common carotid artery
(A') External carotid artery
(A") Internal carotid artery
(B) Vertebral artery
(B') Vertebral artery at the level of
      the atlas

(C) Subclavian artery
(D) Aortic arch
(E) Axillary artery
(F) Brachial artery

(A) Via common carotid artery
      (internal and external)
(B) Subclavian artery
(C) Axillary artery

(D) Brachial artery
(E) Radial artery
(F) Femoral artery
(G) Superficial temporal artery

FIGURE 16-9. Schematics of the percutaneous catheter routes for injection of contrast material in neuroangiography.

CONTRAST AGENTS

The contrast agents used in conventional angiography of the vasculature of the brain and spinal cord have shifted from the ionic water-soluble organic iodine compounds to the nonionic agents. The use of iodinated contrast agents will affect creatinine clearance from the kidneys. Attention to the preliminary blood work, especially the creatinine levels and blood urea nitrogen (BUN) level and the patient's history will help in the identification of those individuals who have a greater risk from the study. Contrast agent reactions and complications are reduced with the use of the nonionic substances. Reference to the package insert accompanying the contrast agents will yield specific information regarding the use and side effects of the material. Table 16-2 lists some representative injection rates for imaging a number of cerebral vessels.

EQUIPMENT

Cerebral angiographic technique requires the use of very short exposure times when rapid serial film changers are used. Modern systems are equipped with radiographic generators capable of both high- and low-capacity requirements. Principles of good radiographic technique must be applied to produce films of high contrast. The kilovoltage used should be just sufficient for penetration of the skull. Use of higher kilovoltage with filtration usually compromises the contrast obtained.

Cerebral angiography requires serial film capture devices to record the passage of the contrast material through the cerebrovascular system. Naturally, the more sophisticated the film changing system, the more information that will be available from the examination. Any variety of serial capture devices may be used.

TABLE 16-2 *Injection Flow Rates and Total Volumes*

Target Vessel	Flow rate (ml/s)	Total Volume (ml)
Internal carotid artery	6	8
External carotid artery	3	5
Vertebral artery	5	8
Common carotid artery	7	11
Aortic arch	22	45

Data from Yousem DM, Trinh BC: *AJNR Am J Neuroradiol* 22(10):1838–1840, 2001.

These can be single-plane or biplane systems, each of which has advantages and disadvantages. When available, a biplane system should be used for cerebral angiography and is considered the method of choice.

In most vascular suites the units are equipped with dual "C" arm systems. This allows the physician to produce any number of different views with the least amount of movement of the patient. Digital subtraction is also a necessity to remove the superimposed bony structures from the image, leaving only the opacified vasculature.

For a differential diagnosis, the arterial, capillary, and venous phases of cerebral circulation must be demonstrated. Each phase is approximately 2 s apart. The exact time between phases is dependent on the circulation time of the contrast agent, which can vary from patient to patient and can be affected by any pathology present.

Needle or catheter insertions are done using sterile techniques. All necessary sterile equipment for cerebral angiography should be prepared ahead and assembled as a sterile tray. This should contain all necessary needles, syringes, drapes, towels, sponges, and receptacles. The equipment to be included in a typical cerebral angiography tray is shown in Box 16-2.

Other equipment that should be available during cerebral angiography includes the following:

1. A head binder or adhesive tape for immobilization of the patient's head
2. Additional sterile catheters and needles in the event of malfunction
3. Various radiation protection devices to ensure a minimum radiation dose to the patient and personnel involved in the procedure
4. An emergency drug cart and oxygen supply to treat possible reactions resulting from the procedure or contrast agent

PATIENT POSITIONING

Relatively few positions are used for recording the events of cerebral angiography. Usually, only anteroposterior and supine lateral views are taken; however, additional views may be requested in certain circumstances.

Anteroposterior View

The anteroposterior view used varies slightly depending on whether a carotid or vertebral arteriogram is being performed. It is necessary to adjust the tube angle specifically for each procedure to

BOX 16-2	*Equipment in a Typical Sterile Cerebral Angiography Tray*
Equipment	**Amount/Size**
Needle	1 ($25 \times \frac{5}{8}$ in)
Needle	1 (22×1 in)
Needle	1 ($20 \times 1\frac{1}{2}$ in)
Needle	1 ($18 \times 1\frac{1}{2}$ in)
Needles	2 (17×2 in)
Luer-Lok control syringe	1 (10 ml)
Luer-Lok control syringe	1 (3 ml)
Luer-Lok syringe	1 (20 ml)
Syringe	1 (2 ml)
Topper sponges	24 (4×4 in)
Towels	3
Monel cups	2
Emesis basin	1
Three-way stopcock	1
Sponge stick	1

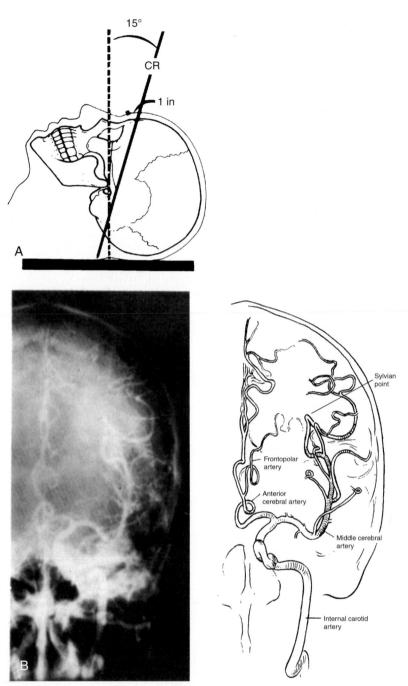

FIGURE 16-10. The standard anteroposterior view for carotid arteriography. **A,** Schematic of the anteroposterior view for carotid arteriography. **B,** Radiograph and labeled tracing of an anteroposterior carotid arteriogram.

demonstrate the desired anatomy in the best way. A caudal tube angle of 15 degrees is used to demonstrate the anatomy during carotid arteriography (Fig. 16-10), whereas a 25–degree angle is needed during vertebral angiography (Fig. 16-11).

In each case, the patient is supine, with the head positioned over the image receptor. The skull must be positioned symmetrically; that is, the median plane of the skull must be perpendicular to the

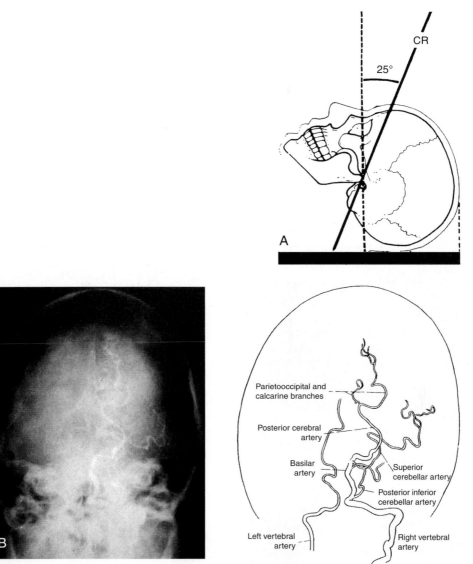

FIGURE 16-11. The standard anteroposterior view for vertebral arteriography. **A,** Schematic of the anteroposterior view for vertebral arteriography. **B,** Radiograph and labeled tracing of an anteroposterior vertebral arteriogram.

film plane to avoid distortion of the anatomy. The chin should be depressed to place the orbitomeatal baseline perpendicular to the film. The tube is then adjusted to the proper caudal angle. The central ray is directed through the frontal bone and external auditory meatus to the center of the image receptor. The field size should be collimated to the size of the head to minimize the production of scattered radiation.

Lateral View

Patient positioning for the routine lateral view is almost identical for both carotid and vertebral angiography. The only difference in the two procedures is the location of the central ray. During carotid angiography, the central ray is directed horizontally at a point approximately 2.5 cm anterior to and

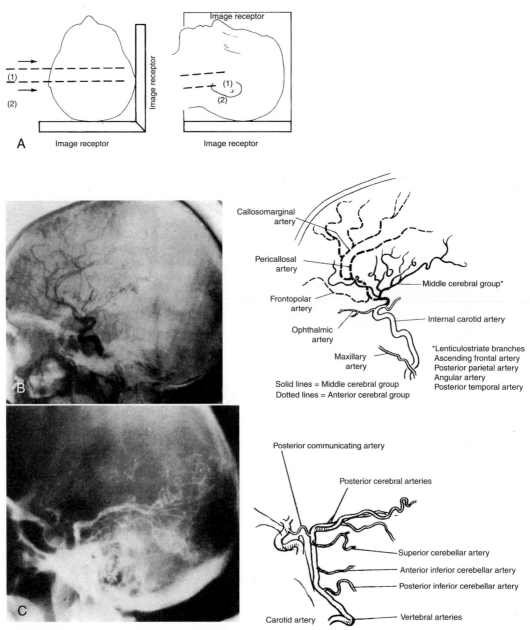

FIGURE 16-12. The routine lateral view. **A,** Schematic of the routine lateral view for carotid (1) and vertebral (2) arteriography. **B,** Radiograph and labeled tracing of a routine lateral carotid arteriogram. **C,** Radiograph and labeled tracing of a routine lateral vertebral arteriogram.

2.5 cm above the external auditory meatus. Vertebral angiography requires that the central ray be directed 2.5 cm posterior to the external auditory meatus (Fig. 16–12).

For the lateral position, the skull must be positioned symmetrically with the orbitomeatal baseline perpendicular to the tabletop. The head should be immobilized to minimize motion. As in the anteroposterior view, the field size should be collimated to just cover the head.

Occasionally, certain pathologic conditions require specialized views to delineate the anatomy. The most common of these is suspected aneurysms, which can be demonstrated best by using the supine

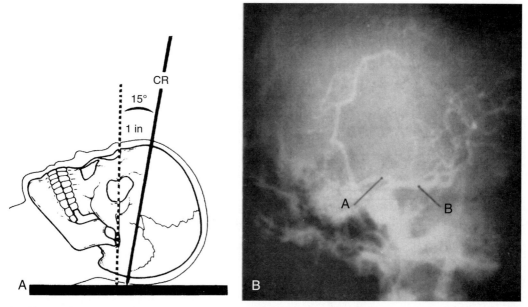

FIGURE 16-13.   The supine oblique view. **A,** Schematic of the supine oblique view. **B,** Radiograph showing the anterior cerebral (*A*) and middle cerebral (*B*) arteries.

oblique view. In cases in which subdural hematoma is suspected, a tangential projection may be used for delineation.

Supine Oblique View

The supine oblique view is accomplished by rotating the patient's head from 30 to 60 degrees away from the injected side or adjusting the "C" arm to a corresponding angle. The central ray is directed through a point approximately 2.5 cm above the supraorbital margin to the midpoint of the film at a caudal angle of from 15 to 20 degrees (Fig. 16-13). Arterial aneurysms in the area of the anterior communicating artery are well delineated with this view.

Transorbital Projection

Another supine oblique view, the transorbital projection, is used to demonstrate arterial aneurysms in the first portion of the middle cerebral artery. The median plane of the skull is rotated approximately 10 degrees toward the injected side. The central ray is then directed cephalad, through the center of the orbit, at an angle of 5 degrees to the center of the film (Fig. 16-14). In all cases, the radiographic field size should be collimated to cover the size of the head.

Tangential Projection

In some instances, it may be necessary to demonstrate a subdural hematoma specifically. This may be accomplished by rotating the median plane of the skull approximately 20 degrees away from the injected side when the hematoma is toward the posterior of the skull and 10 degrees toward the injected side for the hematoma located in the anterior of the skull. The central ray is directed tangentially to the suspected region at right angles to the image receptor (Fig. 16-15). For a summary of cerebral angiographic positioning, see Table 16-3.

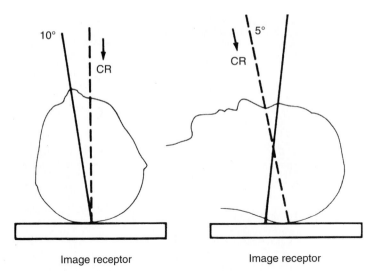

FIGURE 16-14. Schematic of the positioning for the transorbital oblique view.

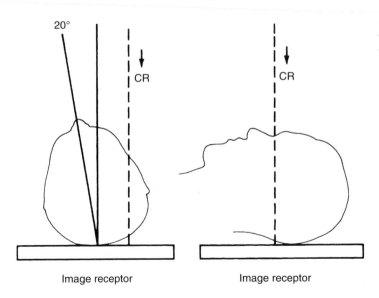

FIGURE 16-15. Schematic of the positioning for the optional tangential view.

COMPLICATIONS

The complications that can arise from cerebral angiography fall under three major headings: contrast agent reactions, mechanical injuries, and physiologic complications. The contrast agent reactions have already been considered in Chapter 6 and will not be repeated here.

Mechanical injuries can result during vessel access or catheter placement. These include hemorrhage, arteriovenous fistula, mechanical obstruction, pseudoaneurysm, vessel lacerations, hematoma at the puncture site, and extravasation of contrast agent.

Physiologic complications can be related to the mechanics of the procedure or occur as a natural response to the procedure. The most common complication is stroke. This can be the result of a dislodged embolus or the introduction of foreign materials during the procedure. Transient ischemic attacks (TIAs) are also a complication resulting from this procedure.

TABLE 16-3   *Cerebral Angiography Positioning*

Procedure	Projection	Position	Central Ray	Anatomy
Carotid angiography	Anteroposterior	OML perpendicular to IR Median plane perpendicular to IR	15 degrees caudal to enter 2.5 cm above glabella	Frontal view of the anterior and middle cerebral arteries
	Lateral	OML perpendicular to table, median plane parallel to IR	Horizontally directed at right angles to film to enter 2.5 cm anterior to and 2.5 cm above external auditory meatus	Lateral view of anterior and middle cerebral arteries and their branches, carotid siphon
	Supine oblique	Median plane 30–60 degrees away from injected side	15 degrees caudal to enter 2.5 cm above supraorbital margin	Anterior and middle cerebral arteries and anterior communicating artery can be delineated with lower angles
	Transorbital	OML perpendicular to IR, median plane 10 degrees toward injected side	5 degrees cephalad to pass through center of orbit	Anterior and middle cerebral arteries, carotid siphon
	Tangential	OML perpendicular to IR, median plane 20 degrees away from or 10 degrees toward injected side	Perpendicular to IR to pass tangentially to region of interest	Subdural hematoma
Vertebral angiography	Anteroposterior	OML perpendicular to IR, median plane perpendicular to IR	25 degrees caudal in median plane, entering at frontal bone and passing through external auditory meatus	Vertebrobasilar system
	Lateral	OML perpendicular to table, median plane parallel to IR	Horizontally directed at right angles to IR to enter 2.5 cm posterior to external auditory meatus	Lateral view of vertebrobasilar system

* OML, orbitomeatal baseline; IR, image receptor.

SUMMARY

Cerebral angiography has undergone many changes since it was first introduced in 1927. The vessels feeding the head and neck originate at the aortic arch, and each of the major vessels can be accessed through the percutaneous puncture method as described by Seldinger. Conventional angiography is performed for the purposes of diagnosis as well as intervention. Magnetic resonance angiography and venography, limited invasive techniques, have increased in use with advances in the equipment.

The indications for the procedure include aneurysms, vascular disease in the neck region, and pre- and postsurgical evaluation. These can vary depending upon whether the procedure is being performed for diagnostic purposes or intervention is the main objective.

The transfemoral percutaneous puncture route is the access point of choice. The contrast agents used in conventional angiography are of the water-soluble organic iodine variety. The nonionic substances are preferred over the ionic agents; however, the ultimate choice is dictated by the radiologist performing the procedure. The complications resulting from this procedure are classified into three major categories: mechanical injuries as a result of catheter manipulations, contrast agent reactions, and physiologic complications such as stroke or transient ischemic attacks.

REFERENCE

1. Yousem DM, Trinh BC: Injection rates for neuroangiography: results of a survey. *AJNR Am J Neuroradiol* 22(10):1838–1840, 2001.

SUGGESTED READINGS

Anzuini A, Chiesa R, Vivekananthan K, Uretsky B, Colombo A, Margonato A, Airoldi F, Rosanio S, Augello G, Birnbaum Y, Magnani G, Esposito G, Melissano G, Moura MR, Briguori C: Endovascular stenting for stenoses in surgically reconstructed brachiocephalic bypass grafts: immediate and midterm outcomes. *J Endovasc Ther* 11(3):263–8, 2004.

Brockow K, Christiansen C, Kanny G, et al: Management of hypersensitivity reactions to iodinated contrast media. *Allergy* 60(2):150–158, 2005.

Chang SD, Levy RP, Marks MP, Do HM, Marcellus ML, Steinberg GK: Multimodality treatment of giant intracranial arteriovenous malformations. *Neurosurgery* 2003; 53:1–11, 2003.

Do HM: Magnetic resonance imaging in the evaluation of patients for percutaneous vertebroplasty. *Top Magn Reson Imaging* 11:235–244, 2000.

Do HM, Marx WF, Khanam H, Jensen ME: Choroid plexus papilloma of the third ventricle: cerebral angiography, preoperative embolization and histology. *Neuroradiology* 43:503–506, 2001.

Goldstein RA, Do HM, Jensen ME, Marks MP: Part 1. Neuroangiographic complications: what to do and when. *Contemp Diagn Radiol* 26:1–6, 2003.

Goldstein RA, Do HM, Jensen ME, Marks MP: Part 2. Neuroangiographic complications: what to do and when. *Contemp Diagn Radiol* 27:1–6, 2003.

Kim HJ, Suh DC, Kim JK, Kim SJ, Lee JH, Choi CG, Yoo B, Kwon SU, Kim JS: Correlation of neurological manifestations of Takayasu's arteritis with cerebral angiographic findings. *Clin Imaging* 29(2):79–85, 2005.

Lee SH, Jung JH, Shim WH: Endovascular treatment of basilar artery stenosis with drug-eluting stent: A case report and literature review. *Catheter Cardiovasc Interv* 64(3):296–300, 2005.

Leibowitz R, Marcellus ML, Chang SD, Steinberg GK, Do HM, Marks MP: Parent vessel occlusion in vertebrobasilar fusiform and dissecting aneurysms. *AJNR AM J Neuroradiol* 24:902–907, 2003.

Matsumoto Y, Hokama M, Nagashima H, Orz Y, Toriyama T, Hongo K, Kobayashi S: Transradial approach for selective cerebral angiography: technical note. *Neurol Res* 22(6):605–608, 2000.

Matsumoto Y, Hongo K, Toriyama T, Nagashima H, Kobayashi S: Transradial approach for diagnostic selective cerebral angiography: results of a consecutive series of 166 cases. *AJNR Am J Neuroradiol* 22(4):704–708, 2001.

Riecker A, Ernemann U, Kastrup A: Cerebellar hemorrhage after angioplasty. *N Engl J Med* 352(6):633–634, 2005.

Sawada M, Kaku Y, Yoshimura S, Kawaguchi M, Matsuhisa T, Hirata T, Iwama T: Antegrade recanalization of a completely embolized vertebral artery after endovascular treatment of a ruptured intracranial dissecting aneurysm. Report of two cases. *J Neurosurg* 102(1):161–166, 2005.

STUDY QUESTIONS

1. The right subclavian and right common carotid arteries are branches of the _____ artery:
   - **a.** brachiocephalic
   - **b.** sternoclavicular
   - **c.** vertebral
   - **d.** basilar

2. The "circulus arteriosus" is another name for _____.
   - **a.** Vieussens' ring
   - **b.** circle of Willis
   - **c.** the sylvian triangle
   - **d.** the conus arteriosus

3. The junction of the superior, sagittal, and occipital sinuses with the right and left transverse sinuses is referred to as the:
   - **a.** conus arteriosus
   - **b.** circle of Willis
   - **c.** confluence of sinuses
   - **d.** isle of Reil

4. Which of the following would be considered as a contraindication to cerebral angiography?
   - **i.** contrast agent sensitivity
   - **ii.** advanced arteriosclerosis
   - **iii.** subarachnoid hemorrhage
   - **a.** i only
   - **b.** ii only
   - **c.** i and iii only
   - **d.** i, ii, and iii

5. The most common approach of vessel access for cerebral angiography is via the:
   - **a.** transfemoral artery
   - **b.** transbrachial artery
   - **c.** transjugular artery
   - **d.** translumbar aortic puncture

6. Another name for the innominate vein is the _____ vein.
   - **a.** internal jugular
   - **b.** superior sagittal
   - **c.** brachiocephalic
   - **d.** inferior sagittal

7. Cerebral angiography is indicated for intervention in all the following cases except:
   - **a.** extracranial blood supply to meningiomas
   - **b.** angiofibromas
   - **c.** arteriovenous malformation
   - **d.** embolization of extracranial lesions

8. In order to image a frontal view of the anterior and middle cerebral arteries the central ray should be directed to _____ at an angle of _____ with the patient in the anteroposterior position.
   - **a.** the nasion, 15 degrees cephalad
   - **b.** a point 2.5 cm above the glabella, 15 degrees caudal
   - **c.** a point 2.5 cm below the inion, 20 degrees caudal
   - **d.** the OML, 40 degrees cephalad

9. Which of the following is not considered to be a mechanical complication of the angiographic procedure?
   - **a.** stroke
   - **b.** extravasation
   - **c.** pseudoaneurysm
   - **d.** hematoma

10. Which of the following projections can be used to demonstrate a subdural hematoma?
    - **a.** supine oblique
    - **b.** anteroposterior
    - **c.** tangential
    - **d.** lateral

17

Vascular Interventional Procedures

CHAPTER OBJECTIVES

After completing this chapter, the reader will be able to perform the following:

- Describe the general interventional techniques used to reduce blood flow

- List the specific indications and contraindications for the reduction of blood flow

- List the various procedures used to reduce blood flow

- Identify the complications inherent in interventional blood flow reduction

- Identify the general interventional techniques used to increase blood flow

- List the specific indications and contraindications for increasing blood flow

- List the various procedures used to increase blood flow

- Describe the complications resulting from interventional vessel dilation

- Explain the techniques used to remove foreign bodies from the vascular system

- Describe the TIPS (transjugular intrahepatic portosystemic shunting) procedure

- Describe vena cava filtration

CHAPTER OUTLINE

TECHNIQUES USED TO REDUCE BLOOD FLOW

    Indications and Contraindications
    Procedure
    Complications

TECHNIQUES USED TO INCREASE BLOOD FLOW

    Indications and Contraindications
    Procedure
    Complications

REMOVAL OF INTRAVASCULAR FOREIGN BODIES

OTHER INTERVENTIONAL PROCEDURES

    Transjugular Intrahepatic Portosystemic Shunting
    Vena Caval Filter Placement

SUMMARY

The term "interventional radiology" was coined by Wallace in 1976 to describe any selective catheter or needle technique used for the diagnosis and treatment of disease. Although the basic techniques had been used for many years, this subspecialty began in 1964 when Dotter and Judkins successfully recanalized arthrosclerotic stenosed femoral arteries. Drawing on their experience as angiographers and using standard equipment, they were able to pass catheters through occluded arterial segments. Their technique used overlapping (coaxial), or telescoping, catheters to compress the plaque. The method improved, and in 1974 Gruntzig developed the double-lumen balloon sheath catheter, which improved the recanalization procedure and reduced trauma to the vascular system at the puncture site. These and other interventional procedures have proved to reduce the cost of treatment without increasing risk to the patient. They have a low mortality rate and, in many cases, are better tolerated by the patient than are more complicated and extensive therapeutic or surgical procedures. In general, interventional radiography encompasses both vascular and nonvascular procedures. The results of an interventional technique can be diagnostic as well as therapeutic. Samples may also be taken for diagnosis to provide histologic, bacteriologic, and biochemical information.

Current catheter systems used for interventional procedures consist of an arterial guiding sheath catheter. This is a catheter with a thinner wall and larger lumen than the typical angiographic catheter. It acts as a guide for the actual interventional catheter. The sheath also provides the means for the injection of contrast agent as well as performing various hemodynamic measurements.

The catheters used can be of different types: the fixed guide wire and the over the guide wire catheter system. Each of these systems has advantages and disadvantages. The fixed guide wire system has the balloon directly attached to a guide wire equipped with a flexible tip. This type of system has the advantage of being able to be manipulated by a single person. Its disadvantage is that it must be completely removed if another size or type of catheter is to be inserted. In the over the guide wire catheter system the catheter rides over a preplaced guide wire. It is a bit more cumbersome to use than the previous system but has increased flexibility in the types of catheters and guide wires that can be accommodated. In this type of system the guide wire remains in its location, facilitating the removal of one catheter and replacement with another without retracing the route with a new guide wire.

There are four major divisions of vascular interventional procedures: those used to reduce or stop blood flow, procedures used to increase blood flow by dilating or recanalizing occluded vessels, interventions used to remove foreign bodies from the vascular system, and other procedures. The first three categories of interventions can be applied in the vasculature of the major organ systems of the body. Certain procedures such as **TIPS** (transjugular intrahepatic portosystemic shunting) are used in specific organ systems and fall in the fourth category, "other interventions." The means of vessel access for these procedures is usually the percutaneous method originally described by Seldinger. Depending upon the target, access may be either arterial or venous.

Box 17-1 illustrates the present scope of interventional radiography for both vascular and nonvascular procedures. The nonvascular interventional procedures will be discussed in Chapter 19 but are listed here for comparison with the vascular interventions. Vascular interventions can be divided into methods that either **reduce** or **increase** blood flow. These techniques are meant to be therapeutic in nature. Vascular interventional radiography procedures use angiography as the primary procedural method for access to the site of the pathologic process. In many cases the percutaneous interventions can save the patient from undergoing a lengthy surgical procedure.

TECHNIQUES USED TO REDUCE BLOOD FLOW

Procedures for reducing blood flow include **embolization** and **balloon occlusion**, **intravascular infusion of vasoconstrictors**, and **intravascular electrocoagulation**. Most of these techniques are performed using percutaneous puncture of the femoral or other superficial arteries. Occasionally, the embolic material is inserted directly into the vessel via an arteriotomy.

Indications and Contraindications

Transcatheter embolization is indicated in cases of posttraumatic hemorrhage, for occlusion of the blood supply to highly vascular neoplasms, and for reduction of bleeding during and after surgical procedures. Because transcatheter embolization is presently used in high-risk cases, there are no

---

BOX 17-1   *Summary of Vascular Interventional Radiography Procedures*

Increase blood flow
    Mechanical methods
    Dilation of stenotic artery (PTA)
    Recanalization of occluded artery
        Laser angioplasty
    Stent* placement
    Removal of embolus
        Atherectomy
    Intra-arterial method
        Infusion of vasodilators

Decrease blood flow
    Mechanical methods
        Embolization
        Balloon techniques
    Intravascular electrocoagulation
    Intravascular method
        Infusion of vasoconstrictors (e.g., posterior pituitary extract)

Removal of Intravascular Foreign Bodies
Other
    Miscellaneous intravascular method
        Infusion of chemotherapeutic agents
    Vena cava filtering
    Renin sampling
    Transjugular intrahepatic portosystemic shunting

---

*A stent is any material used to hold tissue in place while healing is in progress.

---

definitive contraindications to the procedure. Ideally, the embolization method chosen reduces the flow of blood without incurring ischemia of the tissue.

The occlusion of blood vessels can also be accomplished using an electric current to stimulate thrombus formation. Electrocoagulation can be used in cases of diagnosed tumors, hemangioma, and arteriovenous fistulas.

Infusions of vasoconstrictors are indicated in cases of suspected upper gastrointestinal bleeding and as an aid to improving the diagnostic capabilities of angiography in certain areas of the body. If vasoconstrictors are administered during hepatic angiography or peripheral angiography, the diagnostic value of the examination is enhanced. In cases of suspected hepatoma and adenoma, the instillation of vasoconstrictors results in an improved visualization of the neoplasms.

Procedure
Transcatheter Embolization and Balloon Occlusion

Transcatheter intravascular occlusion, the process of closing off or obstructing the inside of blood vessels, is accomplished by placing a foreign substance, tissue, or blood clot into the lumen of a selected vessel through a catheter. Naturally occurring particulate types of embolic materials such as **autogenous** and **autologous** blood clots and tissue fragments (muscle, fat, and so on) have become obsolete with the increased use of synthetic agents that can be delivered through percutaneous catheter methods. The following is a list of the embolic materials that are used for vascular embolization:

Small vessel occluders
   Synthetic agents
      Solid (resorbable)
         Gelatin sponge (Gelfoam)
         Oxidized cellulose (Oxycel)
         Starch microspheres (Spherex)
         Collagen suspensions (Avitene)
            Bovine collagen (Avitene, Angiostat)
            Equine collagen (Tachotop)
      Solid (permanent)
         Polyvinyl alcohol (PVA) sponge
         Silicone beads
         Plastic beads
         Metal microspheres
         Glass microspheres
      Liquid
         Isobutyl-2-cyanoacrylate (IBCA; Bucrylate)
         Ethanol (absolute)
         Hypertonic glucose
         Hot contrast medium
         Iodized oil-based contrast medium (Ethiodol, Lipiodol)
Large vessel occluders
   Mechanical systems
      Coils (stainless steel with threads)
         Plain threads (wool, Dacron, silk)
         Bristle brushes
         Springs
         Wire baffles
         Rashkind double disk occluder
      Balloon systems
      Nondetachable balloon systems*
         Detachable balloon systems
         Controlled leak balloon systems
      Other systems
      Chemoembolization
         Electrocoagulation
         Laser-induced occlusion
         Percutaneous stents (covered)

*These balloons have limited use. In many cases they are used to control blood flow when using another embolic material.

The search for the ideal embolic material has yielded many different products, but none exhibits all of the characteristics of an ideal substance. An ideal embolic material is nontoxic, stable, insoluble in the vascular system, radiopaque, and capable of being shaped, sterilized, and introduced via an angiographic catheter. The material used is determined by the pathology, the patient's clotting ability, and the nature of the blood supply. Occasionally, it is necessary to use a combination of more than one type of embolic material to successfully isolate an area.

The substances used to occlude the blood vessels can be categorized by how long they remain in the vessel—they can be temporary or long lasting. Substances such as Gelfoam, autologous blood clots, muscle tissue clots, and balloon catheters are temporary occluders. These substances are either mechanically removable, such as the balloon catheter, or quickly absorbed by the body through intravascular lysis.

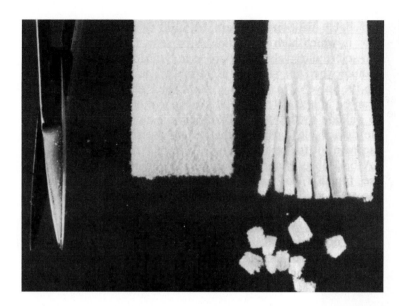

FIGURE 17-1. Sheet of Gelfoam cut for use.

Embolic media such as Gianturco coils, detachable balloon catheters, isobutylcyanoacrylate (IBCA), and polyvinyl alcohol foam are long-term agents used for permanent occlusion of vessels.

Cellulose Sponge Embolic Media. These media include **microfibrillar collagen**, **oxidized cellulose**, and **Gelfoam**, which is the most popular. Gelfoam is manufactured in sheets and in powder (Fig. 17-1). It was first used in 1945 to control hemorrhage during neurosurgery, and it has been successfully used in intravascular occlusion. The powdered form consists of particles ranging from 40 to 60 μm in size. When Gelfoam is used, small fragments (pieces) are cut from the sheet and soaked in normal saline solution, a contrast agent, or both to provide radiopacity. These pieces are then placed into the vessel by injection through an angiographic catheter. The size of the inside lumen of the catheter determines the maximum size of the piece to be used. Gelfoam has the disadvantage of being easily refluxed, causing recanalization of the vessel. This type of embolic medium, when injected into the lumen of a vessel, provides a framework for blood clot formation. Intravascular lysing of this type of material can occur in a relatively short period, but it is much more persistent in a vessel than an autologous blood or tissue clot alone.

Gelfoam powder that has been radiopacified by the addition of tantalum powder is used to produce occlusion at the precapillary level. At this level, recanalization by collateral vessel formation is minimized, making Gelfoam powder an excellent choice for tumor treatment.

This type of embolic medium lasts from less than 48 hours to 30 days.

Balloon Catheter Occlusion. Balloon catheters provide a safe, temporary method of occluding vessels to control or prevent bleeding, as well as isolating vessels for selective infusion of chemotherapeutic agents or placing other types of embolic media (Fig. 17-2). The advantages of using the balloon catheter are that it is retrievable for removal and the position of the balloon can be changed easily.

Four types of balloon catheters are available. The single-lumen type is used with catheter introduction and exchange sheath sets or coaxial catheters. The double-lumen type is constructed to permit contrast injection and balloon inflation in the same catheter. The double-lumen catheter consists of one catheter within a second, larger catheter. The third type—flow-directed detachable miniature balloon catheters—are used for permanent occlusion of high-flow vascular lesions. The controlled-leak balloon catheter systems are also flow-directed catheters that allow the delivery of a liquid embolic material or contrast agent.

Single- and double-lumen catheters are primarily used as temporary occluders. Detachable balloon catheters are used to provide long-term occlusion, especially in areas in which high blood flow is present. Detachable balloon catheters are equipped with self-sealing valves and are usually filled with

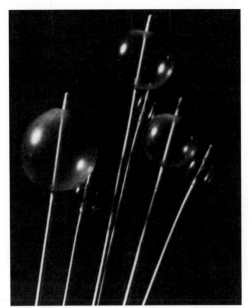

FIGURE 17-2. Occlusion balloon catheters.

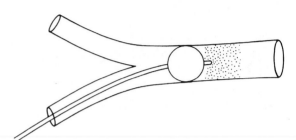

FIGURE 17-3. Schematic of an occlusion balloon catheter used in conjunction with particulate embolic material.

contrast medium or another opaque medium when the study is performed. The catheter has a stainless-steel stem that fits into the valve of the balloon. When the balloon is placed in the vessel to be occluded, it can be inflated. The catheter is then withdrawn, disconnecting the stem and leaving the balloon in the vessel. Detachable balloons can also be flow-guided into position. The detachable balloon catheters are used with coaxial catheter systems to facilitate placement of the miniballoon.

A balloon catheter can be used in conjunction with embolic material and in such cases function like a cork to prevent reflux of the particulate material from the target vessel. Once the particulate embolic material has been firmly set in place, the balloon can be removed (Fig. 17-3).

Occluding Spring Emboli and Other Mechanical Occluders. Occluding springs are mechanical devices of stainless-steel coiled wire about 5 cm long and available in 3-, 5-, 8-, 10-, 12-, and 15-mm diameters. Strands of wool, silk, or Dacron are affixed to the wire to provide a framework for clot formation. The wool-tailed coils are primarily used for larger arteries, whereas the silk- or Dacron-tailed coils are used to occlude smaller arteries. These coils were developed in 1975 by Gianturco, Anderson, and Wallace and are commonly called Gianturco-Anderson-Wallace (GAW) coils (Fig. 17-4).

These devices are supplied uncoiled and braided into an introducer cartridge. To place the coil into the catheter, the introducer cartridge is inserted into the stopcock until it contacts the flared catheter end. The coil is then pushed into the catheter with the stiff end of a guide wire. The distance that the coil should be pushed into the catheter in the loading stage is usually recommended by the manufacturer. In the case of the GAW coil, the manufacturer (Cook, Inc.) recommends leading for a distance of 20 to 30 cm. The guide wire and introducer are removed, and the spring embolus is then pushed through the distal end of the catheter for placement in the vessel. A smaller version of the GAW coil, the minicoil, is also available. This unit is delivered through a 5F catheter.

Occluding spring emboli are considered permanent embolic media because they remain in the vessel for more than 30 days.

The bristle brush has also been successfully used to occlude vessels. This device resembles a miniature chimney cleaning brush and has a central core consisting of a stainless-steel coil with nylon pieces threaded through it. These brushes require the use of large-bore catheters for introduction into

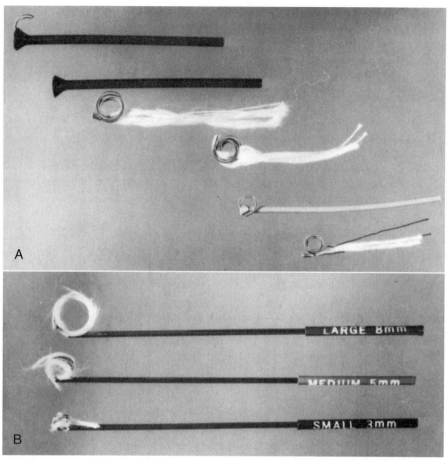

FIGURE 17-4. Stainless-steel Gianturco coils shown as unloaded (**A**) and preloaded (**B**) units.

the target vessel, where they remain to provide a framework for clot formation. They also are considered permanent embolic media.

Liquid Embolic Media. Substances in this category include tissue adhesives (polymerizing agents) such as IBCA and silicon elastomer. These products are long-term embolic media, lasting more than 30 days. These materials are used primarily in life-threatening cases. They solidify (polymerize) when they come into contact with ionizing solutions. Unlike other embolic materials, these substances do not form the framework on which a blood clot is produced; rather, they form a permanent embolus that seals the vessel almost immediately.

IBCA is used for direct vessel occlusion but has not yet been approved by the Food and Drug Administration (FDA) for unrestricted use. A permit must be secured for any use of this material in human beings.

The silicon elastomer embolic medium is a low-viscosity substance that exhibits a more controlled polymerization time than IBCA, making it a better choice for occlusion of extensive arteriovenous malformations. Silicon elastomer can be mixed with iron microspheres, which allows an externally applied magnet to control the position of the material until the polymerization process is complete. This procedure was devised to prevent the embolic material from moving to a nontarget vessel.

The technique for placement of these liquid emboli substances requires the use of coaxial catheters. These are specially paired catheters comprising a larger outer catheter and a smaller inner catheter. These sets come with a correctly sized guide wire and are complete for use during

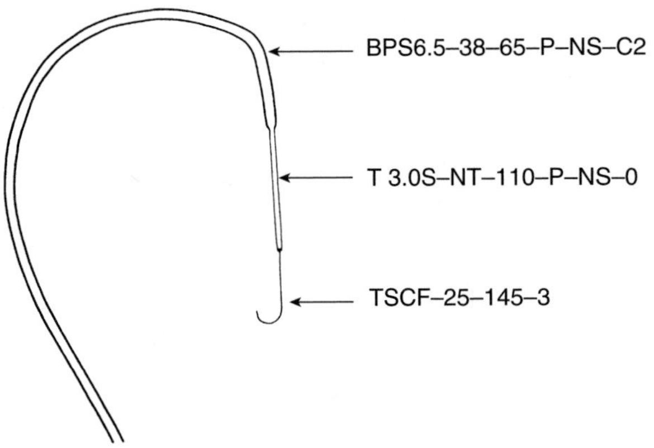

FIGURE 17-5. Coaxial catheter system.

BPS6.5–38–65–P–NS–C2

T 3.0S–NT–110–P–NS–0

TSCF–25–145–3

intravascular embolization procedures (Fig. 17-5). The large outer catheter is passed through the vessel to the approximate site of occlusion. A small amount of sterile silicon grease can be applied to the tip of the small inner catheter, which is then passed through the outer catheter into the specific vessel to be occluded. The application of the silicon grease helps to prevent adhesion of the catheter tip to the vessel wall after injection of the embolic medium.

The liquid tissue adhesive, mixed with a contrast agent, is then injected into the site. It is important for the inner catheter to be removed as soon as the injection is complete to avoid adhesion of the catheter tip to the vessel wall. Because the substances polymerize when in contact with an ionic solution, the catheters cannot be flushed with normal saline solution. The flushing may be accomplished with a 10% solution of dextrose and water.

Embolization by percutaneous catheter delivery of absolute ethanol has proved to be safe and efficient. Its main mode of action is by damaging the endothelium and stimulating the coagulation systems that cause the vascular occlusion. It is generally used with one of the nondetachable balloon systems. The balloon helps to control reflux of the absolute ethanol. This substance has several advantages such as availability, lack of toxicity, low cost, and low complication rate. Ethanol can also be mixed with one of the nonionic contrast agents to monitor and control the embolization procedure.

Routine angiography is usually performed at the beginning of the procedure to localize the site of bleeding and again after injection of the material to confirm occlusion of the vessel. Use of liquid embolic substances can cause a mild histiocytic reaction in the vessel lumen that does not involve the vessel walls or adjoining parenchyma.

Intravascular Electrocoagulation

Intravascular electrocoagulation, as the name implies, produces a thrombus in the vessel as a result of the application of a direct electric current. Its use was initially limited because of the problems associated with the technique. Early electrocoagulation devices used a stainless steel anode that was subject to destruction due to the passage of an electric current (electrolysis). The breakdown of the stainless steel often caused the anode tip to become detached inside the vessel. The use of stainless steel and the length of time required to produce a clot in larger vessels restricted the procedure to the occlusion of vessels less than 5 mm in diameter. The lengthy procedure resulted in tissue injury from the heat of the ground plate that was placed in contact with the patient. Modern devices use a platinum anode that resists the corrosive effects of electrolysis and a special lubricated grounding pad that prevents skin burns. This allows thrombus formation in larger vessels while protecting the patient from mechanical injury.

The Guglielmi detachable embolization coil is an example of a device that combines electrocoagulation with a detachable mechanical device to achieve satisfactory results.[1] Once in place, the electric current promotes thrombus formation, and detachment of the coil aids in the occlusion process through electrolysis of its soft stainless-steel connector. The procedure time is shortened, and the device can be manufactured in various lengths and coil sizes for use in a variety of vessel lumens.

Transcatheter Infusion Therapy

The slow infusion of vasoconstrictors such as vasopressin into a vessel through a catheter is a useful therapeutic technique for the control of bleeding. Vasoconstrictors cause contraction of the muscles associated with the arteries and capillaries, resulting in an increase in the resistance to the flow of blood with a corresponding increase in blood pressure.

Transcatheter infusion therapy is used extensively in the gastrointestinal tract to create controlled ischemia. Transcatheter infusion of vasopressin is made selectively at a rate of 0.2 unit per minute for 20 minutes followed by a repeat angiogram. The dose can be increased to 0.4 unit per minute for an additional 20 minutes if bleeding continues; however, if the bleeding does not stop at this dose infusion, therapy should be discontinued and alternative embolization procedures used. If the bleeding is successfully controlled, the dose should be continued for 12 to 24 hours followed by a 50% reduction in dose for an additional 24 hours. The patient should remain stable for at least 12 hours after the treatment before the catheter is removed. During this period, an infusion of normal saline or dextrose solution should be administered.

In most cases, the treatment will stop arterial or mucosal bleeding without any further intervention. Selective infusion of vasoconstrictors is also a valuable adjunct to mechanical transcatheter embolization by helping to prevent the reflux of the embolic material during placement of the embolic material.

The most popular pharmacologic agent currently used for this procedure is vasopressin. It is supplied as an aqueous solution of the substance pressor that is synthesized from the posterior pituitary gland. Vasopressin has been very successful when used to control bleeding in the gastrointestinal tract, primarily because it causes bowel constriction as well as arterial constriction in this anatomic area. Both of these actions combine to provide a reduction in the flow of blood, allowing clot formation at the site of the bleeding. Other agents such as norepinephrine and propranolol have also been investigated, but the complication and reaction rates are higher than those with vasopressin. These agents also do not create a sustained effect and have not been extensively used.

Complications

Use of transcatheter vascular embolization produces certain reactions, including localized transient pain accompanied by a mild fever, malaise, increased pulse and respiration rates, restlessness, irritability, loss of appetite, and insomnia for a period of 24 to 48 hours after embolization. Other complications may occur, such as embolization of nontarget organs, because of reflux of the embolic medium, ischemia, nerve palsy, infection, and possibly death. It should be remembered that these procedures are performed on patients who present a great surgical risk and on patients who are in life-threatening situations. As with any radiographic procedure, it should be determined that the benefit of performing any interventional procedure outweighs the risks presented by the procedure.

Intravascular electrocoagulation can cause damage to the vessel in which the thrombus is formed. Perforation is another risk associated with this technique.

When a vasoconstrictor such as vasopressin is used to control bleeding, it is important to monitor the patient because vasopressin is a potent diuretic that can cause water retention or have a direct depressive effect on the myocardium.

TECHNIQUES USED TO INCREASE BLOOD FLOW

Interventional procedures can also be applied to increase the flow of blood in a particular vessel. Four types of procedures are used: percutaneous transluminal angioplasty (PTA), vascular stent placement, intravascular thrombolysis, and intra-arterial infusion of vasodilators. These procedures provide relatively safe methods of increasing blood flow without the necessity of extensive surgery. These studies are usually done using the percutaneous approach. The arterial cut-down approach is occasionally used, and the necessary sterile tray should be available in the radiography suite. Box 17-2 summarizes some common approaches used for angioplasty.

BOX 17-2	*Summary of Catheter Approaches for Angioplasty*
Approach	**Target Vessels**
Percutaneous	
Retrograde femoral catheterization	Iliac artery, renal artery
Left axillary catheterization	Visceral vessels, renal artery with acute angle
Antegrade femoral catheterization	entry
	Superficial femoral artery, popliteal artery
Arterial cutdown	
Retrograde brachial cutdown	Coronary arteries

Indications and Contraindications

Interventional procedures for increasing blood flow are used to either **dilate stenotic vessels** or **recanalize obstructed vessels**. Percutaneous transluminal angioplasty (PTA) encompasses both dilation and recanalization. It is used to treat stenotic arterial disease primarily in medium- to large-sized vessels. Coronary, renal, and peripheral arteries are prime candidates for PTA. The lesions treated are usually localized and contain either fibromuscular or complicated plaque (atheroma). Fibromuscular plaque affects the intima by the production of smooth muscle cells, collagen, elastic fibrils, and some lipids. Complicated plaque is actually a fibromuscular plaque encased in a thin fibrous cap. The lesions should be short (not more than 10 cm) for successful angioplasty. Congenital coarctation, Takayasu's arteritis, and fibromuscular dysplasia can also be treated with PTA.

One drawback to PTA is the potential for restenosis of the vessel by the procedure due to intimal hyperplasia or elastic recoil of the vessel wall. The use of intravascular **stents** has reduced the negative aspects of percutaneous transluminal balloon angioplasty and provides a method of maintaining the dimension of the vessel lumen as well as its overall patency.

Intravascular thrombolysis is used to treat arterial thromboemboli. The areas that benefit most from this technique are the coronary, peripheral, visceral, and pulmonary vascular sites.

Infusion of vasodilators is useful in treating cases of vessel spasm or constriction and has been successful in the treatment of atherosclerosis obliterans, a common cause of vascular occlusion.

There are no defined contraindications to the use of these procedures. In most cases, the patients are usually candidates for surgery, and attempts at treatment with these techniques usually outweigh the risks involved. When percutaneous transluminal coronary angioplasty is done, a surgical team and an operating room should be available for immediate coronary bypass surgery if complications occur. The only other contraindication is if the anatomy precludes the passage of a dilation catheter.

Procedure
Percutaneous Transluminal Angioplasty

Percutaneous transluminal angioplasty is a nonsurgical procedure defined as the process of accessing a blood vessel through a puncture in the skin and performing a procedure through the blood vessel to reshape or repair the inside diameter of the vessel through balloon inflation. This procedure was first performed in 1964 by Dotter and Judkins; they used a coaxial catheter system (telescoping catheter) to recanalize a stenosed femoral artery. In 1974, Gruntzig developed the double-lumen balloon catheter, which reduced the complication rate at the puncture site. Currently, there are many different balloon lengths and diameters available for use during PTA (Fig. 17-6).

The objectives of this procedure can be summarized as follows: improvement of blood flow (increase in lumen size), maintenance of long-term vessel patency, creation of a smooth inner surface, production of no distal emboli, and minimal disturbance of the vascular wall structure. Basically, the

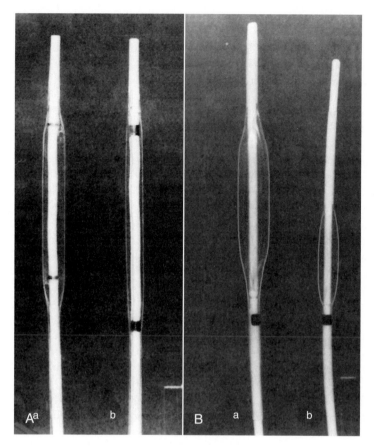

FIGURE 17-6. Balloon dilation catheters. **A**, 7F catheter with polyvinyl chloride balloon: *a*, 3 cm long, 6 mm diameter; *b*, 4 cm long, 4 mm diameter. **B**, Polyethylene balloon: *a*, 8F catheter, 8-mm diameter balloon 2 cm from catheter tip; *b*, 7F catheter, 2-cm long, 5-mm diameter balloon 3 cm from catheter tip.

procedure should permanently improve blood flow in a vessel and result in minimum complications. Obviously, not all of these objectives are achieved in all cases.

Angioplasty has also been used as an adjunct to surgery and can be performed in the operating suite. Intraoperative transluminal angioplasty is useful in reaching lesions that are outside the surgical field.

The technique of catheter introduction during PTA is the same as that used for routine angiography. Usually, a routine angiogram is performed to define the anatomy. Once this has been accomplished, the coaxial or balloon catheters are introduced, at which time the angioplasty guide wire is advanced through the lesion. When the guide wire has successfully traversed the lesion, the appropriate catheter is advanced over it through the lesion. The balloon is then inflated, and dilation of the vessel is accomplished.

The preceding is an oversimplification of the angioplasty procedure. Difficulties may arise in passing the guide wire and catheter through the lesion because of anatomic variations. This is the most critical part of the procedure; most complications occur at this stage. The amount of force required to open the vessel successfully varies with the type of lesion and its flow characteristics. The amount of pressure applied should be sufficient to achieve the objectives of angioplasty, as stated earlier. The fluoroscopic image of the balloon indicates when a successful dilation has been accomplished—the balloon becomes tube-shaped. Balloon catheters have been designed to provide maximum dilatation force on inflation and enhanced ability to cross the blockage as well as those having multiple levels of inflation so that catheter exchange during a procedure is minimized.

After dilation, a postprocedural angiogram is usually performed to assess the results. If dilation has been successful, the catheter is removed.

Antithrombotic medication both before and after the procedure is being used in many institutions. Several medications and methods of administration have been used:

1. Aspirin (acetylsalicylic acid) and dipyridamole (Persantine), 24 to 48 hours before angioplasty
2. Heparin, 5000 units intra-arterially during angioplasty
3. Nitroglycerin, 1% lidocaine, or oral calcium antagonists after arterial catheterization
4. Intravenous heparin drip 24 to 48 hours after angioplasty
5. Long-term administration (3 to 6 months) of aspirin and Persantine
6. Long-term administration (1 to 3 months) of warfarin (Coumadin)

The theory behind the use of these agents is that foreign materials (e.g., catheters, guide wires) introduced into the body are thrombogenic in nature. PTA itself is disturbing to the vascular system, and its flow pattern creates a situation in which complicating thrombosis is a possibility. Preprocedural administration of antithrombotic agents usually reduces the likelihood of thrombus formation. Postprocedural regimens have been recommended for the same reasons as well as to improve long-term patency rates. The physician performing the angioplasty selects the agent(s) to be used.

Balloon PTA has several limitations in permanently treating atherosclerotic disease. Restenosis of the vessel is the major limiting factor to the procedure. The development of adjunct procedures has provided the physician with the means to increase the success rate of this interventional procedure; among these techniques are laser-assisted balloon angioplasty, atherectomy, and stent placement.

Percutaneous Laser Angioplasty

Recent innovations in fiberoptic technology have provided the mechanism to link laser systems with angiographic catheter systems. This allows the treatment of vascular lesions that are not amenable to treatment by current technology. Several laser systems are used both clinically and experimentally for this procedure.

The laser system converts light (electromagnetic radiation) into a highly amplified form of radiation that differs from ordinary light in several ways. The laser beam is composed of monochromatic radiation that travels in the same phase. It also possesses a small amount of divergence and therefore tends to travel in a straight line. Laser radiation systems are capable of producing considerable energy. This energy is expressed in watts per square centimeter. Different laser systems vary in wavelength, energy levels, whether they are pulsed or continuous, and the amount of tissue penetration and interaction that they produce. The laser systems currently available can be divided into two categories—**thermal** and **nonthermal**.

The thermal laser systems destroy tissues by converting the solid material into a gas. This process is also called thermal vaporization. These systems can cause vascular burn injury and vascular spasm. They are usually equipped with a small orifice, which minimizes the amount of area that can be treated.

The nonthermal laser systems are of the excimer (excited dimmer) variety and use argon, krypton, or xenon associated with a halogen such as chlorine or fluorine. Examples of this type of laser include the 193-nm argon-fluoride, 248-nm krypton-fluoride, 351-nm xenon-fluoride, and the 308-nm xenon-chloride, which is used primarily in dermatology for nonablative phototherapy. These systems cause vaporization through the ionization of the atoms with subsequent dissociation of the molecules of the tissue. Unlike the thermal systems, they do not cause vascular burn injury or vascular spasms. Table 17-1 presents a summary of the laser systems currently in use.

Other components of the system are the optical fibers that transmit the laser beam to its target. The light-transporting portion of the fiberoptic system is usually quartz enveloped in a refractive coating that reflects light back toward the quartz core. An external sheath of inert material such as Teflon surrounds the fiberoptic system. The fiberoptic component is covered by a heat-generating element at its tip (Fig. 17-7); the tip provides the laser-tissue interaction.

The tip of the optical fiber can be open or capped with metal or a lens; the metal-tipped fiber is used most extensively. For all systems, an external power unit is used to provide energy.

The open-tipped laser system uses tissue absorption of the energy to effect the angioplasty. It has not been as successful as the other systems. The metal-tipped fiber uses the heat produced by the laser

TABLE 17-1   *Laser Systems*

System and Description	Type	Use

Neodymium: yttrium aluminum garnet (Nd:YAG)
  Near-infrared spectral emission (1060 nm)
  60 mm depth of tissue penetration
  Much tissue scatter
  High level of thermal vascular trauma
  Continuous wave or pulsed wave application
	Thermal	This laser system is used for some endoscopic procedures. It penetrates more deeply into tissue than CO_2 systems. The Nd:YAG laser can coagulate blood vessels at low power densities and is able to vaporize tumors at high power densities. Useful in the treatment of esophageal carcinoma.

Argon laser system
  Visible (blue-green) spectral emission
  (488 to 514 nm)
  1000 mm depth of tissue penetration
  Moderate tissue scatter
  High level of thermal vascular trauma
  Continuous wave or pulsed wave application
	Thermal	Argon laser is primarily absorbed by pigmented tissue such as hemoglobin and melanin.

CO_2 laser system
  Far-infrared spectral emission (10,600 nm)
  0.03 mm depth of tissue penetration
  Little tissue scatter
  Limited thermal vascular trauma
  Continuous wave or pulsed wave application
	Thermal	This system has found use in cardiac surgery as well as treating stenosis, and in myocardial revascularization.

Excimer laser system
  Ultraviolet spectral emission (308 nm)
  0.001 mm depth of tissue penetration
  Minimal tissue scatter
  Minimal thermal vascular trauma
  Pulsed wave application
	Nonthermal	Excimer lasers are used in cardiovascular procedures, particularly angioplasty.

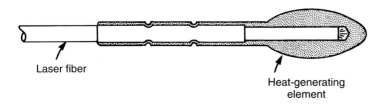

Laser fiber

Heat-generating element

FIGURE 17-7.   The basic laser probe design.

energy to interact with the tissue. Temperatures of 400° to 600° C can be reached in a short period of time. The lens–tipped fiber is able to focus the laser beam for more precise treatment. This type of system is still in the investigative stage.

The procedure can be performed in the angiographic or special procedure suite. It is currently used in conjunction with balloon angioplasty to treat peripheral obstructions that cannot be resolved with conventional PTA.

The percutaneous catheterization procedure is the same as for other interventional procedures. An angiogram is done to localize the site of the obstruction. The laser probe is advanced through the catheter, positioned at the point of occlusion, and confirmed by fluoroscopy. The laser is activated, and the tip is advanced through the occlusion until penetration of the obstruction has been achieved (Fig. 17-8).

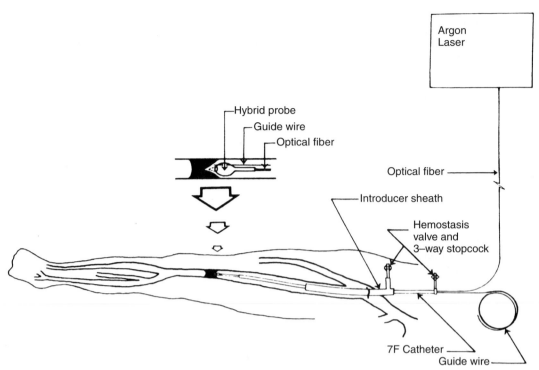

FIGURE 17-8. Laser recanalization using the "hybrid" probe. The probe tip is shown in proximity to a lesion totally occluding the superficial femoral artery. The probe is extended from a 7F catheter that is inserted via a sheath in the common femoral artery. A guide wire is also passed alongside the probe. The 300-µm core optical fiber is connected to the probe from the 7F catheter to the argon laser system. A magnification of the contact site between the probe tip and the arterial occlusion shows the beam vaporizing a channel in the obstruction and widening the vascular lumen.

Angiography confirms the opening of the vessel. Balloon angiography is then performed to further dilate the vessel.

Laser systems have recently been combined with balloon catheter systems to reduce elastic recoil and cellular proliferation (Fig. 17-9). These factors contribute to the restenosis of the treated vessel that can occur after conventional balloon angioplasty. The complications associated with this procedure are the same as those of conventional angioplasty, and postprocedural treatment of the patient is similar to that of other percutaneous interventional procedures.

Transmyocardial Revascularization

Transmyocardial revascularization (TMR) is performed when interventional techniques have not been effective and surgery is contraindicated. It consists of establishing channels within the heart muscle for the purpose of renewing the blood supply (angiogenesis). A CO_2 heart laser system is used to create between 20 and 40 1-mm–wide channels in the left ventricle of the heart. This has the effect of bringing oxygen-rich blood to the myocardium and has been shown to be an effective method of providing direct blood flow to the heart muscle. It has been shown that the channels remain open on the inside of the heart but heal on the outside. Revascularization (angiogenesis) also occurs at the site. The procedure affords relief from angina symptoms, providing an alternative for patients who are at risk for angioplasty or coronary bypass surgery. The laser produces channels that remain patent for an extended period of time and do not exhibit the restenosis associated with angioplasty.

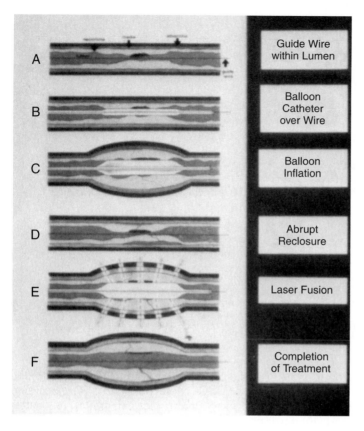

A

B

C

D

E

F

| Guide Wire within Lumen |
| Balloon Catheter over Wire |
| Balloon Inflation |
| Abrupt Reclosure |
| Laser Fusion |
| Completion of Treatment |

FIGURE 17-9. Schematic drawing of the treatment of acute closure (**D**) after percutaneous transluminal coronary angioplasty (**A** to **C**) with laser balloon angioplasty (**E**). Thermal fusion of separated tissue layers, dehydration of thrombus, and reduction of arterial recoil with successful laser balloon angioplasty results in a relatively wide, smooth, thrombus-free lumen (**F**).

Atherectomy

This procedure involves the removal of plaques (atheromas) containing fatty or lipid material that form in and occlude the lumen of blood vessels. Atherectomy is accomplished using specialized catheters. The catheters that are available to excise and remove the plaque can be divided into the directional or "pull back" variety and the circumferential systems (Box 17-3). All of the procedures use the same techniques of the catheter introduction that are employed in balloon PTA.

Directional Atherectomy. The equipment used for this type of procedure includes the directional atherectomy system (Eli Lilly Company.). This type of system is designed so that the resection window in the cutting head is less than 360 degrees. There is a nonflexible cutting/collection assembly at the distal portion of the catheter system (Fig. 17-10). The cutting assembly is offset on one side by a balloon. Once the cutting head is positioned across the area of the stenosis, the balloon is

---

BOX 17-3	*Atherectomy Catheter Systems*
Type of Excision	**Type of Removal**
Directional	Cutting window less than 360 degrees with mechanical removal of plaque
Circumferential	Grinding of plaque with irrigation and antegrade dispersion of pulverized material
	Cutting through plaque with mechanical removal of material
	Cutting through plaque with suction removal of material

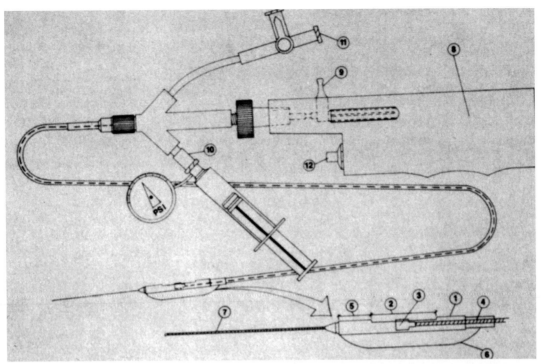

FIGURE 17-10. Peripheral atherectomy catheter system. Components include the cylindric housing (1), longitudinal opening (2), cutter (3), cutter drive cable (to motor) (4), specimen collection area (5), balloon support mechanism (6), fixed guide wire (7), motor (8), cutter advance lever (9), balloon inflation port (10), flush port (11), and on/off switch for motor (12).

inflated, forcing the cutting assembly against the plaque. Some of the plaque protrudes into the resection window. The rotational cutter is manually advanced, cutting through the plaque. The distal tip of the assembly, or nose cone, is hollow to collect the material being cut away. The procedure is repeated, turning the cutting head from 20 to 45 degrees. The excised plaque is mechanically removed from the vessel by withdrawing the catheter. Patency of the vessel is confirmed by follow-up angiography and can be accomplished through the introducer sheath after the cutting assembly has been withdrawn proximal to the lesion. Figure 17-11 illustrates the procedure followed for peripheral atherectomy using a directional (pull-back) catheter system. Complications from this procedure are relatively few and include distal embolization, delayed vessel occlusion, and arterial tears.

Circumferential Atherectomy. These systems are similar in that the cutter or "burr" that removes the plaque rotates to grind or pulverize it (Fig. 17-12). The small particles are then physiologically eliminated from the body. The burr tip rotates at speeds ranging from 100,000 to 150,000 rpm. This action grinds or pulverizes the plaque into microparticles. In each case the microparticles are removed through antegrade flow into the vascular system; these particles are small enough to pass through the capillaries without causing embolization. The circumferential atherectomy systems are considered to be nonextraction systems.

Extraction Atherectomy. The transluminal extraction catheter (TEC) system (Fig. 17-13, *A*) is designed to be used over a guide wire. It is equipped with a conical distal tip that encloses rotating cutting blades. TEC catheters are available in a variety of sizes: 5F, 6F, 7F, 8F, 9F, 10F, 12F, 14F, and 15F (Fig. 17-13, *B*) to accommodate different vessel diameters. The battery-driven blades rotate slowly at approximately 750 rpm, cutting the plaque into very fine particles (Fig. 17-13, *C*). The slow rotation of the blades allows for improved cutting control. It also eliminates the heat buildup that is characteristic of high-energy systems. The cutting assembly is hollow and is connected to an externally located

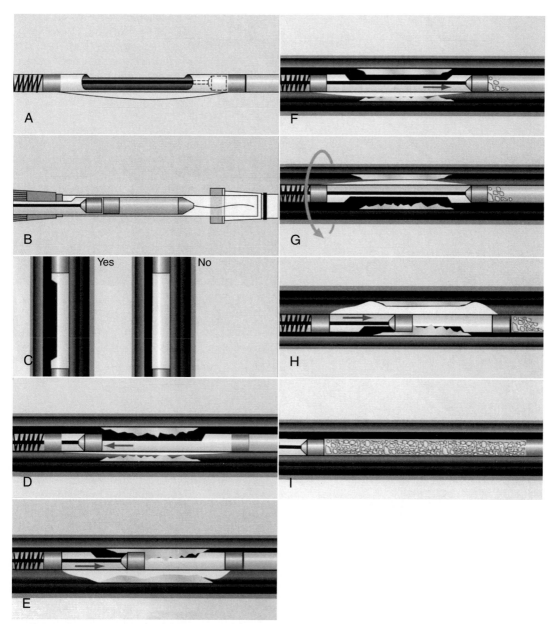

FIGURE 17-11. Steps in peripheral atherectomy. **A,** Distal tip of the catheter showing the cutter assembly completely forward in the system. **B,** The catheter is introduced into the introducer sheath. The catheter is advanced with the cutter housing positioned across the lesion. **C,** Cutter position is confirmed by fluoroscopic imaging. The cutter should be viewed in the medial or lateral plane to determine correct placement. **D,** The cutter assembly is retracted and the balloon is inflated to 20 to 40 psi. **E,** The cutter head is advanced under fluoroscopic control, cutting through the lesion and packing the debris into the collection chamber. **F,** The cutter head is maintained in its most distal position and the balloon is deflated. **G,** The catheter is rotated from 20 to 45 degrees. **H,** The balloon is reinflated and the cutting procedure repeated. (Repeat the foregoing sequence to cut the lesion at the different angles.) **I,** When the collection chamber is full, the cutter head is positioned against the collecting chamber, the balloon deflated, and the catheter removed from the vessel.

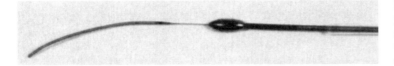

FIGURE 17-12. Distal portion of the "Rotoblator" atherectomy catheter. The "burr" rotates and creates very small particles of plaque which are carried away by the blood.

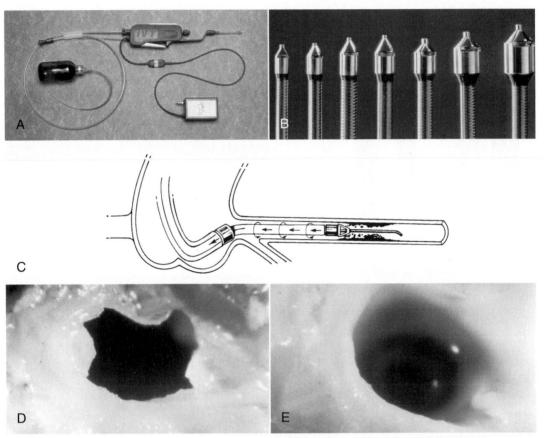

FIGURE 17-13. **A,** The TEC peripheral extraction atherectomy catheter system. **B,** Size range of TEC catheters. **C,** The flexible steerable guide wire is shown passing through a lesion in the coronary artery with simultaneous excision and extraction of the plaque through the center of the TEC torque tube. **D,** Vessel before transluminal endarterectomy. **E,** Same vessel after transluminal endarterectomy.

vacuum device that aids in the removal of the excised plaque. Before and after illustrations of an artery treated with TEC are shown in Figure 17-13, *D* and *E*.

Vascular Stent Placement

Percutaneous transluminal balloon angioplasty has been successfully used in the recanalization of stenosed vessels since the late 1970s. Although results of the procedure have been positive, the major drawbacks are the restenosis of the vessel after a period of time and a weakening of the vessel wall due to the pressure of the balloon expansion. One drawback that can occur when the wall has been weakened by

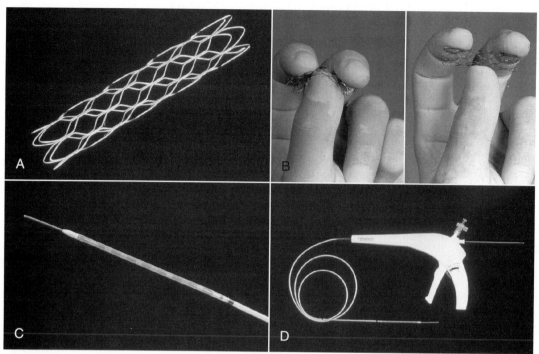

FIGURE 17-14. **A,** The Symphony Nitinol stent. **B,** The Nitinol stent showing its memory. **C,** The Symphony stent loaded onto the catheter system. **D,** The catheter guidance system.

the procedure is its collapse. This usually occurs during or immediately after the angioplasty when the patient is in the recovery room. Surgical bypass correction of the collapsed area is one method used to correct the problem.

In a substantial number of cases the patients would present recurrent chest pain as a result of a renarrowing at the site of treatment. This process is known as **restenosis**. Restenosis is a complex reaction that is thought to have some connection with hyperplasia of the intima after the procedure. The result of the restenosis would be repeat intervention or ultimately surgical repair.

The complication of vessel wall collapse and to some degree restenosis after PTA has been somewhat overcome by the use of intravascular stenting. A **stent** is any device that can supply support for a tubular structure functioning as a scaffold to strengthen the wall and reduce the occurrence of restenosis. Stents function to maintain the patency of vessels and have been successfully used in coronary arteries, peripheral vessels, and the biliary and urinary systems. In theory, a stent is delivered to a specified location, expanded, and left in place to provide a scaffolding or internal support. They serve to maintain the patency of the vessels while opposing the elastic recoil of the vessel walls that is partially responsible for restenosis. Figure 17-14 shows a stent and its delivery system.

Intraluminal stenting, in which the internal opening of a vessel is supported, is accomplished using the same general procedures as percutaneous transluminal angioplasty (Fig. 17-15). Stents are supplied in a compressed form and expanded at the site of the stenosis. They can be bare metal or coated with a drug whose action will reduce the natural restenosis that can occur. Generally stents are expanded across the blockage by means of a balloon or in some cases are self-expanding. The coated stents are a relatively new innovation in the application of stents. In fact at this writing there are only two FDA-approved drug-eluting stents on the market. These are the Cordis Cypher sirolimus-eluting stent and the Boston Scientific Taxus paclitaxel-eluting stent system. In these systems the outer surface is coated with a thin polymer containing a pharmacologic agent that can prevent the formation of scar tissue at the site of the intervention. The Cordis Cypher coating consists of the drug known as **sirolimus**. This

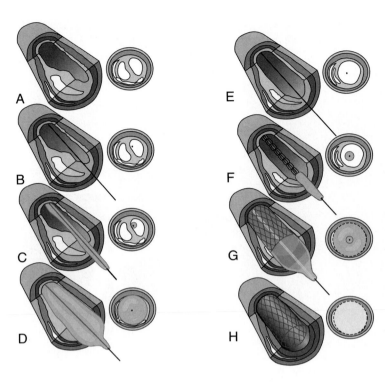

FIGURE 17-15. A, Atherosclerotic artery with compromised lumen. **B,** Guide wire passed through the blockage. **C,** The balloon catheter is advanced through the blockage. **D,** The balloon is inflated. **E,** The deflated balloon is withdrawn. **F,** A new balloon catheter (with stent) is advanced over the guide wire through the blockage. **G,** This expands the stent compressing it against the vessel wall. **H,** When the balloon is deflated the stent remains and the balloon catheter can be withdrawn from the vessel.

drug has been successfully used to prevent rejection following organ transplantation. The use of drug-eluting stents dramatically reduces restenosis when compared to bare metallic stents.

Stents can be classified in many different ways. The currently available stents can be grouped into two distinct categories by their expansion mechanism: the balloon expandable and the self-expanding type. They can also be categorized by their makeup (e.g., the type of material that they are made of) Stents can be manufactured from stainless steel, cobalt-based alloy, tantalum, nitinol, inert coating, active coating, or biodegradable. Some manufacturers classify their stents by the design characteristics: mesh structure, coil, slotted tube, ring, multidesign, or custom design. Table 17–2 summarizes some of the stents that are available for use. The general area in which the stent is applied is also listed. This does not mean that the particular stent is not useful in other areas of the body. Many of the stents come in a

TABLE 17-2 *Summary of the Stents Currently on the Market*

Stent	Material	Category	Use
Palmaz Stent	Stainless steel	Balloon expandable	Short segment lesions
Perflex	Stainless steel	Balloon expandable	Iliac arteries—long segments
AVE 5670	Stainless steel	Balloon expandable	Coronary arteries
Intrastent	Stainless steel	Balloon expandable	Iliac arteries
Herculink	Stainless steel	Balloon expandable	Renal arteries
Strecker	Tantalum	Balloon expandable	Iliac arteries/renal arteries
Multilink Pixel	Stainless steel	Balloon expandable	Small coronary vessels
Racer	Cobalt-based alloy	Balloon expandable	Biliary stent system
Wallstent	Stainless steel	Self-expanding	Long segment lesions
Bard Luminexx	Nitinol	Self-expanding	Biliary stent system
Symphony	Nitinol	Self-expanding	Iliac arteries
Smart Stent	Nitinol	Self-expanding	Aortic/iliac arteries
AVE SE	Nitinol	Self-expanding	Coronary arteries
Dynalink	Nitinol	Self-expanding	Coronary arteries

variety of sizes. This enables them to be used in a wider array of locations. Work is in progress to perfect the biodegradable stent. The stent is constructed of a special polymer that allows it to biodegrade after a period of time. The stent can also contain a wide variety of pharmacologic agents that can be used to administer medication to a specific site. Stenting is commonly performed in coronary revascularization. A discussion of the specific procedure will be presented in Chapter 18.

Balloon Expandable Stents. These systems are constructed so that the stent is mounted in some fashion over the balloon end of the catheter. The method for holding the stent to the catheter varies with the manufacturer. The Palmaz intraluminal stent is held in place by an outer sheath, which is withdrawn prior to the expansion of the stent with the balloon. The catheter is guided into place across the stenosis, the outer sheath is removed, and the balloon is expanded, deforming the stent and fixing it to the wall of the vessel. If it is determined by repeat angiography that the stent has not been sufficiently expanded, the balloon can be expanded again to correct the problem.

Self-Expanding Stents. This type of stent falls into two distinct categories: stents that expand as a result of a simple spring action and those that are made from thermal memory materials. Regardless of the type of mechanism used for self-expansion of the stent, further dilation using a balloon catheter to fix the stent to the vessel wall will be necessary.

Spring Action Stents. The Wallstent (Boston Scientific, Inc.) is an example of the spring-loaded stent. After preliminary balloon angioplasty, the coaxial catheter system, consisting of an interior tube with the compressed stent fixed in place by the exterior tube, is placed across the area of stenosis. As sterile saline is injected between the interior and exterior tubes, the delivery system becomes operable. The exterior tube can then be easily retracted, releasing the compressed stent end, allowing it to expand.

The Gianturco Z Stent (Cook, Inc.) is another type of spring-loaded stent. It is compressed over the introducer catheter, and a second outer catheter holds the stent in place. After positioning across the stenosis, the outer catheter is withdrawn, allowing the stent to return to its original diameter and shape.

Thermal Memory Stents. These stents are manufactured using a nickel titanium alloy that expands in response to a change in temperature. Once the stent is placed across the stenosis, body heat will trigger expansion to its original configuration. The specific temperature at which the device will expand can be controlled during the manufacturing process.

Intravascular Thrombolysis (Fibrinolysis)

Initially, pharmacologic thrombolytic therapy was accomplished systemically by introducing specific thrombolytic agents intravenously. Through advances in interventional techniques, equipment, and the fibrinolytic process, the procedure has become an accepted interventional technique. Selective and subselective applications of the pharmacologic agents have been accomplished in a shorter time span with minimal side effects.

The substances available for use in intravascular thrombolysis include streptokinase, a nonenzymatic protein derived from β-hemolytic streptococci; urokinase, which is derived from human kidney cultures; and tissue-type plasminogen activator, a serine protease that is produced commercially. There are differences among these agents that do not affect the efficacy of either substance. Research is continuing in this area, and several new fibrinolytic agents have been tested for use in coronary interventional procedures.

The success of treatment is dependent on the age, size, and location of the lesion. Single-vessel clots that are less than 7 days old and located in vessels with a flow pattern that can provide good runoff of the thrombolytic agent are prime targets for this procedure. As the age of the thrombus approaches and exceeds 7 days, it becomes increasingly resistant to treatment by the thrombolytic agent. If the clot is too extensive, complete removal becomes more difficult, and the chance for successful treatment is diminished. In totally occluded vessels that provide no runoff, retrograde clot formation can occur along the path of the catheter.

Intravascular thrombolysis is performed after general angiography has confirmed the diagnosis. A guide wire is usually passed through the occlusion followed by the infusion catheter. There are two

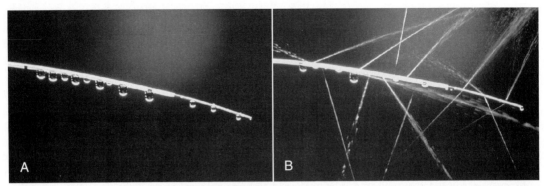

FIGURE 17-16. **A,** The Katzen infusion wire inside the Mewissen infusion catheter, illustrating "weep" (infusion) delivery of the thrombolytic agent. The position of the wire in the catheter allows for variable infusion lengths. **B,** Multiple holes in a spiral array deliver the thrombolytic agent in a "pulse-spray" delivery, which delivers the thrombolytic agent over a large surface area.

major methods used for thrombolysis—infusion and pulse-spray pharmacomechanical methods (Fig. 17-16). In both cases the thrombolytic agent is infused into the clot over a period of time, and the catheter is advanced through the clot as lysis is accomplished. The major advantage of the pulse-spray method over the infusion method is the forceful infusion of urokinase through a catheter designed with many small slits or side holes allowing simultaneous treatment of the entire clot. This method appears to enhance the dissolution of the clot. In both cases the progress of the procedure is checked by means of follow-up angiography.

The patient should be closely monitored for complications and improvement throughout the course of the infusion. Considering the length of an infusion procedure, the patient should be monitored in an intensive care unit, and repeat angiography should be performed every 2 to 6 hours to oversee both dose and catheter position. Complications from this procedure are those normally associated with angiography as well as hemorrhage and rethrombosis.

Infusion of Vasodilators

Infusion of a vasodilator such as prostacyclin, reserpine, papaverine, prostaglandin E, and sodium nitroprusside is used primarily to treat vascular spasm or nonocclusive acute mesenteric ischemia, although it can be used to dilate stenotic vessels. However, most occlusive vascular problems are managed with one of the techniques previously discussed.

Complications

All of these procedures can engender complications. Many reported problems associated with the percutaneous approach are those associated with the catheterization itself, such as flow disturbances, vessel occlusion, localized hemorrhage, and systemic embolization.

PTA presents the risks of vessel dissection or perforation, thrombotic occlusion, distal embolization caused by debris from the lesion, vessel spasm caused by the movements of the catheter, and guide wire and balloon rupture caused by overinflation.

In all the procedures discussed, the principle of benefit versus risk is applicable. Patient selection is made with the possible hazards in mind, and patients should be closely monitored before, during, and after the study to minimize the risk of complications.

REMOVAL OF INTRAVASCULAR FOREIGN BODIES

In 1964, Thomas described a nonsurgical procedure for the removal of foreign bodies from intravascular locations. Since then, various devices have been developed to remove foreign bodies from

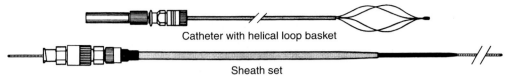

Catheter with helical loop basket

Sheath set

FIGURE 17-17.   The Dotter intravascular retriever set.

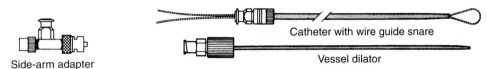

Catheter with wire guide snare

Side-arm adapter

Vessel dilator

FIGURE 17-18.   The Curry intravascular retriever set.

these sites. These materials arise from accidental loss or breakage of intravascular equipment such as guide wires or catheters. It is important to remove these from the vascular system before serious complications occur. Before Thomas's use of this technique, they had to be surgically removed.

Several types of devices have been developed, including helical loop basket sets, grasping devices, hook-shaped catheter and guide wire sets, snare loop catheter sets, and balloon-tip retrieval catheters. The helical loop basket catheters, such as the Dotter Intravascular Retriever Set, is used to snare foreign fragments and move them to peripheral vascular locations, where they are easily removed (Fig. 17-17).

Snare loop catheter sets, such as the Curry Intravascular Retriever Set, are used to retrieve lost catheters (Fig. 17-18). This is accomplished by catching a free end of the lost catheter in the snare loop and maneuvering it to a location from which it can be withdrawn from the vessel. In some cases, both ends of the lost device may be lodged in a vessel, and it is necessary to free one end before using the snare loop catheter. This can be accomplished with a hook-shaped catheter, which pulls one end of the catheter from the vessel.

Balloon-tip retrieval catheters pull fragments from locations when retrieval by one of the other methods is not possible. The balloon tip is passed beyond the fragment, inflated, and then carefully withdrawn under fluoroscopic supervision, moving the fragment along its path. When the foreign body is in a suitable location, one of the other devices is used for complete removal.

Grasping devices are not usually designed for intravascular use and present the risk of vessel trauma, but they can be used, if necessary, to remove fragments through arterial cutdown. These devices are used only when other methods are not successful. Figure 17-19 shows one type of grasping device.

Complications arising from the use of this type of interventional procedure are very rare. The possibility of complications depends on the length of time the foreign body has been in place, the patient's disposition toward mechanical stimulation, and the ultimate location of the foreign body.

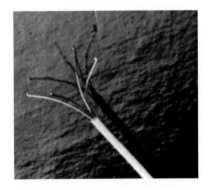

FIGURE 17-19.   MPF 20/55 multipurpose forceps.

OTHER INTERVENTIONAL PROCEDURES

Interventional radiology is an expanding field. Minimally invasive therapeutic procedures are being pioneered, building on the general principles of percutaneous vascular catheterization and endoscopic techniques. Some of the procedures do not fit the categories relegated purely to vascular interventions, which are the increase and decrease of blood flow or the removal of foreign bodies. Two procedures have proved to be successful in treating specific pathologic conditions: transjugular intrahepatic portosystemic shunting (TIPS) and vena cava filtration.

Transjugular Intrahepatic Portosystemic Shunting

Portal hypertension has traditionally been treated through invasive surgery to place shunts to decompress the pressure in the portal system. The results of this approach have not been encouraging owing to the stenosis of the vessels used in the shunt procedure. The development of the stent to stabilize vessels and provide longer term patency enabled the physician to successfully treat portal hypertension and gastrointestinal bleeding by means of a percutaneous interventional procedure that provides for a connection between the portal and hepatic venous systems. Although bare metallic stents have an extended duration of patency, stenosis of the shunt is still a viable possibility. Drug-eluting stents may offer the key to successful long-term patency of the portosystemic shunt.

The indications for the TIPS procedure include Budd-Chiari syndrome (BCS), portal vein thrombosis, bleeding anorectal varices secondary to portal hypertension, acute variceal hemorrhage, hepatorenal syndrome, portal vein thrombosis, and as a palliative treatment for hepatopulmonary syndrome. The procedure is contraindicated in cases of severe liver failure, biliary obstruction, polycystic liver disease, systemic infection, heart disease such as congestive heart failure, and pulmonary hypertension.

The procedure follows the standard process for percutaneous vessel access. TIPS needle kits are available containing a long TIPS sheath (9 to 10 French), an angled needle, curved tip, guide catheter equipped with a 16-gauge access needle.

The right jugular vein is the usual approach, although if this route is compromised, the left jugular approach is a viable option. It is also possible to perform the procedure using a transhepatic, transfemoral, external jugular, or vena cava access. When using the transjugular approach, a 9 to 10 French TIPS sheath is inserted into the vessel and advanced to the right atrium. At this point the potential for arrhythmias and the patient should be monitored carefully. A curved catheter is used to select the right hepatic vein; at this time wedged venography can be performed to confirm patency of the portal vein. The needle is then tunneled through the hepatic parenchyma on the underside of the liver and through the chosen portal vein. A guide wire is then passed from the hepatic vein through the liver parenchyma into the portal vein and subsequently into the splenic or superior mesenteric vein. Portal and hepatic vein pressures are measured to provide the portosystemic gradient. Once accomplished, an 8- to 10-mm diameter angioplasty balloon is advanced through the liver parenchyma to span the hepatic and portal veins. The balloon catheter is used to enlarge the tract through the parenchyma. Once the tract has been enlarged, stents or stent-grafts are used to line the parenchymal tract. The stents should extend into both the hepatic and portal veins. Repeat hepatic and portal vein pressures are taken. Ideally, the reduction of the portosystemic gradient to ≤12 mm Hg is critical to the success of the procedure, especially in cases of esophageal variceal bleeding. Once the procedure has been completed the catheters and guide wires can be removed. Figures 17-20 and 17-21 illustrate the TIPS procedure.

The complications and risks of the procedure include potential puncture of the bile ducts, hepatic capsule, or gallbladder; renal failure; heart attack; and death. Although there are a number of complications that can occur as a result of the procedure, the two most common are restenosis or occlusion of the shunt and hepatic encephalopathy. Other complications include recurrent variceal bleeding, intra–abdominal hemorrhage, pneumothorax, portal vein thrombosis, and hematoma. It is recommended that the patient undergo a diagnostic ultrasound within 24 hours of the procedure to ensure the successful procedure and to establish a baseline measurement for routine follow–up monitoring.

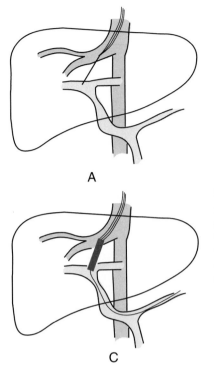

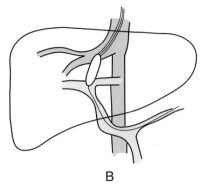

FIGURE 17-20. Schematic drawing showing the TIPS (transjugular intrahepatic portosystemic shunting) procedure. **A,** The approach is from the internal jugular vein into the right hepatic vein. **B,** Once pressure measurements are taken, a pathway through the liver parenchyma to the portal vein is created. Once again, pressure measurements are taken and the pathway is dilated. **C,** A metallic stent is then placed in the pathway and secured; the stent is expanded until the pressure readings are below 12 mm Hg. The catheter is then removed.

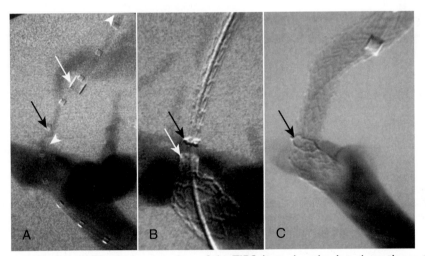

FIGURE 17-21. Radiographic demonstration of the TIPS (transjugular intrahepatic portosystemic shunting) procedure. **A,** The white arrow shows the distal end of the TIPS sheath in the right hepatic vein. The white arrowheads show the pathway between the hepatic vein and the portal vein. The black arrow indicates a catheter that is used to inject the contrast medium for venography. **B,** The sheath has been positioned through the pathway. The black arrow indicates the end of the TIPS shunt pathway, and the white arrow indicates that the sheath is being pulled back, releasing the stent. **C,** Venogram illustrating a correctly placed stent graft (*black arrow*).

Vena Caval Filter Placement

The primary purpose for the insertion of a filter in the vena cava is to reduce or prevent the possibility of a pulmonary embolus. The device used is simply a filter to trap an embolus before it reaches the pulmonary circulation. It will not prevent the formation of emboli, nor will it eliminate any of the

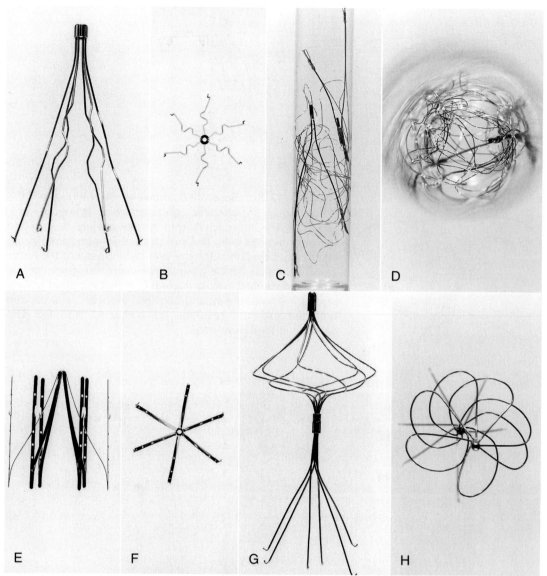

FIGURE 17-22. Schematic drawings of several types of vena caval filters shown in the frontal and top views. **A** and **B**, Greenfield filter — stainless steel. **C** and **D**, Bird's nest filter. **E** and **F**, LGM Vena Tech filter. **G** and **H**, Simon Nitinol filter.

emboli that are trapped. Most of these devices are designed to be permanently placed in the vena cava; however, a number of them are removable. There are currently several types of vena caval filters available; these include the Greenfield filters (stainless steel, titanium, and stainless steel alternating hook), the "Bird's Nest" filter, the Simon nitinol filter, the Vena Tech filter, the Gunther Tulip, the Recovery, and the OptEase. Table 17-3 summarizes the properties of the vena caval filters listed. Figure 17-22 illustrates some of the vena caval filters that are currently available.

The major indication for the procedure is deep vein thrombosis (DVT) or pulmonary embolus (PE) complicated by a contraindication to anticoagulant therapeutic agents. The broader range of indications revolves around DVT and PE. Vena caval filtering would be indicated if documented DVT is present in cases in which anticoagulant therapy must be discontinued or is no longer medically

TABLE 17-3 *Properties of Vena Caval Filters*

Filter	Material	Sheath French Size O.D.	Permanent	Removable
Bird's nest	Stainless steel	12	X	
Greenfield 12-F	Stainless steel	15	X	
Greenfield 24-F	Stainless steel	28	X	
Greenfield titanium	Titanium*	14	X	
Gunther tulip	Elginoy[†] nonparamagnetic alloy A	10		X
OptEase	Nitinol*	8.5		X
Recovery	Nitinol*	9		X
Simon Nitinol	Nitinol*	9	X	
TrapEase	Nitinol*	8.5	X	
VenaTech	Phynox nonparamagnetic alloy A	12.9	X	

*Nonferromagnetic material: cobalt-chromium-nickel alloy.
[†]Elginoy is a registered name for the metal Phynox. It is a cobalt-chromium-nickel alloy that exhibits an excellent fatigue life. It demonstrates corrosion resistance in numerous environments and is nonmagnetic.

effective. It is also indicated in cases of massive pulmonary embolus requiring surgical intervention. Patients who present with a history of DVT and are candidates for surgical procedures that have a high risk of DVT would also be considered for this procedure. There are relatively few contraindications to the procedure. These would be primarily patency and access related. If the vena cava is totally thrombosed, placement of the filter would be impractical. Also, the inability to gain access to the vena cava would prevent the procedure from being done.

The percutaneous method of vessel access is used to introduce the filter into the vena cava. Depending upon the type of filter that is chosen and patient anatomy, a variety of routes can be used. The primary access routes would be via either the femoral or internal jugular vein. Other routes include translumbar catheterization of the vena cava, percutaneous puncture of the subclavian vein or through one of the veins of the upper extremity. The filter is usually placed in the inferior vena cava, although in cases of upper extremity vein thrombosis it will necessarily be placed in the superior vena cava. In either case the apex of the filter should be oriented toward the heart.

In the inferior vena cava the ideal position for the filter is inferior to the renal veins. Suprarenal placement of the filter is warranted when there is a history of renal vein thrombosis. The transfemoral approach is usually favored. Once the catheter is in place in the femoral vein, an injection of contrast agent should be made to determine the status of the inferior vena cava (IVC). Once it has been determined that the IVC is satisfactory, the sheath can be advanced to a position that will place the filter in the infra renal vein position (Fig. 17-23). Each of the types of filters has its own method of introduction and discharge. The materials that accompany the filter kit should be read before the procedure in order to become familiar with its deployment. It is important that the filter be placed in the IVC in the proper orientation for the collection of thrombi. Once the filter is in place, another injection of contrast agent is given to document the placement of the filter.

Placement of a filter in the superior vena cava (SVC) generally uses either the jugular approach or one of the upper extremity veins. The apex of the filter should be oriented toward the heart; however, the apex should not be placed within the right atrium. This procedure is not as common as filter placement in the IVC. It is usually indicated when pulmonary embolus from the upper extremity is documented.

General complications from the procedure are usually associated with the percutaneous introduction of the filter delivery system. This can be expected when the larger delivery systems are used. The recently

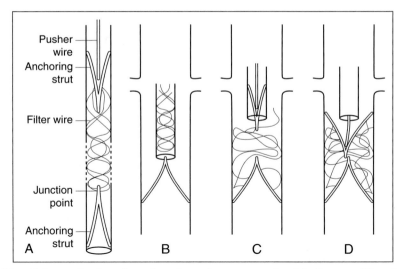

FIGURE 17-23. Schematic drawing showing placement of a bird's nest filter in the inferior vena cava. **A,** Filter in delivery sheath showing the various parts of the system. **B,** The filter is advanced in the sheath until the anchoring struts are deployed. **C,** The filter wires are advanced and placed in the inferior vena cava. **D,** The distal anchoring struts are deployed, and the catheter sheath can be withdrawn.

developed vena caval filters have smaller delivery systems, and complications have been reduced correspondingly. Other complications include tilting or malpositioning of the filter, making it ineffective. In these cases if the filter is of the removable type, it can be removed and another can be inserted. In the case of permanent filters another filter can be placed above it. Migration of the filter can also occur. The potential for caval perforation also exists with certain types of filters; however, the consequences of this complication are generally not of major significance. The establishment of a baseline venogram demonstrating the filter position is important for follow-up in cases of recurrent symptoms.

SUMMARY

Interventional radiography has proved to be a relatively safe and inexpensive method for treating various vascular problems. In many cases, it has obviated the necessity for complicated surgical procedures.

Vascular interventional radiography can be classified into procedures that increase or decrease blood flow, extraction of foreign bodies, and other types of therapeutic procedures, such as transjugular intrahepatic portosystemic shunting and vena caval placement. Several mechanical devices have been developed that are used in conjunction with basic angiographic techniques to provide the desired therapeutic result.

REFERENCE

1. Guglielmi G, Vinuela F, Duckwiler G, et al: Endovascular treatment of posterior circulation aneurysms by electrothrombus using electrically detachable coils. *J Neurosurg* 77:515, 1992.

SUGGESTED READINGS

Vascular Occlusion
Baglivo E, Boudjema S, Pieh C, et al: Vascular occlusion in serpiginous choroidopathy. *Br J Ophthalmol* 89(3):387–388, 2005.

Ebeid MR, Braden DS, Gaymes CH, et al: Closure of a large pulmonary arteriovenous malformation using multiple Gianturco-Grifka vascular occlusion devices. *Catheter Cardiovasc Interv* 49(4):426–429, 2000.

Ebeid MR, Gaymes CH, Smith JC, et al: Gianturco-Grifka vascular occlusion device for closure of patent ductus arteriosus. *Am J Cardiol* 87(5):657–660, 2001.

Grifka RG, Mullins CE, Gianturco C, Nihill M, O'Loughlin MR, Slack MC, Clubb FJ, Myers TJ: New Gianturco-Grifka vascular occlusion device: initial studies in a canine model. *Circulation* 91:1840–1846, 1995.

Miyachi S, Negoro M, Handa T, et al: Histopathological study of balloon embolization: silicone versus latex. *Neurosurgery* 30:483, 1992.

Moldenhauer JS, Gilbert A, Johnson A: Vascular occlusion in the management of complicated multifetal pregnancies. *Clin Perinatol* 30(3):601–621, 2003.

Vascular Dilation

Allen K, Dowling R, DelRossi A, Realyvasques F, Lefrak E, Pfeffer T, Fudge T, Mostovych M, Schuch D, Szentpetery S, Shaar C: Transmyocardial laser revascularization combined with coronary artery bypass grafting: a multicenter, blinded, prospective, randomized, controlled trial. *J Thorac Cardiovasc Surg* 119:540–549, 2000.

Allen K, Dowling R, Fudge T, Schoettle P, Selinger S, Gangahar D, Angell W, Petracek M, Shaar C, O'Neill W: Comparison of transmyocardial revascularization with medical therapy in patients with refractory angina. *N Engl J Med* 341:1029–1036, 1999.

Biamino G: The excimer laser: science fiction fantasy or practical tool? *J Endovasc Ther* 11(Suppl 2):II207–II222, 2004.

Fowkes FGR, Gillespie IN: Angioplasty (versus nonsurgical management) for intermittent claudication (Cochrane Review). In The Cochrane Library, Issue 2. Chichester, UK, 2004, John Wiley & Sons.

Horvath KA, Aranki SF, Cohn LH, et al: Sustained angina relief 5 years after transmyocardial revascularization with a CO_2 laser. *Circulation* 104(Suppl I):81–84, 2001.

Huikeshoven M, van der Sloot JA, Tukkie R, van Gemert MJ, Tijssen JG, Beek JF: Improved quality of life after XeCl excimer transmyocardial laser revascularization: results of a randomized trial. *Lasers Surg Med* 33(1):1–7, 2003.

Koster R, Kahler J, Brockhoff C, Munzel T, Meinertz T: Laser coronary angioplasty: history, present and future. *Am J Cardiovasc Drugs* 2(3):197–207, 2002.

Laird JR Jr, Reiser C, Biamino G, Zeller T: Excimer laser assisted angioplasty for the treatment of critical limb ischemia. *J Cardiovasc Surg (Torino)* 45(3):239–248, 2004.

Steinkamp HJ, Rademaker J, Wissgott C, et al: Percutaneous transluminal laser angioplasty versus balloon dilation for treatment of popliteal artery occlusions. *J Endovasc Ther* 9(6):882–888 2002.

Tcheng JE, Volkert-Noethen AA: Current multicentre studies with the excimer laser: design and aims. *Lasers Med Sci* 16(2):122–129, 2001.

Wissgott C, Scheinert D, Rademaker J, Werk M, Schedel H, Steinkamp HJ: Treatment of long superficial femoral artery occlusions with excimer laser angioplasty: long-term results after 48 months. *Acta Radiol* 45(1):23–29, 2004.

Vascular Stents

Bessoud B, de Baere T, Denys A, Kuoch V, Ducreux M, Precetti S, Roche A, Menu Y: Malignant gastroduodenal obstruction: palliation with self-expanding metallic stents. *J Vasc Interv Radiol* 16(2 Pt 1):247–253, 2005.

Dagenais F, Normand JP, Turcotte R, Mathieu P: Changing trends in management of thoracic aortic disease: where do we stand with thoracic endovascular stent grafts? *Can J Cardiol* 21(2):173–178, 2005.

Messer RL, Wataha JC, Lewis JB, Lockwood PE, Caughman GB, Tseng WY: Effect of vascular stent alloys on expression of cellular adhesion molecules by endothelial cells. *J Long Term Eff Med Implants* 15(1):39–47, 2005.

Palmaz JC: Intravascular stents in the last and the next 10 years. *J Endovasc Ther* 11(Suppl 2):II200–II206, 2004.

Pillai B, Smith J, Hasan A, Spencer D: Review of pediatric airway malacia and its management, with emphasis on stenting. *Eur J Cardiothorac Surg* 27(1):35–44, 2005.

Richter GM, Stampfl U, Stampfl S, Rehnitz C, Holler S, Schnabel P, Grunze M: A new polymer concept for coating of vascular stents using PTFEP (poly(bis(trifluoroethoxy)phosphazene) to reduce thrombogenicity and late in-stent stenosis. *Invest Radiol* 40(4):210–218, 2005.

Intravascular Infusion

Idell S, Coagulation, fibrinolysis, and fibrin deposition in acute lung injury. *Crit Care Med* 31(4 Suppl):S213–220, 2003.

Pilloud J, Rimensberger PC, Humbert J, Berner M, Beghetti M: Successful local low-dose urokinase treatment of acquired thrombosis early after cardiothoracic surgery. *Pediatr Crit Care Med* 3(4):355, 2002.

Transjugular Intrahepatic Portosystemic Shunt

Boyer TD, Haskal ZJ: American Association for the Study of Liver Diseases. The role of transjugular intrahepatic portosystemic shunt in the management of portal hypertension. *Hepatology* 41(2):386–400, 2005.

Haskal ZJ, Martin L, Cardella JF, Cole PE, Drooz A, Grassi CJ, et al: Quality improvement guidelines for transjugular intrahepatic portosystemic shunts. *J Vasc Interv Radiol* 12(2):131–136, 2001.

Helton WS, Maves R, Wicks K, Johansen K: Transjugular intrahepatic portasystemic shunt vs surgical shunt in good-risk cirrhotic patients. *Arch Surg* 136(1):17–20, 2001.

Quaretti P, Michieletti E, Rossi S: Successful treatment of TIPS-induced hepatic failure with an hourglass stent-graft: a simple new technique for reducing shunt flow. *J Vasc Interv Radiol* 12(7):887–890, 2001.

Perello A, Garcia-pagan JC, Gilabert R, Suarez Y, Mointinho E, Cervantes F, et al: TIPS is a useful long-term derivation therapy for patients with Budd-Chiari syndrome uncontrolled by medical therapy. *Hepatology* 35(1):132–139, 2002.

Rosado B, Kamath PS: Transjugular intrahepatic portosystemic shunts: an update. *Liver Transplant* 9(3):207–217, 2003.

Salvalaggio PR, Koffron AJ, Fryer JP, Abecassis MM: Liver transplantation with simultaneous removal of an intracardiac transjugular intrahepatic portosystemic shunt and a vena cava filter without the utilization of cardiopulmonary bypass. *Liver Transplant* 11(2):229–232, 2005.

Sanyal AJ, Genning C, Reddy KR, Wong F, Kowdley KV, Benner K, et al: The North American study for the treatment of refractory ascites. *Gastroenterology* 124(3):634–641, 2003.

Van Ha TG, Funaki BS, Ehrhardt J, Lorenz J, Cronin D, Millis JM, Leef J: Transjugular intrahepatic portosystemic shunt placement in liver transplant recipients: experiences with pediatric and adult patients. *AJR Am J Roentgenol* 184(3):920–925, 2005.

Vena Cava Filter Placement

Athanasoulis CA, Kaufman JA, Halpern EF, et al: Inferior vena caval filters: review of a 26-year single-center clinical experience. *Radiology* 216(1):54–66, 2000.

Blebea J, Wilson R, Waybill P, et al: Deep venous thrombosis after percutaneous insertion of vena caval filters. *J Vasc Surg* 30:821–829, 1999.

Couch GG, Johnston KW, Ojha M: An in vitro comparison of the hemodynamics of two inferior vena cava filters. *J Vasc Surg* 31(3):539–549, 2000.

Geerts WH, Heit JA, Clagett GP, et al: Prevention of venous thromboembolism. *Chest* 119(1 Suppl):132S–175S, 2001.

Ku GH, Billett HH: Long lives, short indications. The case for removable inferior cava filters. *Thromb Haemost* 93(1):17–22, 2005.

Mano A, Tatsumi T, Sakai H, Imoto Y, Nomura T, Nishikawa S, Takeda M, Kobara M, Yamagami T, Matsubara H: A case of deep venous thrombosis with a double inferior vena cava effectively treated by suprarenal filter implantation. *Jpn Heart J* 45(6):1063–1069, 2004.

Mozes G, Kalra M, Carmo M, Swenson L, Gloviczki P: Extension of saphenous thrombus into the femoral vein: a potential complication of new endovenous ablation techniques. *J Vasc Surg* 41(1):130–135, 2005.

Stone PA, Aburahma AF, Hass SM, Hofeldt MJ, Zimmerman WB, Deel JT, Deluca JA: TrapEase inferior vena cava filter placement: use of the subclavian vein. *Vasc Endovasc Surg* 38(6):505–509, 2004.

STUDY QUESTIONS

1. Which of the following would *not* be a means of interventional dilatation of a blood vessel?
   - **a.** laser angioplasty
   - **b.** embolization
   - **c.** intravascular stent placement
   - **d.** atherectomy

2. In cases of suspected upper gastrointestinal bleeding the following interventional procedure would not be employed.
   - **a.** intravascular electrocoagulation
   - **b.** intravascular injection of vasopressin
   - **c.** laser embolectomy
   - **d.** balloon angioplasty

3. Which of the following would not be used as an embolic agent to reduce blood flow?
   - **a.** Gelfoam
   - **b.** bird's nest filter
   - **c.** detachable balloons
   - **d.** Gianturci coil

STUDY QUESTIONS (*cont'd*)

4. _____ is added to Gelfoam to make it radiopaque.
   a. tantalum powder
   b. nitinol
   c. microfibrillar microcapsules
   d. butyl acrylic

5. The process of accessing a blood vessel through a puncture in the skin and performing a procedure through the blood vessel to reshape or repair the inside diameter of the vessel is referred to as:
   a. intravascular ablation
   b. shunting
   c. transluminal angioplasty
   d. transformational reconstruction

6. Which of the following laser systems is considered to be a nonthermal system?
   a. argon laser
   b. excimer laser
   c. Nd:YAG laser
   d. krypton laser

7. The process of establishing channels within the heart muscle for the purpose of renewing the blood supply to create the development of new blood vessels (angiogenesis) is referred to by these initials:
   a. TMR
   b. PTA
   c. TIPS
   d. TRA

8. Which of the following is considered to be anticoagulant medication?
   i. aspirin
   ii. vasopressin
   iii. nitroglycerin
   a. i only
   b. i and ii only
   c. i and iii only
   d. i, ii, and iii

9. Lost catheter fragments can be retrieved from the vascular system using a _____ system.
   a. Greenfield filter
   b. recovery filter
   c. TIP shunt
   d. snare loop catheter

10. One result from the performance of a TIPS procedure would be to reduce the portosystemic gradient to a level of _____ mm Hg.
    a. ≤ 8
    b. ≤ 10
    c. ≤ 12
    d. ≤ 15

18 *Cardiac Interventions*

CHAPTER OBJECTIVES

After completing this chapter, the reader will be able to perform the following:

- List the percutaneous coronary interventional techniques
- List and describe the various cardiac intervention procedures that can be performed
- Identify the indications and contraindications for the various procedures
- Identify the complications associated with each procedure
- Describe balloon angioplasty
- Describe stent placement in the coronary vasculature
- Define the debulking techniques
- Explain the methods used for cardioversion

CHAPTER OUTLINE

The conventional diagnostic angiographic techniques used to demonstrate the anatomy of the heart have already been discussed in Chapter 12. In this chapter we will discuss some of the **interventional** techniques that are in use today. Interventional cardiology primarily focuses on several major areas: hemodynamic studies, techniques to improve the flow of blood to the myocardium, techniques to improve valve performance, extraction techniques (biopsies, foreign body removal), and electrophysiologic procedures. The techniques for transseptal left-sided heart catheterization as well as hemodynamic measurements have also been discussed in Chapter 12. These techniques can be considered as diagnostic rather than therapeutic (interventional).

Cardiac catheterization is a specialty area that is used for the diagnosis, assessment, and treatment of abnormalities of the heart and great vessels. The procedures are accomplished with standard angiographic catheterization techniques. They are relatively safe and, as we have already seen, may be used as diagnostic studies to determine the nature of the anatomy and any pathology and in conjunction with interventional procedures to effect a nonsurgical treatment.

PERCUTANEOUS CORONARY INTERVENTIONS

Coronary artery disease results from a buildup of plaque in the vessels supplying the heart muscle with blood. This is referred to as the stenosis or narrowing of the vessel lumen. Coronary bypass surgery is the invasive method for treatment of this disease. The process of plaque buildup is no different in the heart than it is in any of the vessels that we have already discussed in previous chapters. The development of percutaneous interventional techniques and selective and subselective catheterization equipment has made percutaneous coronary interventional cardiology possible.

Percutaneous Transluminal Angioplasty

Percutaneous transluminal angioplasty is the interventional technique of enlarging the lumen of a stenosed vessel. Three methods are used to recanalize the vessel: balloon angioplasty, balloon angioplasty with stent placement, and transluminal atherectomy. The procedural technique for the three methods is similar. The thoracic aorta is catheterized using the transfemoral approach and an arterial sheath catheter. The guiding sheath is placed in the orifice of the intended coronary artery, and a guide wire is introduced through it into the coronary artery. The guide wire is passed through the area of stenosis, and the angioplasty catheter is placed across the stenotic area. The method may vary slightly depending upon the type of catheter system that is used.

The angioplasty catheter can be a simple balloon catheter arrangement or a balloon-stent catheter system. The delivery system for the angioplasty catheter will be either over the guide wire or fixed guide wire system. Once the balloon is determined to be in the correct position, it is inflated a number of times. The inflation can last from several seconds to minutes. This action has the result of compressing the plaque against the lumen wall, restoring the flow of blood through the vessel. The expansion of the balloon has the effect of stretching and weakening the vessel wall. Some of the elasticity of the vessel is lost; however, after a period of time the diameter of the vessel lumen can shrink, causing restenosis. This is referred to as "recoil." The restenosis caused by this phenomenon can be reduced by the use of the balloon-stent system because the stent provides additional support for the arterial wall.

The **balloon-stent**, as its name implies, has the balloon encased in a metallic stent. The process is slightly different from the balloon catheter alone. The initial expansion of the plaque is usually accomplished by means of a separate balloon catheter, which is subsequently removed once the amount of compression has been achieved and replaced by a "stent over balloon" catheter. When this catheter is placed in the expanded lumen and the balloon is inflated, the stent is compressed into the plaque, providing a firmer support for the compressed plaque. The stent remains in place and the deflated balloon catheter can be removed, leaving a patent vessel (Fig. 18-1). Another type of stent is the **self-expanding** stent. This type of stent is mounted over the catheter and held in a compressed state by a sheath or membrane. When placed in the area of stenosis the covering sheath or membrane can be removed, allowing the stent to expand to its full diameter. This type of stent is held in place by means of its own expansion force against the vessel wall. Figure 18-2 illustrates the placement of a typical self-expanding stent.

Restenosis of the vessel is possible with either system; however, stents have the added advantage of supporting the vessel wall in cases in which the expanding balloon may have caused it to be weakened. The newer "drug eluting" stent systems show promise in reducing the incidence of restenosis of the vessel. As discussed in Chapter 17, these stents are coated with certain drugs that reduce the incidence of restenosis.

Transluminal atherectomy has already been discussed in Chapter 17. Atherectomy, also referred to as "debulking," has the advantage over simple transluminal angioplasty of accomplishing the physical removal of the plaque from the artery. This would decrease the probability of rapid restenosis of the vessel. The procedure has some drawbacks. Among these is the relative size of the catheter system compared to angioplasty. Atherectomy systems are much larger and therefore require a larger access sheath. This fact

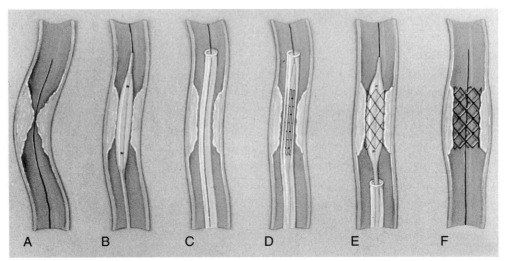

FIGURE 18-1. Schematic illustration of the procedure used to restore patency to a stenosed vessel using both the balloon catheter and the balloon/stent catheter combination. **A,** Guide wire passed through area of stenosed vessel. **B,** Balloon catheter passed through the stenosed area over the guide wire and expanded to allow the balloon/stent sheath to pass through the area. **C,** Balloon/stent sheath passed through stenosed area. **D,** Balloon/stent positioned across the stenosis within the sheath. **E,** The sheath is withdrawn and the balloon/stent is inflated, further expanding the vessel's lumen. **F,** The sheath and balloon catheter are withdrawn, leaving the stent in place, and finally the guide wire is removed.

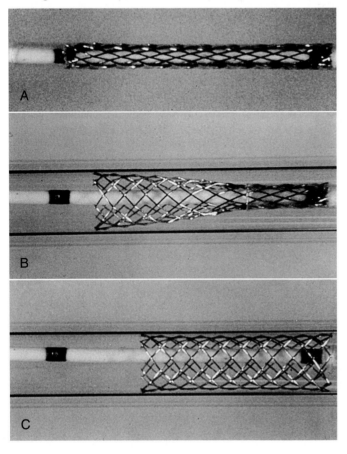

FIGURE 18-2. Photographs of the balloon/stent combination showing the following: **A,** The balloon and stent compressed and enclosed in its sheath. **B,** The sheath is partially withdrawn showing the stent expanding. **C,** The fully expanded stent is shown against the vessel wall.

can increase the potential for severe complications in certain at risk patients. This procedure is best utilized in cases in which the vessel lumen is larger or the stenosis is confined to the vessel orifice. Atherectomy is generally not the method of choice and is rarely applied today in the recanalization of stenotic vessels.

Percutaneous Balloon Valvuloplasty

Percutaneous balloon valvuloplasty is similar to the procedure previously described in percutaneous transluminal angioplasty. The difference is that angioplasty is used to repair stenotic vessels and valvuloplasty is used to repair heart valves that are poorly functioning due to stenosis and scarring. The scarring of the valve leaflets cause it to open incompletely, restricting the flow of blood. When the valve is compromised the heart works harder to push the blood through the stenosed valve. There is also a buildup of pressure in the pulmonary circulation due to the backup of blood which can lead to dyspnea. As the scarring progresses it fuses the leaflets at the point where they touch, increasing the narrowing and exacerbating the symptoms. Some symptoms of compromised valve function include dyspnea accompanied by wheezing or coughing, hemoptysis, fluid retention in the lower extremities or lungs, cardiomegaly, atrial fibrillation or other irregular heart rhythms, thrombosis, stroke, and possibly death from severe heart failure.

The point at which the leaflets of the valve fuse is referred to as a "commissure," and the repair procedure is commonly called a "commissurotomy." The process causes a breaking of the bond holding the valve leaflets and allows it to operate in a much improved fashion. Originally the repair methods included surgical separation of the leaflets via open heart surgery or valve replacement with a mechanical or animal (pig) valve. In most cases percutaneous valvuloplasty will eliminate the necessity for surgical intervention. Valvuloplasty is commonly employed when there is stenosis of the mitral valve; however, it is also used to relieve tricuspid valve stenosis, aortic valve stenosis, and pulmonary stenosis as well as some congenital valvular diseases.

The procedure is similar to that discussed for percutaneous angioplasty and heart catheterization. The balloon expansion technique is used to achieve repair of the valve. The route of the catheterization varies depending on the valve that is to be repaired.

Percutaneous Balloon Mitral Valvuloplasty

The mitral valve must be accessed from an antegrade position via a transseptal approach to facilitate the valvuloplasty. The catheter can be inserted either in an upper extremity vein or more commonly through the femoral vein. Once in the right atrium the catheter is passed through an interatrial opening (either naturally occurring or created and enlarged enough to admit the catheter). If the opening between the atria must be created, a Brockenbrough needle is used and dilation of the opening is accomplished using a tapered dilator. Measurements of the cardiac output are made using the thermodilution or green dye dilution methods once the catheter is in the left atrium.

A specially designed "Inoue balloon catheter" is usually used for the procedure. The catheter is made from polyvinyl chloride with a balloon at its distal end. The balloon has a latex band around its center so that it restricts the inflation of the center of the balloon. When it is fully inflated it will resemble an hourglass shape (Fig. 18-3).

Once the opening into the left atrium has been accomplished and dilated, the deflated Inoue catheter is placed in the atrial chamber. The distal end is expanded, and the catheter is allowed to float across the valve opening. Additional inflation is applied, the proximal end begins to expand, and the balloon engages the valve. When the balloon resembles an hourglass the catheter is in place across the valve and ready for the valvuloplasty. The balloon is expanded further against the valve to complete the procedure (Fig. 18-4).

Percutaneous Balloon Aortic Valvuloplasty

The principle behind this procedure is the same as in percutaneous balloon mitral valvuloplasty as previously described. A balloon catheter passed through the aortic valve is used to achieve commissural

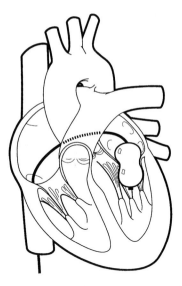

FIGURE 18-3. The placement of the Inoue balloon catheter across the mitral valve.

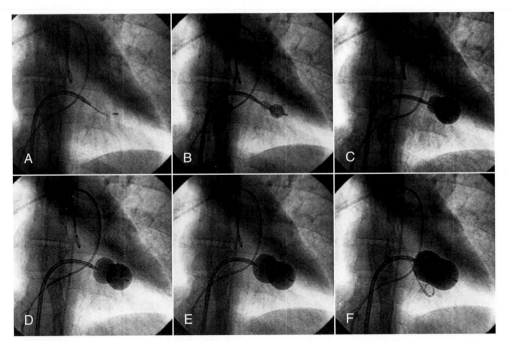

FIGURE 18-4. Radiographic representation of a percutaneous mitral valvuloplasty. **A,** Catheter in place by the mitral valve. **B,** Front half of catheter is floated across the mitral valve. **C,** Catheter is retracted to place the distal portion against the mitral valve. **D,** The rear portion of the balloon is inflated showing the hourglass shape. **E,** Additional inflation of the balloon enlarges the mitral valve opening. The inflated central portion of the balloon separates the commissures. **F,** The balloon is almost fully inflated, concluding the procedure.

separation. The catheter is passed retrograde from a peripheral artery. The most common route is via the femoral artery; however, in cases of severe peripheral vascular disease the brachial route can be used. If the upper extremity approach is required, smaller diameter catheters are generally used.

The balloon catheter is passed through the aorta and across the aortic valve. The dilation process is accomplished using several different size catheters in succession, gradually increasing their size through the procedure. It is important that the patient's cardiac rhythm be monitored, and pressure measurements should also be observed during the inflation portion of the procedure. The objective of the procedure is to reduce the pressure gradient between the left ventricle and the aorta to below 30 mm Hg, with a corresponding increase in the diameter of the aortic valve.

Pulmonary Valvuloplasty

The procedure can also be used to relieve pulmonary valve stenosis. This intervention does not differ significantly from that discussed earlier. The route of catheter placement is through the femoral vein. It is passed across the pulmonary valve and expanded to reduce the stenosis. As in the previous procedures the objective is the reduction in the gradient across the pulmonary valve. The procedure holds the same risks and complications as in the mitral and aortic valvuloplasty procedures, and restenosis is always a possibility.

Complications of Percutaneous Valvuloplasty

The complications of this procedure are varied and can range from a mild vasovagal reaction to death. The possibility that the procedure will not provide the patient with any mitigation of the stenosis as well as the possibility of restenosis are risks attendant with this procedure. The following list is a summary of some of the complications that can be the result of percutaneous valvuloplasty.

- Vasovagal reaction
- Mechanical complications
  - Failure to pass the catheter through the valve
  - Vascular injury
  - Failure or malfunction of the balloon catheter system
  - Failure to advance the catheter through the vascular system to the valve
  - Injury or perforation of the myocardial wall
  - Valvular damage
  - Embolization resulting from valve fragments, air, or thrombus formation
  - Valvular regurgitation
  - Hematoma at the entry site
- Infection
- Cardiac arrhythmias
- Transient ischemic episodes
- Congestive heart failure
- Pulmonary edema
- Myocardial infarction
- Respiratory arrest
- Renal failure
- Contrast agent allergic reactions
- Death

Catheter Ablation

Ablation is a general term referring to the process of destroying and removing tissue. This procedure is commonly accomplished using radiofrequency waves. There are several different energy sources that can be used for catheter ablation besides radiofrequency energy. These include direct electrical stimulation, microwave, laser, cryoablation, ultrasound (US), and chemical. Box 18-1 summarizes the type of energy used and its effect on tissue.

Ablation is a technique used in various parts of the body to necrose and remove tumor tissue. Ablation can also be used in the treatment of bone metastases. Also, cardiac electrophysiology has

BOX 18-1	*Energy Source and Effect on Tissue*
Type of Stimulation	**Result on Tissue**
Chemical	Cytotoxic reaction which selectively destroys the tissue
Ultrasound	Localized hyperthermia at predictable depths
Radiofrequency	Tissue destruction by conductive and resistive heating
Microwave	Dielectric heating—does not require contact with tissue to provide heat
Laser	Thermal heating with tissue vaporization—strength and depth of heating dependent upon the type of system
Cryoablation	Freezing and thawing of tissue

adapted catheter ablation to interrupt arrhythmias, specifically atrial fibrillation, atrial flutter, and various other tachyarrhythmias. Transcatheter ablation was originally accomplished using direct current; however, radiofrequency waves in the range of 300 to 1200 kHz are now being used. Radiofrequency waves are a combination of electric and magnetic energy. It occurs naturally as visible light, radio waves, and microwaves. The electromagnetic energy that is used in catheter ablation is produced by a radiofrequency generator. The energy is directed to a specific focal point by means of the special catheter electrodes that are used. An advantage of radiofrequency ablation over direct current ablation is that it permits a more focused destruction of tissue.

Indications

The cardiac rhythm is maintained by its electrical system. In the normal state the electrical rhythm begins at the sinoatrial node, the cardiac pacemaker, which is located in the right atrium close to the ostium of the superior vena cava. The activity of the sinoatrial node produces a steady rhythm heart muscle to contract approximately 70 to 80 times per minute. The electrical impulse then passes through the atrioventricular node, the atrioventricular bundle of His entering the ventricular septum. As the impulse travels down the ventricular septum it passes through the Purkinje fibers that give off many smaller branches into the cardiac muscle stimulating the ventricular muscle to contract. If the impulses are interrupted, delayed, or sent down the wrong path, the heart beat may become irregular. This irregularity can be either too fast or too slow and is termed an arrhythmia. Cardiac ablation is indicated when the irregularity causes a rhythm that is too fast (tachycardia).

Some indications for catheter ablation are the following:

- Atrial fibrillation
- Atrial flutter
- Atrial tachycardia
- Atypical ventricular tachycardia
- Wolff-Parkinson-White syndrome
- Supraventricular tachycardia (SVT)

Procedure

The technique is similar to a standard electrophysiologic study. An intravenous line is established for the purpose of administration of medication. The patient care may include antibiotic treatment and administration of anticoagulant (heparin) during the procedure. All antiarrhythmic medication should be discontinued, and a cardiac monitoring system is necessary if mapping is to be carried out.

Because both electrophysiologic studies and ablation are accomplished from the right side of the heart, the catheters are introduced in the same manner as right cardiac catheterization. The access routes can be from the femoral, internal jugular, subclavian, or antecubital veins. Specialized catheters are used that are equipped with electrodes at the distal end (Fig. 18-5). Generally two catheters are

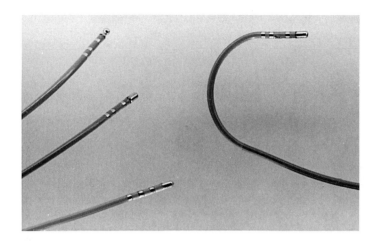

FIGURE 18-5. Examples of catheters equipped with distal electrodes for ablative interventions.

introduced per vein. The total number of catheters required depends upon the type of study being performed.

One of the catheters is placed in the region of the sinus node; another is introduced into the right ventricle and placed in close proximity to the bundle of His. In cases of ventricular tachycardia the left side of the heart must be catheterized. This is accomplished through the femoral artery, placing the catheters into the left side of the heart.

When the catheters have been satisfactorily placed an electrophysiologic baseline study is performed. This is done to identify the specific location of the abnormality. Once this is completed the mapping and ablation procedure can be done. The specific techniques for the catheter placement and administration of the radiofrequency waves differ with the specific pathologic condition and are beyond the scope of this text.

At the conclusion of the ablation process a final electrophysiologic study is performed. The study will demonstrate whether the procedure is successful or if the arrhythmia recurs. The catheters are then removed and pressure is applied to the entry site. The patient is then monitored for a period of 24 hours to determine if the arrhythmia recurs or if any complications appear.

Complications

Complications include mechanical damage to the heart or blood vessels due to the placement of the catheters; damage from the heat generated by the catheters is also a possibility. Coughing, chest pain, and hemoptysis are also possible risks from the procedure. Major complications include stroke, heart attack, and death.

Endomyocardial Biopsy

This procedure is used to obtain a small sample of myocardial tissue for analysis. It is accomplished by the use of an instrument referred to as a bioptome. This is a catheter system with a set of movable jaws at the distal end. Once in position within the heart the sample can be taken. There are three general categories of instruments: stiff shaft, variable flexible, and flexible shaft systems. The length of the bioptome is dependent upon the route of access to the heart.

Indications and Contraindications

There are several indications for this procedure; however, the major reason for its use is to determine the success or rejection of a heart transplant. Other indications include pathologic processes such as sarcoidosis, amyloidosis, hemachromatosis, myocarditis, chest pain, arrhythmia, neoplasm, and anthracycline cardiotoxicity.

The relative contraindications for the procedures are abnormalities that would prevent the introduction of the bioptome. Anticoagulation is also a contraindication for the procedure.

Procedure

The patient is prepared in the same manner as for right cardiac catheterization. The femoral vein and the internal jugular are the common routes used. The percutaneous insertion of the catheter is the accepted method for its introduction.

In the case of the femoral approach, once the vessel is punctured a guide wire is inserted. The dilator and catheter sheath are introduced. The sheath is advanced over the guide wire until it is placed in the right atrium. Once accomplished the bioptome is advanced through the sheath into the right ventricle for the actual biopsy. A small segment of the ventricular septum is removed for microscopic evaluation. The variable flexible catheter has the advantage in the femoral approach over the other types of systems in that it can be made flexible when entering the heart to prevent the sheath from being dislodged from the right atrium. Once in place it can be stiffened to obtain the actual biopsy.

A shorter bioptome system is used when the internal jugular approach is used. The Seldinger technique is used to introduce the dilator/sheath combination over a guide wire. In this case the stiff shaft bioptome system is preferred. The bioptome is introduced into the right atrium and then advanced into the right ventricle. Using a slight twisting motion the bioptome head is placed so that a sample can be removed from the ventricular septum.

At the conclusion of the procedure pressure is placed over the entry site, and the patient is monitored for complications.

Complications

The complications from endomyocardial biopsy are similar to those for any heart catheterization. Mechanical problems resulting from the introduction of the catheter system at the access site as well as the potential for perforation of the ventricular septum are possible. Stimulation of cardiac arrhythmias and conduction abnormalities are also a risk. In rare instances death can occur.

Foreign Body Extraction

During the performance of intravascular procedures it is possible for the equipment to fail. Portions of catheters and guide wires have broken off and become lodged in blood vessels or the heart. The procedure for the removal of these fragments follows a relatively simple procedure. The process is made possible by the use of specially designed extraction catheters (Fig. 18-6). These usually employ a "loop and snare" system. Several types of catheters have been designed for this purpose.

The procedure is relatively simple. It involves the placement of the extraction catheter close to the foreign body. The loop is extended and the catheter is manipulated so that the fragment is snared by the loop. The loop is then tightened around the fragment and it is gently withdrawn (Fig. 18-7).

The major complication from this procedure is the possibility that the sharp end of the fragment could tear or perforate the blood vessel as it is being withdrawn. If at all possible, the extraction loop is placed at the distal end of the fragment so that the sharp end is trailing as it is removed.

Intra-aortic Balloon Placement

This procedure is a short-term intervention that acts as a circulatory assist device. The purpose of the device is to increase the myocardial oxygen supply while simultaneously decreasing the myocardial oxygen demand. Patients with severe heart disease or individuals awaiting a heart transplant are the primary beneficiaries of this procedure. The intervention is also referred to as intra–aortic balloon counterpulsation. The timed inflation and deflation of the balloon serves to increase the diastolic pressure while decreasing "afterload." The afterload is intimately related to the aortic pressure and can be described as the systemic vascular resistance to the flow of blood ejected by the left ventricle. The

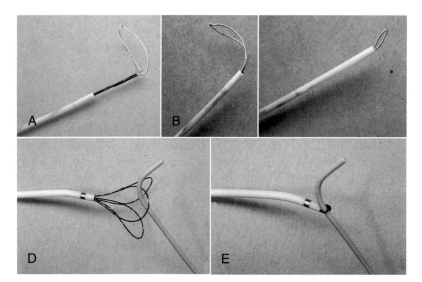

FIGURE 18-6. Photographs of the Amplatz gooseneck snare and the EnSnare systems. **A,** The Amplatz snare in the fully opened position. **B,** Midpoint position and **C,** The fully closed position. **D,** The EnSnare is capturing a catheter in the opened position. **E,** The EnSnare closed and in the retrieval position.

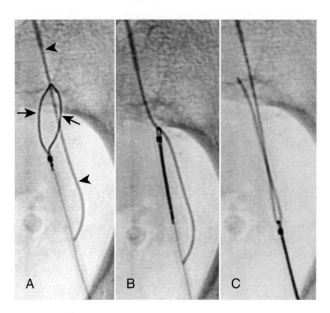

FIGURE 18-7. Radiographs of the Amplatz gooseneck snare catheter retrieving a guide wire. **A,** The opened snare encircles the guide wire. **B,** The guide wire is secured by tightening the snare loop. **C,** The guide wire is being withdrawn into the snare's sheath for removal.

reduction in afterload through the use of the intra-aortic balloon pump also leads to a reduction in ventricular wall stress and better perfusion of the myocardium through the coronary arteries. The reductions in afterload and ventricular wall stress lead to a fall in myocardial oxygen consumption.

Counterpulsation is accomplished by having the intra-aortic balloon inflate when the heart muscle relaxes and then deflate just prior to the next heart beat. The intra-aortic balloon is placed in the lumen of the thoracic aorta, and the inflation and deflation sequence is controlled by a computer.

Indications and Contraindications

The indications for this procedure include cardiogenic shock, severe left main coronary artery stenosis, intractable angina, complications from acute myocardial infarction, ventricular tachycardia, and therapy after percutaneous transluminal coronary angioplasty, especially in high-risk cases. Intra-aortic balloon placement is also indicated in patients awaiting cardiac transplant. The procedure has also been used in patients subsequent to coronary bypass surgery.

The procedure is contraindicated when there is uncontrolled bleeding, abdominal aortic aneurysm, uncontrolled sepsis, aortic dissection, abnormalities of the femoral artery or severe bilateral peripheral vascular disease, aortic regurgitation, arteriovenous shunting, and patent ductus arteriosus.

Procedure

Once the contraindications for the procedure have been ruled out the intra-aortic balloon (IAB) catheter is percutaneously inserted into a femoral artery using a modified Seldinger technique. The process involves the percutaneous puncture of the femoral artery. A J-shaped guide wire is then inserted through the needle into the aorta. The needle is removed, and the puncture site is dilated with a dilator sheath combination. The dilator is then removed, and the balloon catheter is threaded over the guide wire into the descending aorta. The balloon should be deflated completely prior to insertion. The tip of the balloon should be placed in the descending aorta slightly inferior to the top of the aortic arch just distal to the left subclavian artery. The distal end of the balloon should be placed so that it is above the origins of the renal arteries. Once deployed in the correct position the balloon catheter is connected to the operating console and counterpulsation begins. Aortic pressure measurements are taken through the catheter lumen, and if proper position and function are confirmed, the catheter is held in place with sutures.

The inflation and deflation of the balloon must be correctly synchronized with the patient's cardiac cycle. This can be accomplished through direct pressure readings, monitoring the patient's electrocardiogram, or using an intrinsic pump rate. The ideal method is through the use of direct pressure readings; however, if the patient's cardiac cycle is used the intra-aortic balloon is triggered to initiate inflation in the middle of the T wave, and deflation should be accomplished just before the end of the QRS complex at or before the R wave.

Although the femoral approach is the most common route of entry, the subclavian, axillary, and iliac arteries have also been successfully used for this procedure.

Removal of the balloon catheter is accomplished either through a surgical intervention or via the closed method. The closed method involves complete deflation of the balloon.

Complications

The complications resulting from this procedure can be categorized as either vascular or nonvascular. They are summarized as follows:

Vascular Complications
- Vascular dissection
- Arterial obstruction and ischemia in the lower extremity
- Arterial laceration
- Hemorrhage

Nonvascular Complications
- Cholesterol embolization
- Hemolysis and platelet destruction
- Cerebral ischemia
- Balloon rupture
- Infection at the puncture site
- Visceral ischemia

Pericardiocentesis

This procedure can be used as an emergency procedure to relieve the cause of **cardiac tamponade** (fluid or blood accumulation in the pericardial space that puts pressure on the heart). This prevents the ventricles of the heart from expanding fully. Cardiac tamponade is an acute

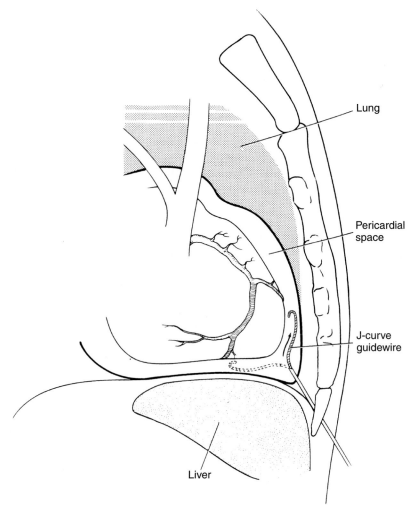

FIGURE 18-8.   Schematic drawing of the pericardiocentesis procedures. The catheter is being placed in the pericardial space to remove a fluid accumulation.

condition resulting from pericarditis, myocardial infarction, aortic dissection or aneurysm, and cardiac trauma.

Pericardiocentesis can also be performed to diagnose and treat chronic **pericardial effusions** (excess fluid accumulation around the heart). This can be caused by cancer, inflammation or infections, kidney failure, and cardiac surgery.

Procedure

The goal of the procedure is to tap into the pericardium to extract some or all of the excess fluid collection (Fig. 18-8). If continuous drainage is desired, a catheter can be placed in the pericardium. Regardless of the expected outcome the patient should be monitored throughout the procedure. Electrocardiographic tracings should be continuously obtained.

Initial needle entry can be performed at one of several sites on the chest wall. One of the most common sites is just inferior to the xiphoid process. The patient is placed in the recumbent position for the procedure. A long pericardiocentesis needle, approximately 6 inches in length, is positioned at the left xiphocostal angle, 3 to 5 mm below the costal margin. The puncture is made by directing the needle toward the inner aspect of the ribcage toward the left shoulder.

There are several methods of needle guidance during the initial insertion: two-dimensional echocardiography, electrocardiographic, and hemodynamic monitoring. The choice of guidance methods is determined by the hospital protocol and physician preference. This is the most important portion of the procedure, and the complication of myocardial puncture or pneumothorax is possible.

Fluid removal can immediately be initiated in emergency situations by attaching a syringe to the needle hub. If longer term drainage is warranted, a catheter can be introduced following the percutaneous insertion method. Once the puncture is accomplished and confirmed, a guide wire is placed through the needle into the pericardial space. The needle is removed and a dilator sheath is passed over the guide wire to enlarge the opening. A multiple side hole pigtail catheter is then placed over the guide wire and inserted into the pericardium. The process is complete when the pericardial sac is emptied of fluid.

Boston Scientific markets a pericardial fluid aspiration procedure kit. This kit, called the PeriVac, contains all the necessary instruments and supplies for pericardiocentesis in one presterilized package.

Complications

Possible complications from this procedure are the perforation of either the right atrium or ventricle, laceration of the myocardium, laceration of a coronary artery, pneumothorax, cardiac arrhythmias, and puncture of the stomach or colon.

Cardioversion

The normal electrical sequence of the cardiac cycle has been discussed in the section on intracardiac ablation. In some cases the electrical cycle becomes short–circuited, causing it to loop continuously, stimulating the heart and creating an abnormal rhythm. This phenomenon is referred to as reentry. Cardioversion is the application of high-energy direct current to change an irregular heart rhythm into one that is normal. In other words it converts the electrical loop into a normal electrical cycle.

The technique can be applied externally, internally, and surgically. In many cases external cardioversion will be sufficient to return the heart to its normal rhythm. Surgical cardioversion is accomplished with the chest wall surgically opened. Internal cardioversion provides the electrical stimulation by means of the placement of special catheters into the heart. Cardioversion is similar to defibrillation in that the procedure is used to return the heart to its normal rhythm. Defibrillation differs from cardioversion in that it uses a much higher level of electricity to administer the shock and it is nonsynchronized with the cardiac rhythm. Defibrillation is used in emergency situations to convert much more severe arrhythmias.

Cardioversion is a procedure that can be performed either externally or internally. External cardioversion is accomplished using electrodes applied to the chest. Internal cardioversion involves the placement of catheter electrodes, and the impulse is given endocardially.

External cardioversion is indicated for the conversion of abnormal cardiac rhythms that have not been successfully treated medically. The most common abnormality treated with external cardioversion is atrial fibrillation with duration of greater than 48 hours. Cardioversion can be used to treat a variety of tachycardias.

External cardioversion is used to treat hemodynamically stable patients. The patient's electro-cardiogram should be monitored. Paddles are placed on the anterior chest wall. The exact position is dependent upon the type of arrhythmia being treated. It is important that the impulse be delivered at the peak of the QRS complex, and proper synchronization should be accomplished prior to administering the shock. Sedation of the patient is initiated prior to the administration of the electrical impulse. Several impulses of increasing strength may have to be delivered before a successful cardioversion is achieved.

Internal Cardioversion

This procedure is indicated in cases of failed external cardioversion or to assess the feasibility of an implantable cardioverter-defibrillator (ICD). Atrial fibrillation is the primary reason for internal cardioversion.

The patient is normally under general anesthesia or conscious sedation during the procedure. Specially designed electrode catheters are introduced percutaneously into the right atrium and coronary sinus. A bipolar catheter is placed in the right ventricle and is used to achieve the proper timing of the shock. Additional impulses may be necessary in order to convert the abnormal rhythm.

Complications

Complications resulting from external cardioversion include transient depression of myocardial function due to tissue necrosis, asystole, ventricular tachycardia or fibrillation, cardiac dysfunction, and transient hypotension.

The complications of internal cardioversion are specific to the mechanics of right cardiac catheterization. Some other complications that can occur include initiation of arrhythmias, pericardial effusion, and decreased cardiac output.

SUMMARY

The procedures discussed in this chapter primarily involve the establishment of vessel patency through the use of balloon expansion, stent placement, or a combination of both procedures. The use of these methods has been well documented. Percutaneous transluminal angioplasty has commonly been used to reestablish blood flow in a wide variety of vessels including the coronary vasculature. Stents are applied in cases in which restenosis of the vessel has occurred or presents a viable possibility. The procedure involves the use of the Seldinger method of vessel access and makes use of a specialized catheter system that includes an expandable balloon. The balloon is used to compress the plaque in the vessel and increase the internal diameter of the vessel.

The percutaneous balloon techniques are also applied in cases in which the valves of the heart become compromised. The balloon is used to open compromised valves in the heart, restoring an adequate blood flow. Balloon devices have also been used to function as a temporary circulatory assist device. In these cases the balloon is placed in the aortic lumen and inflated and deflated in conjunction with the cardiac cycle to provide an assist in maintaining circulatory pressure.

The destruction of specific areas of cardiac tissue by chemical, electrical, laser, cryogenics, and radiofrequency can reestablish the proper cardiac rhythm. The technique is referred to as catheter ablation. This is also a percutaneous procedure that has provided relief to many patients with cardiac arrhythmias.

Percutaneous biopsy, foreign body extraction, and pericardial puncture are also techniques that have proved to be important interventional procedures. The use of the percutaneous method has proved its usefulness in aiding in the nonsurgical removal of foreign bodies in the vascular system.

Finally, internal cardioversion or maintenance of the proper cardiac rhythm using an implantable electrode to stimulate the cardiac rhythm through percutaneous placement has found its place as a viable thoracic interventional procedure. Cardioversion is used after failure of external defibrillation or to assess the feasibility of an implantable pacemaker.

SUGGESTED READINGS

Percutaneous Balloon Valvuloplasty

Das P, Prendergast B: Imaging in mitral stenosis: assessment before, during and after percutaneous balloon mitral valvuloplasty. *Expert Rev Cardiovasc Ther* 1(4):549–557, 2003.

Prendergast BD, Shaw TRD, Iung B, Vahanian A, Northridge DB: Contemporary criteria for the selection of patients for percutaneous balloon mitral valvuloplasty. *Heart* 87(5):401–404, 2002.

Rudzinski A, Werynski P, Krol-Jawien W, et al: Percutaneous balloon valvuloplasty in the treatment of pulmonary valve stenosis in children—late results. *Acta Cardiol* 59(2):230–231, 2004.

Yetkin E, Erbay AR, Turhan H, et al: Changes in plasma levels of adhesion molecules after percutaneous mitral balloon valvuloplasty. *Cardiovasc Pathol* 13(2):103–108, 2004.

Intra-aortic Balloon Pump Placement

Abid Q, Rao PS, Kendall SW: Use of intraaortic balloon pump in left ventricle rupture after mitral valve replacement. *Ann Thorac Surg* 74(6):2194–2195, 2002.

Baskett RJF, Ghali WA, Maitland A, Hirsch GM: The intraaortic balloon pump in cardiac surgery. *Ann Thorac Surg* 74(4):1276–1287, 2002.

Christenson JT, Cohen M, Ferguson JJ III, Freedman RJ, Miller MF, Ohman EM, Reddy RC, Stone GW, Urban PM: Trends in intraaortic balloon counterpulsation complications and outcomes in cardiac surgery. *Ann Thorac Surg* 74(4):1086–1090, 2002.

H'Doubler PB Jr, H'Doubler WZ, Bien RC, Jansen DA: A novel technique for intraaortic balloon pump placement via the left axillary artery in patients awaiting cardiac transplantation. *Cardiovasc Surg* 8(6):463–465, 2000.

Lonergan-Thomas H, Brennan S, Cianci P, et al: Enhanced external counterpulsation: bringing the concept of the intraaortic balloon pump to the outpatient setting. *Dimens Crit Care Nurs* 23(3):119–121, 2004.

Overwalder PJ: Intra aortic balloon pump (IABP) counterpulsation. *Internet J Thorac Cardiovasc Surg*, 1999.

Sheah K: Intraaortic balloon pump mimicking catheter tip fracture. *AJR Am J Roentgenol* 183(5):1522–1523, 2004.

Catheter Ablation

Bruce CJ: Intracardiac echocardiography guiding successful ablation. *Eur J Echocardiography* 4:4–5, 2003.

Ernst S, Ouyang F, Lober F, et al: Catheter-induced linear lesions in the left atrium in patients with atrial fibrillation. *J Am Coll Cardiol* 42:1271–1282, 2003.

Hsu LF, Jais P, Sanders P, et al: Catheter ablation for atrial fibrillation in congestive heart failure. *N Engl J Med* 351(23):2373–2383, 2004.

Jais P, Sanders P, Hsu LF, et al: Catheter ablation for atrial fibrillation. *Heart* 91(1):7–9, 2005.

Katritsis D, Giazitzoglou E, Korovesis S, Zambartas C: Comparison of the transseptal approach to the transaortic approach for ablation of left-sided accessory pathways in patients with Wolf-Parkinson-White syndrome. *Am J Cardiol* 91:610–613, 2003.

Pai RK, Boyle NG, Child JS, et al: Transient left recurrent laryngeal nerve palsy following catheter ablation of atrial fibrillation. *Heart Rhythm* 2(2):182–184, 2005.

Endomyocardial Biopsy

Benvenuti LA, Moreira LF, Aiello VD, et al: Sequential histologic analysis of the myocardium after dynamic cardiomyoplasty: a study based on right ventricular endomyocardial biopsies. *J Heart Lung Transplant* 23(12):1438–1440, 2004.

Frustaci A, Pieroni M, Chimenti C: The role of endomyocardial biopsy in the diagnosis of cardiomyopathies. *Ital Heart J* 3(6):348–353, 2003.

Jones RL, Miles DW: Use of endomyocardial biopsy to assess anthracycline-induced cardiotoxicity. *Lancet Oncol* 6(2):67, 2005.

Veinot JP: Diagnostic endomyocardial biopsy pathology—general biopsy considerations, and its use for myocarditis and cardiomyopathy: a review. *Can J Cardiol* 18(1):55–65, 2002.

Vorlat A, Conraads VM, Vrints CJ: Deep vein thrombosis after transfemoral endomyocardial biopsy in cardiac transplant recipients. *J Heart Lung Transplant* 22(9):1063–1064, 2003.

Pericardiocentesis

Ceron L, Manzato M, Mazzaro F, Bellavere F: A new diagnostic and therapeutic approach to pericardial effusion: transbronchial needle aspiration. *Chest* 123(5):1753–1758, 2003.

Luckraz H, Kitchlu S, Youhana A: Haemorrhagic peritonitis as a late complication of echocardiography guided pericardiocentesis. *Heart* 90(3):e16, 2004.

Mangi AA, Torchiana DF: Pericardial disease. *Card Surg Adult* 2:1359–1372, 2003.

Quraishi AR, Khan AA, Kazmi KA, et al: Clinical and echocardiographic characteristics of patients with significant pericardial effusion requiring pericardiocentesis. *J Pak Med Assoc* 55(2):66–70, 2005.

Tsang TS, Seward JB: Pericardiocentesis under echocardiographic guidance. *Eur J Echocardiogr* 2(1):68–69, 2001.

Implantable Cardioversion

Berger JT: The ethics of deactivating implanted cardioverter defibrillators. *Ann Intern Med* 142(8):631–634, 2005.

Gorenek B, Kudaiberdieva G, Goktekin O, et al: Detection of myocardial injury after internal cardioversion for atrial fibrillation. *Can J Cardiol* 20(2):165–168, 2004.

Sinha SK, Mehta D, Gomes JA: Prevention of sudden cardiac death: the role of the implantable cardioverter-defibrillator. *Mt Sinai J Med* 72(1):1–9, 2005.

Swerdlow CD, Schwartzman D, Hoyt R, et al: Determinants of first-shock success for atrial implantable cardioverter defibrillators. *J Cardiovasc Electrophysiol* 13(4):347–354, 2002.

Young JB, Abraham WT, Smith AL, et al: Combined cardiac resynchronization and implantable cardioversion defibrillation in advanced chronic heart failure: the MIRACLE ICD Trial. *JAMA* 289(20):2685–2694, 2003.

STUDY QUESTIONS

1. The narrowing of the internal lumen of a vessel is referred to as:
   a. transluminization
   b. endomyocardium
   c. revascularization
   d. stenosis

2. The process by which a stent has the ability to release medication after placement in a vessel is referred to as:
   a. dilution
   b. marginalizing
   c. elution
   d. exfoliation

3. The point at which the leaflets of a valve meet is referred to as a _____.
   a. commissure
   b. plasty
   c. margin
   d. stricture

4. The procedure by which a cardiac valve is repaired is referred to as a _____.
   a. pericardiocentesis
   b. valvulostenosis
   c. valvuloplasty
   d. angioplasty

5. In the normal state the electrical rhythm of the heart begins at the _____.
   a. cardiac ostium
   b. bundle of His
   c. sinoatrial node
   d. Purkinje fibers

6. The process of destroying and removing tissue using radiofrequency waves is called:
   a. angioplasty
   b. ablation
   c. centesis
   d. revascularization

7. Which of the following are complications related to percutaneous valvuloplasties?
   i. infection
   ii. death
   iii. hematoma
   a. i only
   b. i and iii only
   c. ii and iii only
   d. i, ii, and iii

8. Endomyocardial biopsy is usually taken from the _____ of the heart.
   a. right ventricular septum
   b. right atrial wall
   c. left atrial wall
   d. pulmonary artery

9. Which of the following approaches are used in performing an endomyocardial biopsy?
   i. femoral vein
   ii. antecubital vein
   iii. internal jugular vein
   a. i only
   b. ii only
   c. iii only
   d. i and iii only

10. The procedure that is used to increase the myocardial oxygen supply while simultaneously decreasing the myocardial oxygen demand is called:
    a. pericardiocentesis
    b. intra-aortic balloon pump
    c. valvuloplasty
    d. angioplasty

19 Nonvascular Interventional Procedures

CHAPTER OBJECTIVES

After completing this chapter, the reader will be able to perform the following:

- Identify the anatomy and pathophysiology of the gastrointestinal system
- Identify the anatomy and pathophysiology of the biliary system
- Identify the anatomy and pathophysiology of the urinary system
- Describe the general methodology used for needle biopsies
- Explain the general methodology of puncture and drainage procedures
- Describe the general methodology for percutaneous calculi removal procedures
- Explain the general methodology of endoscopic retrograde cholangiopancreatography
- Describe extracorporeal shock wave lithotripsy

CHAPTER OUTLINE

ANATOMY AND PATHOPHYSIOLOGY

    Gastrointestinal System
    Urinary System

GENERAL METHODOLOGY OF PROCEDURES

    Needle Biopsy
    Puncture and Drainage Methods
    Percutaneous Calculi Removal
    Endoscopic Retrograde Cholangiopancreatography
    Extracorporeal Shock Wave Lithotripsy

SUMMARY

Nonvascular interventional radiography encompasses a wide range of procedures, and an in-depth discussion of all of them is beyond the scope of this text. However, some major areas—notably, percutaneous needle biopsy, puncture, and drainage procedures and percutaneous removal of calculi—merit discussion. Because each of these procedures can be used in many different areas of the body, a brief discourse on the anatomy and pathophysiology of the more common areas treated by these methods is warranted. It is expected that most of the normal anatomy will already have been covered in previous course work; therefore a cursory reminder of the anatomy will be sufficient, along with a summary of some major pathophysiologic conditions. The interventional treatments that are used in each of these areas will also be discussed.

BOX 19-1   *Upper and Lower Divisions of the Gastrointestinal System*

Upper Division
Mouth
Esophagus
Stomach

Lower Division
Small intestine
Large intestine (colon)
Sigmoid, rectum, and anus

ANATOMY AND PATHOPHYSIOLOGY

Gastrointestinal System

The gastrointestinal system can be compared to a hollow tube that begins at the mouth and ends at the rectum. It consists of several accessory organs, notably the pancreas, gallbladder, liver, and salivary glands. It can be divided into an upper portion and a lower portion. Box 19-1 summarizes the components of each of the divisions.

The gastrointestinal system functions to process food and fluids that are taken in through the mouth. The accessory organs of the gastrointestinal (GI) tract serve to aid in the processing of the material, or in some cases they can change the makeup of the ingested product to yield different substances as they are needed. For example, the salivary glands add fluid and enzymes to the material and begin the breakdown of carbohydrates. The liver utilizes amino acids that are produced in the GI tract to produce new proteins. Bile from the gallbladder, along with pancreatic and intestinal secretions, digests fats and carbohydrates. The nutrients, electrolytes, and water that are produced by this process are absorbed into the bloodstream, where they are carried to and used by the various cells in the body.

The stomach is not well suited to the absorption of the ingested products. Absorption is accomplished along the path of the intestines. The by-products of digestion are ultimately stored in the rectum and finally eliminated by defecation. The wall of the GI tract is composed of several layers. These are listed from the interior layer to the exterior: mucosa, submucosal layer, smooth muscle fibers (circular and then longitudinal), and the visceral peritoneum or serous layer. The peritoneum is a double membrane; the visceral portion provides the covering of the outer wall of the GI tract, and the parietal peritoneum covers the abdominal wall. The peritoneal structures are thin-walled and quite vascular. Double-layered folds of the peritoneum form the mesentery. This provides blood vessels and nerves to the wall of the intestine and provides support for the jejunum and ileum of the small intestine.

The blood supply for the abdominal viscera arises from the aorta as the celiac, superior, and inferior mesenteric arteries (Fig. 19-1). All these vessels are clearly demonstrated on an abdominal aortogram.

Angiography of these arteries is accomplished for a variety of pathologic conditions including mesenteric ischemia caused by stenosis or thrombosis, acute gastrointestinal bleeding, celiac artery compression, aneurysms, vasculitis, and arteriovenous malformations. Diagnostic as well as interventional procedures for the vasculature of the GI system have been discussed in previous chapters.

Box 19-2 lists some of the disorders that can affect the GI system. In some cases therapies such as drug therapy, diet alteration, and stress reduction are successful; however, many pathologic conditions have been treated utilizing interventional techniques.

Accessory Organs

The liver, gallbladder, and pancreas are in intimate contact with the duodenum (the first part of the small intestine). These organs provide substances that aid in the digestive process.

The liver is one of the heaviest organs in the body. One of the functions of the liver is to maintain a normal concentration of blood glucose, which is necessary to carbohydrate metabolism. It also plays a

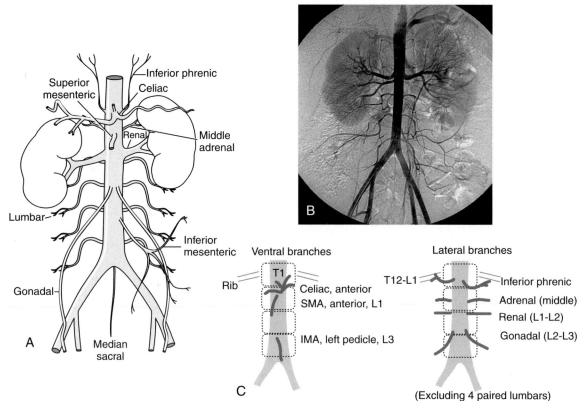

FIGURE 19-1. **A,** Illustration of the major vessels originating from the descending aorta. These vessels supply the abdominal viscera with blood. **B,** Aortogram demonstrating the vessels as they appear radiographically. **C,** Major branches of abdominal aorta in relationship to vertebral column.

BOX 19-2	*Gastrointestinal System Disorders*
Pathology	**Interventional Procedure**
Chronic mesenteric ischemia	Percutaneous balloon angioplasty
	Stent placement
Acute gastrointestinal (GI) bleeding	Intra-arterial infusion of vasopressin (Pitressen)
	Transcatheter embolization
Gastrointestinal decompression	Percutaneous gastrostomy
Nutritional support	Percutaneous gastrojejunostomy
Upper GI tract stricture	Balloon angioplasty
Esophageal and duodenal strictures	Stent placement
Achalasia	
Cecal dilatation	Percutaneous cecostomy
Acute bowel obstruction	Colonic stenting

part in lipid metabolism by synthesizing fats that are stored in adipose tissue in the body. The liver also converts some amino acids into other types of amino acids.

One of the primary functions of the liver is to produce bile. This substance aids in the digestion of fats and is secreted into the duodenum via the bile duct. It is produced in the hepatic cells and secreted into the bile canals in the liver. The bile canals empty into the right and left hepatic ducts, which become the common hepatic duct. The common hepatic duct and the cystic duct join to form the common bile duct, which leads to the duodenum. The bile is secreted in response to the presence of proteins and fats in the small intestine.

Although the liver appears to be a single large structure, it has been described by Claude Couinaud, a French surgeon, as being segmental with each of the segments having its own outflow, inflow, and biliary drainage.[1] He described eight areas according to a concept of plates and vasculobiliary sheaths (Fig. 19-2). The performance of the diagnostic and interventional procedures performed is dependent upon an accurate knowledge of the relationships between the intrahepatic ducts. A standard anatomic description is present in approximately 60% of individuals, and the physician must determine the exact nature of the patient's anatomy in order to perform a successful procedure.

Normally bile collects in the common bile duct until needed. Excess bile backs up the duct and enters the gallbladder, where it is stored and concentrated. In cases of blockage/obstruction of the ducts, bile accumulates in the liver, causing the bile salts and pigments to enter the bloodstream. This increase of bilirubin in the blood causes a condition referred to as jaundice. The body tissues become yellow as a result of the buildup of the pigments. One common reason for the blockage can be a large amount of fluid being absorbed from the bile or precipitation of the cholesterol in the bile. In both of these cases the result is the production of gallstones (biliary calculi), which can lodge in the ducts and create the blockage. Jaundice can be caused by other pathologic factors such as hepatitis, cirrhosis, trauma, biliary surgery, biliary cancer, tumors, and choledochal cysts. Box 19-3 summarizes the common interventions used to treat certain pathologic conditions affecting the biliary tract.

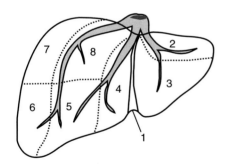

FIGURE 19-2. A schematic illustration of the eight segments of the liver.

BOX 19-3	*Summary of Common Interventions for the Biliary System*
Pathology	**Interventional Procedure**
Biliary obstruction	Endoscopic retrograde cholangiopancreatography
	Percutaneous biliary drainage
Benign biliary stricture	Percutaneous balloon dilation
	Metallic stent placement
Common bile duct stones	Endoscopic retrograde cholangiopancreatography
	Percutaneous T-tube tract stone removal

BOX 19-4	*Results of Abnormal Plasma Renin Activity Levels*
Decreased Levels	**Increased Levels**
Hypertension	Salt retention
Renal artery stenosis	Antidiuretic hormone therapy
Cirrhosis	
Addison's disease	
Hypokalemia	
Renal tumors	
Hemorrhage	
Renovascular hypertension	

Urinary System

The urinary system is an integral part of the excretory mechanism. It consists of a pair of kidneys that help to maintain the proper chemical makeup of the blood, regulate the pH, and produce a hormone that stimulates red blood cell production in the bone marrow. They also maintain body fluid levels and produce **renin**, which helps to regulate the blood pressure.

Renin is an enzyme released by the kidneys into the renal veins to regulate the blood pressure, fluid balance, and the body's sodium/potassium equilibrium. This substance activates the renin-angiotensin system, which is a vasoconstrictor that also stimulates aldosterone production from the adrenal glands. Aldosterone regulates the sodium and potassium levels in the blood. These elements will affect the blood pressure. Renin also helps to maintain the electrolyte balance in the body. These minerals are necessary for fluid balance and the maintenance of cardiac function, muscle contraction, and brain activity.

Renin levels are usually checked by means of a blood test. This is known as a plasma renin activity (PRA) test and is usually done fasting. All medications must be discontinued for a period of 2 to 4 weeks. The normal values vary with age and body position. Renin collection can be accomplished by means of sampling directly from the renal vein. Usually, samples from both kidneys are taken and compared to determine which kidney is affected. Abnormal findings from the PRA test can indicate several pathologic conditions. Box 19-4 lists some of the conditions that can be diagnosed.

The urinary system also includes a pair of ureters, the urinary bladder, and the urethra. The physiology related to the kidney function should be well known and will not be discussed here.

The kidneys are located against the dorsal body wall in the retroperitoneum at about the level of T11–T12 to L2–L3. The right kidney lies about 1 to 2 cm lower than the left owing to its position in relation to the liver. It is important to remember that because of their relationship with the pleura a danger of pneumothorax exists when percutaneous interventions are performed. The kidneys are surrounded by fat, which helps in maintaining their customary position. Each kidney has an upper pole, a lower pole, and an indentation on its medial aspect called the hilum. The blood and lymphatic vessels, nerves, and the ureter enter the kidney at the hilum.

Internally the kidney is divided into three sections: the cortex, medulla, and a flat cavity called the renal pelvis. It should be noted that there is a relationship between the location of the blood vessels and the renal pelvis. The renal vein is situated anteriorly followed by the renal artery and then the renal pelvis. Therefore, the renal pelvis presents itself when the patient is in the prone position. The renal pelvis narrows to leave the kidney as the ureter. This structure transports the urine to the urinary bladder.

The ureters descend behind the parietal peritoneum, running a parallel course with the vertebral column. As they approach the common iliac artery they run slightly medially and then posterolaterally, where they enter the pelvic cavity. The ureters then turn medially to enter the bladder. Each ureter

TABLE 19-1   *Summary of Nonvascular Interventions of the Urinary System*

Pathology	Interventional Procedure
Obstruction (malignant)	Antegrade pyelography
Strictures	Percutaneous nephrostomy
Stones	
Ureteral leaks	
Fistulas	
Staghorn calculi	Percutaneous lithotripsy
	Percutaneous nephrolithotomy
Benign ureteral stricture	Balloon dilatation
Malignant ureteral stricture	Ureteral occlusion
	Coils
	Glue
	Gelfoam
Acute urinary retention	Suprapubic cystostomy
Ureteropelvic junction obstruction	Endopyelotomy
Renovascular hypertension, renal artery stenosis	Renin sampling

narrows naturally in three places along its route: the junction between the ureter and the renal pelvis, at the level of the common iliac artery, and at the junction of the ureter with the bladder.

The urinary bladder is a muscular organ that serves to temporarily store urine. It lies primarily behind the symphysis pubis when empty. As it fills it expands superiorly. As it expands it displaces the bowel out of the pelvic cavity. The structure that carries the urine outside the body is the urethra. The urethra differs in length in the two sexes. The male urethra is approximately 20 cm (8 in) long while the female urethra is about 4 cm (1½ in) in length. Two valves, the internal and external urethral sphincters, control the release of the urine.

Table 19-1 summarizes some of the currently applied nonvascular interventions for pathology of the urinary system.

GENERAL METHODOLOGY OF PROCEDURES

Needle Biopsy

Indications and Contraindications

Needle biopsy is performed for diagnostic purposes in many areas of the body, including the thyroid; intracranial and intraorbital structures; spinal cord; lungs; abdomen; abscessed regions; genitourinary, lymphatic, and biliary systems; soft tissues; and bone. Each technique varies with the anatomy involved and information desired. The specific needles used also vary with the type of anatomic structure being biopsied, as well as with the type of procedure being performed. Two basic methods of biopsy are used and are classified by the type of needle used to do the biopsy. Specimens are obtained with the large-gauge core-type needle method or the percutaneous fine needle aspiration approach.

With the large-gauge core needle method, a "plug" of tissue is cut for analysis. Its advantage is that it produces a larger specimen for analysis, but this method also entails a greater risk of complications than does the fine needle technique. Because of the anatomy, as for bone biopsy, for example, or the type of specimen required, certain procedures or conditions require the use of the cutting or core biopsy method. Histologic analysis or study of the tissue structure requires the large-gauge core technique. Specimens for cytologic analysis or the study of tissue cells can be collected with the fine needle aspiration method.

Complications resulting from needle biopsies are infrequent. In most cases they are nonfatal and cause no permanent damage. Complications vary depending upon the type of procedure, location of

> **BOX 19-5** *Guidance Methods Used for Interventional Radiographic Biopsy Procedures*
>
> | Guidance Method | Anatomic Area |
> | --- | --- |
> | Ultrasonography | Lymph nodes |
> | | Breast |
> | | Abdominal viscera |
> | | Liver |
> | | Extremities |
> | | Intrathoracic lesions |
> | | Vertebral column |
> | Computed tomography | Lymph nodes |
> | | Brain lesions |
> | | Abdominal viscera |
> | | Kidneys |
> | | Bone lesions |
> | | Mediastinal masses |
> | | Breast |
> | Conventional fluoroscopy | Lymph nodes |
> | | Lung |
> | | Kidney |
> | | Mediastinal masses |
> | Magnetic resonance imaging | Brain lesions |
> | | Bone lesions |
> | | Breast |

the lesion, and possibly needle size. Hemorrhage and sepsis are common complications of needle biopsy. Some other complications that have been reported are peritonitis, pancreatitis, pneumothorax, and tumor seeding. Use of computed tomography (CT) or ultrasonic guidance reduces the complication rate if all necessary precautions are taken. Some possible complications are infection, bleeding, formation of fistulas, and tumor seeding. It should be remembered that the percutaneous biopsy procedure replaces surgical biopsy, which has considerably higher complication and mortality rates.

Guidance Methods

To successfully localize the lesion, the procedure must be guided. This guidance is accomplished with ultrasonography, CT, conventional fluoroscopy, or magnetic resonance imaging. These modalities are used alone or in combination to provide the maximum diagnostic information about the components of the lesion and its location. Each of the modalities has advantages and disadvantages. The choice of method depends on the physician's preference, equipment availability, and hospital protocol. Box 19-5 provides a summary of the types of modalities and some of the anatomic areas where they have been used.

Most needle biopsies require ultrasound or CT to guide the biopsy needles precisely. These techniques pinpoint the lesion's location and allow a high degree of accuracy in sampling. The two guidance methods achieve the same results, but there are some basic differences between them. The use of ultrasound to guide the needle is both more cost-effective and safer for the patient than CT. Ultrasonographic equipment is considerably more economical to purchase and install. This method eliminates the need for exposure to radiation during the localization phase of the procedure. Equipment design also permits faster lesion location and puncture. Specialized puncturing transducers are available that accurately guide the puncture needle. In addition, the use of real-time ultrasonographic equipment permits visual guidance of the needle.

Although the use of ultrasound appears to be the best method of needle guidance, there are situations in which the use of ultrasonography is contraindicated or impossible. Indications for using

CT for guided needle biopsy include the following:
1.   Extremely obese patients
2.   Presence of overlying gas
3.   Presence of overlying bone
4.   Skin pathology that precludes transducer contact
5.   Pathology that contraindicates skin compression
6.   Necessity for three-dimensional resolution
7.   Unsuccessful ultrasonographic guidance

One disadvantage to the use of CT as the guidance method is that the length of the procedure is usually extended. CT requires several manipulations of the needle, especially for small lesions. The specific organ to be biopsied also governs the choice of guidance method.

Magnetic resonance imaging guidance methods have not been widely used clinically and are still undergoing evaluation.[2]

Ultrasonography. Ultrasonic guidance is performed with either the static or the dynamic scanning technique.[3] Static scanning is the older of the two methods. The target lesion is initially located and referenced with two planes perpendicular to each other. The puncture route should always be the shortest distance possible. The scan continues by manipulating the transducer to show on the television monitor the ultrasonic beam running along the chosen puncture path. At this point, the skin surface is marked, the patient is prepped for the puncture procedure, and the physician introduces a local anesthetic. The scan is repeated using a special puncture transducer, which has a central canal that accepts the puncture needle. The central canal allows the needle to follow the direction of the ultrasonic beam. These types of transducers accept several different needle sizes with the use of special adapters. The distance from the skin surface to the lesion is measured from the image on the television monitor. The needle stop is then set for the scan depth plus the length of the transducer. When this is done, the punctures can proceed.

Dynamic scanning has been made possible with the use of real-time ultrasonic scanners. These units show the movement as it is occurring, which increases the accuracy of the puncture considerably because moving target lesions can be continuously monitored during puncture. Small changes in direction or distance can be compensated for with direct visual control of the needle. The basic procedures for lesion location and needle introduction are the same as those for static scanning. Equipment designs for dynamic scanners will have variations, usually in the type of transducer used for the scan.

Computed Tomography. When the use of ultrasonography is contraindicated, CT may be used for localization and needle guidance for lesion puncture. Spiral (helical) CT, rapid image reconstruction, and the use of stereotactic CT devices can facilitate needle placement and biopsy. As in ultrasonography, the same basic rule applies to needle puncture with CT assistance; that is, the route chosen should be as short as possible. This pathway is marked on the skin during a preliminary CT scan. The patient is prepped for the puncture by sterilizing and draping the skin, the local anesthetic is applied, and the needle is inserted along the predetermined pathway to the desired depth. The patient is then rescanned to determine whether the needle has been accurately inserted into the lesion. There are several different methods of needle insertion; the ultimate choice of insertion technique is made by the radiologist performing the procedure.

Once the needle has been successfully placed in the lesion, material may be removed for cytologic analysis. The aspiration technique is the most frequently used biopsy method. This is done by attaching an empty syringe to the needle hub and withdrawing the plunger. A small sample of tissue or fluid is then aspirated into the needle and prepared for cytologic diagnosis.

The same method can be used to facilitate needle placement for cyst and abscess drainage. These studies are usually performed with minor modifications in the equipment and techniques used.

Puncture and Drainage Methods

This group of procedures includes the percutaneous needle puncture technique for diagnosis of cystic masses and the percutaneous drainage of fluid accumulations. These methods have proved to be safe procedures, with relatively low complication rates. The following outline summarizes the types of puncture and drainage procedures currently being performed:

- Genitourinary system
  - Percutaneous nephrostomy techniques
    - Catheter inserted through needles
    - Catheter-sheathed needle
    - Angiographic system
    - Trocar-cannula-catheter system
  - Percutaneous catheter drainage of renal and extrarenal fluid collections
  - Cyst puncture
  - Fluid drainage procedures
- Biliary system
  - Periductal fluid drainage procedures
    - T tube or Penrose drain access
    - Percutaneous puncture, dilation, and drainage
  - Biliary system drainage
    - Percutaneous transhepatic biliary drainage after fine needle transhepatic cholangiography
    - Percutaneous choledochoplasty
- Abdomen
  - Percutaneous abscess drainage techniques
    - Angiocatheter system
    - Trocar-catheter system
- Pelvis
  - Percutaneous drainage techniques
    - Transrectal approach
    - Transperineal approach
    - Transsciatic notch approach
- Thorax
  - Percutaneous fluid drainage techniques
    - Trocar method
    - Angiocatheter method

Percutaneous Puncture

The percutaneous puncture of identified renal masses is an example of this type of procedure. After the mass has been localized, it must be determined whether it is a cyst or tumor. Several methods of diagnosing the mass are available, including ultrasonography, nephrotomography, arteriography, and needle puncture. Percutaneous needle puncture procedures provide samples of aspirate for cytologic analysis and can help demonstrate the mass radiographically by using a contrast agent. If the mass is shown to be solid when punctured, arteriography is then used to demonstrate it successfully for diagnosis.

Procedure. The percutaneous puncture method is relatively simple and does not require much sophisticated equipment for successful lesion puncture. Ultrasonographic guidance can be used to precisely guide the needle to the mass. The localization requires the use of a special transducer (discussed previously). It also necessitates fluoroscopy to demonstrate the mass radiographically.

The setup for a percutaneous puncture examination includes an assortment of syringes, anesthesia and puncture needles, contrast agent, and anesthetic. The actual puncture setup varies slightly with the anatomic area of interest and the puncture method used. A typical equipment grouping for a renal cyst puncture is shown in Figure 19-3. The percutaneous puncture technique is considered a minor

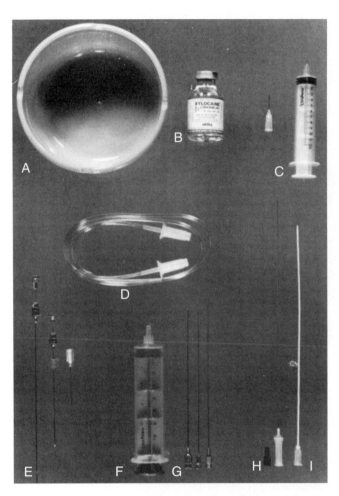

FIGURE 19-3. Typical grouping of equipment for renal mass puncture. *A,* Bowl for contrast material. *B,* Local anesthetic agent. *C,* Syringe and 25-gauge needle for shin anesthesia. *D,* Extension tube. *E,* 22-gauge needles for deeper anesthesia and puncture. *F,* 35-ml syringe for aspirating and opacifying large cysts. *G,* Cuatico needle with side holes. *H,* Trocar-sleeve assembly. *I,* Standard 20-gauge and Teflon-sheathed needles.

operative procedure and should be carried out under aseptic conditions. Preparation of the patient also varies with the location of the lesion.

Renal cyst puncture requires the patient to be in the prone position for preparation and puncture. The lesion is then localized with either fluoroscopy or ultrasonography. If ultrasound is used, the needle follows the path presented by the special puncture transducer. This method shortens the actual procedure time. When fluoroscopy is used, the lesion is first localized and marked, and the needle insertion is then tracked as it is being inserted into the lesion. Once the lesion has been localized by the physician, the puncture needle is inserted through the segment of anesthetized tissue parallel to the path of the x-ray beam. In this method, the needle is advanced slowly with fluoroscopic monitoring of the needle's progress. Successful puncture is confirmed by the aspiration of cystic fluid.

Once the cyst has been entered, cytologic analysis of the aspirated fluid and radiographic examination of the interior of the cyst are performed. The contrast agent used for the internal examination of the cyst can be any of the water-soluble preparations.

Cytologic analysis is essential in the determination of the nature of the cyst. When the diagnostic portion of the examination has been completed, interventional treatment of the cyst can be initiated. In most cases, the cystic fluid is aspirated, and some type of sclerosing agent is then injected (Fig. 19-4).

Complications. Percutaneous puncture procedures do not entail a great risk to the patient. Complications usually occur as a result of the needle insertion procedure—for example, a needle might pass through the wall of the kidney and cause hemorrhaging. Another possible complication is extravasation of the contrast agent when a thin-walled cyst is encountered.

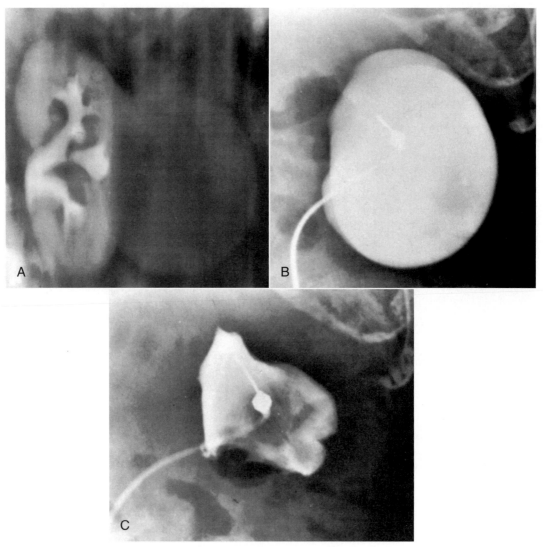

FIGURE 19-4. **A,** Cyst localization by CT. **B,** Contrast-filled renal cyst after percutaneous puncture. **C,** Partially aspirated renal cyst showing collapsed cyst wall.

Percutaneous Drainage

The drainage of fluid collections—abscesses in the urinary system, biliary system, and abdominal cavity—can be done with the percutaneous catheter drainage method. The use of this technique also enables physicians to dilate stenotic channels, occlude areas of leakage, close off fistulas, infuse substances to dissolve or remove calculi, and perform biopsies. The obvious advantage of this technique is that fewer surgical procedures must be performed to achieve these results. Other benefits to the patient are reduced hospital costs and a reduced complication rate.

There are three phases to a successful percutaneous puncture: access to the fluid collection, aspiration of fluid to confirm position, and placement of the drainage catheter. It is important during percutaneous access that precise guidance is provided between the entry point and the fluid accumulation to avoid passing the puncture needle through the bowel or other organ, or a major blood vessel. Drainage can also be accomplished through cannulation of the sinus tract associated with the abscess. The two most commonly used procedures for drainage catheter placement are the trocar-cannula and modified Seldinger methods.

Percutaneous Nephrostomy

A representative type procedure for the external drainage of the urinary system is percutaneous catheter nephrostomy (PCN). This procedure provides the temporary drainage of an obstructed urinary system. It is primarily used to relieve the obstruction resulting from a urinary calculus. The relief from urinary obstruction can enable the system to heal leaks or fistulas and cyst decompression. PCN relies on the placement of a catheter within the renal pelvis using a percutaneous insertion technique. The trocar-cannula method is the most popular. This system allows a catheter of relatively large diameter to be passed into the kidney. Once the trocar has been inserted, various procedures can be performed. The following outline is a summary of the applications of PCN:

- Drainage
  - Generalized obstruction (external drainage)
  - Selected obstruction (internal release)
  - Leaks and fistulas
  - Renal-perirenal fluid collections
    - Infected cyst
    - Abscess
    - Urinoma
    - Seroma
    - Lymphocele
- Drug instillation
  - Treatment of bacterial infection with antibiotics
  - Treatment of fungal infection with antifungal agents
  - Chemical dissolution of calculi
  - Chemotherapy
- Special instrument insertion
  - Steerable basket catheters
  - Steerable biopsy brushes
  - Nephroscope insertion
  - Dilating balloon catheters

Procedure. PCN patients are mildly sedated and well hydrated before beginning the procedure. After the patient is prepared and draped, the kidney is localized by using either intravenously injected contrast agents followed by fluoroscopic localization or ultrasonography or CT. Once the position of the kidney has been determined, a local anesthetic is administered, and the kidney is punctured with a 22-gauge spinal needle (Fig. 19-5). The puncture is done in a manner similar to that used for previously discussed studies—that is, it normally parallels the x-ray beam. When the needle punctures the kidney and enters the collecting system, it can be attached to a flexible connecter tube. Pressure measurements can be made and urine samples taken for analysis prior to performing any other interventional procedure.

After these preliminary steps have been completed, an antegrade pyelogram is obtained. This is necessary to determine if a PCN is necessary. It is important to instill an amount of contrast agent equal only to the amount of urine that has been aspirated to avoid the possibility of trauma to the urinary system if an obstruction exists. Radiography during this phase is directed by the radiologist performing the procedure. If the antegrade pyelogram indicates the necessity for PCN, the physician chooses the catheter size as determined from the information obtained with the antegrade pyelogram—usually an 8F or 12F Silastic catheter that is either soft or stiff (Fig. 19-6).

The antegrade pyelogram is used to determine the need for PCN as well as identify the renal calyx that will be used to implant the catheter. The choice of calyx will be determined by the pathology present and the procedure that is being done. The general procedure for the placement of the nephrostomy tube using the Cope nephrostomy kit is as follows:

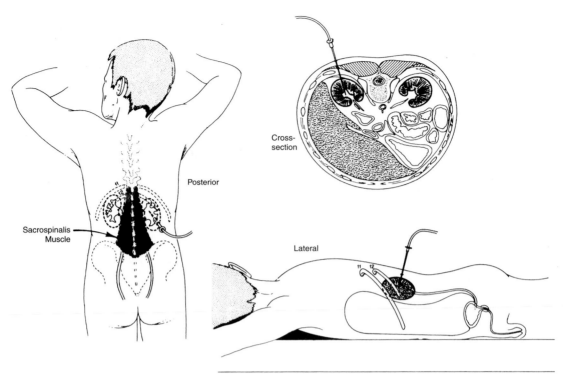

FIGURE 19-5. Schematic of anatomy of percutaneous puncture.

- Place the patient in the prone oblique position with the affected side elevated 45 degrees.
- Prepare the site for the puncture.
- Anesthetize the area using a local anesthetic.
- Make a small nick in the skin at the point of entry.
- Using a 22-gauge (15-cm) needle, advance it toward the chosen calyx.
- Once the collecting system has been entered, remove the stylet, and adjust the needle position to ensure that urine can be aspirated.
- The guide wire can then be introduced into the ureter.
- The skin nick can be widened using a dilator to enlarge the opening to accept the nephrostomy catheter.
- Introduce a trocar to facilitate the passage of the catheter into the collecting system.
- When the catheter is in place the trocar can be removed and the catheter can be put in the shape necessary to anchor it in the kidney. This will cause the catheter to become larger than the pathway used to insert it, thereby anchoring it firmly in the renal collecting system. Two types of locking catheters are available:
  - A pigtail (locking-loop or Cope-loop) catheter: This system forms a loop that locks in the kidney after placement.
  - The Malecot catheter also locks in place by making the distal end larger than the insertion path. This is accomplished by retracting the catheter tip, which makes the distal end larger. This catheter can be used when the renal pelvis is small or when a large calculus is present. Distal end is shaped somewhat like a tulip.

Continued

(cont'd)
- The catheter can be anchored externally either through the use of an ostomy device or simply attaching it directly to the patient's skin. In both cases the catheter is first wrapped with adhesive tape, which forms the external anchor. The adhesive tape is then sutured to the ostomy or the patient's skin.
- External drainage should be continued until decompression is achieved. Occasionally the catheter must be changed as a result of an obstruction that cannot be cleared. Catheters can also be dislodged requiring replacement. This can be accomplished easily by returning the distal portion of the catheter to its original shape or size, removing it, and exchanging it for a new system.

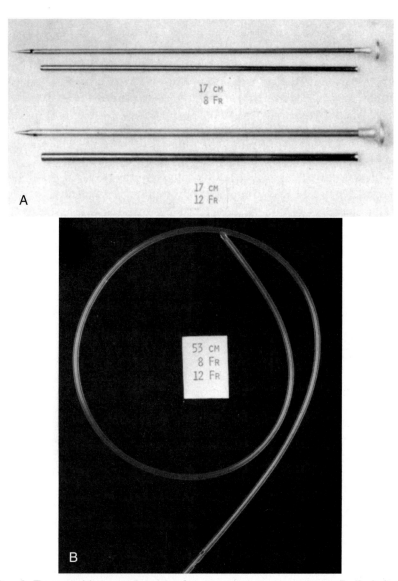

FIGURE 19-6. **A,** Trocar with cannula units for percutaneous puncture. **B,** Soft flexible silicone catheter used for percutaneous nephrostomy.

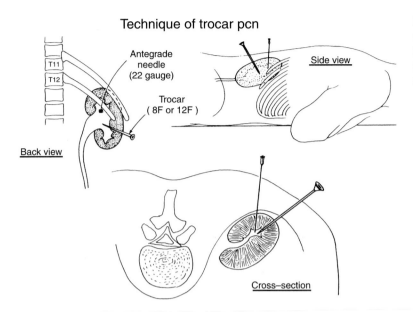

Technique of trocar pcn

FIGURE 19-7. Schematic of the relation between the fine puncture needle and the trocar-cannula unit.

When the catheter has been firmly attached, it is prepared to accept a stopcock assembly and drainage bag. At this time, follow-up radiographs can be performed, or decompression treatment can be initiated.

A second method of catheter insertion is the trocar-cannula method. The trocar-cannula unit is inserted somewhat laterally to a previously inserted 22-gauge spinal needle (Fig. 19-7). This is accomplished by making a small nick in the skin (approximately 2 cm deep) with a scalpel. The trocar-cannula unit is then inserted under fluoroscopic monitoring until the kidney is punctured. When the trocar is removed, the appropriate catheter is inserted into the kidney through the cannula (Fig. 19-8). After the catheter position is confirmed, the cannula is removed over the catheter and secured to the skin to prevent accidental removal from the kidney. If other procedures are to be performed, they are done before removal of the cannula. Other therapeutic procedures that can be performed after trocar-cannula puncture of the kidney are shown in Figures 19-9 to 19-12.

Complications. The complication rate from PCN is relatively low. Possible complications include infections, catheter dislodgement, catheter obstruction, and hemorrhage.

Percutaneous Calculi Removal

Residual calculi can be removed nonsurgically from either the genitourinary or the biliary system. This can be accomplished percutaneously or subsequent to an initial operative procedure. The risks associated with percutaneous calculi removal are minimal compared with those of surgery. These procedures are usually performed on an outpatient basis.

Renal calculi can be removed percutaneously from the renal pelvis, calyx, or ureter using the procedure described for percutaneous catheter nephrostomy (PCN). Extracorporeal shock wave lithotripsy (ESWL) is used in a majority of cases involving renal or upper ureteral calculi. Another method of removing large calculi is percutaneous ultrasonic lithotripsy (PUL) or electrohydraulic lithotripsy, which utilizes a small (5F) probe and a flexible endoscope to fracture the stones for subsequent removal.

Biliary calculi can be removed after surgery through a T tube, percutaneously after transhepatic biliary drainage, or by means of endoscopic retrograde cholangiopancreatography (ERCP).

Percutaneous Nephrolithotomy

As mentioned, renal calculi can be removed percutaneously with the procedure described previously for PCN. Once the percutaneous nephrostomy cannula is positioned, a steerable catheter system with a

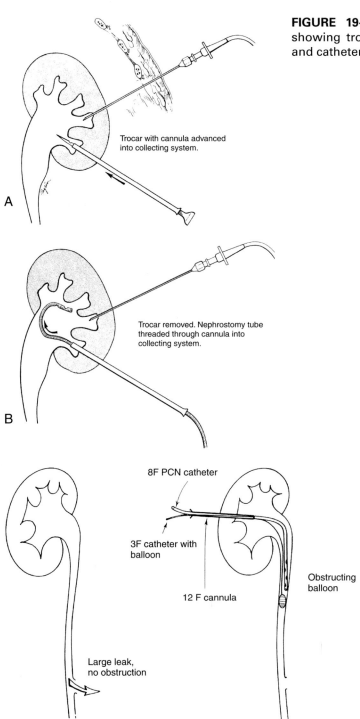

FIGURE 19-8. Schematic of the kidney, showing trocar-cannula unit placement (**A**) and catheter placement (**B**).

Trocar with cannula advanced into collecting system.

A

Trocar removed. Nephrostomy tube threaded through cannula into collecting system.

B

8F PCN catheter

3F catheter with balloon

12 F cannula

Obstructing balloon

Large leak, no obstruction

FIGURE 19-9. Mechanism for diverting the urine in case of a leak in the ureter, using a balloon catheter and an external drainage catheter.

stone basket can be introduced into the kidney. Many variations of this system are available, and the ultimate choice remains with the radiologist. The catheter with a stone basket is inserted through the cannula and positioned close to the calculus. The stone basket is then advanced in a fully opened position and maneuvered to engage the calculus. The basket is retracted until it contacts the catheter tip, which has the effect of closing the basket over the calculus (Fig. 19-13). Both the catheter and the stone basket are then removed together through the cannula. When all of the calculi are removed, a

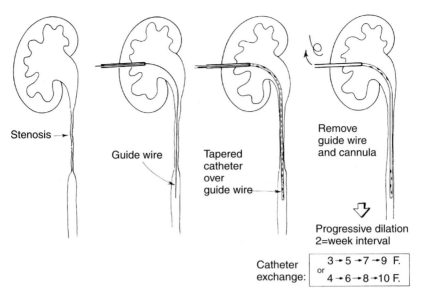

FIGURE 19-10. Mechanism for progressive dilation of a stenosed ureter using graduated catheters.

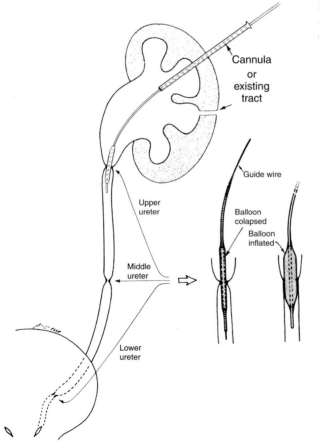

FIGURE 19-11. Mechanism for dilating a stenosed ureter using a balloon catheter.

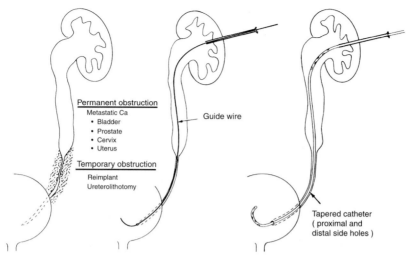

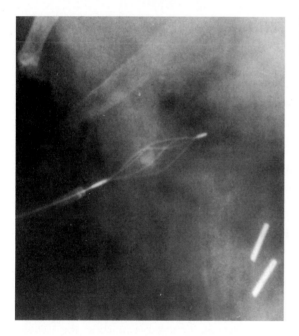

FIGURE 19-12. Mechanism for stent placement through the trocar-cannula unit in an obstructed or leaky ureter.

FIGURE 19-13. Radiograph of a renal calculus caught in a stone basket and ready for removal through the trocar-cannula unit.

nephrostomy catheter is placed into the kidney and secured in place. Several days after stone removal, radiographs should be taken, using contrast medium, to determine the patency of the urinary tract and the presence or absence of calculi.

Calculi can be removed from the biliary tree either after surgery through a T tube or percutaneously after transhepatic biliary drainage. Both methods require the use of a steerable catheter system with a stone basket catheter insert. Percutaneous transhepatic biliary calculi removal is usually performed on patients who are poor candidates for surgery.

Postoperative Biliary Calculi Removal

This procedure is performed from 4 to 6 weeks after surgery to allow biliary T-tube tract preparation. Medication is limited to minor doses of drugs to relieve anxiety, such as diazepam, and to an antibiotic regimen to reduce the possibility of infection.

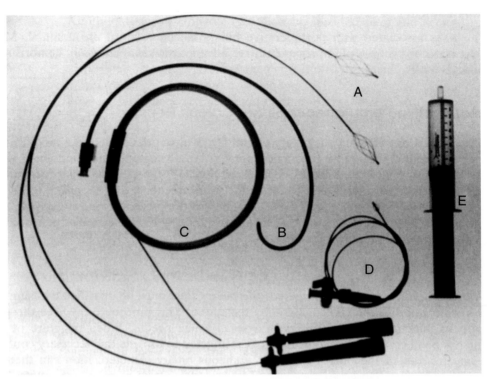

FIGURE 19-14. Basic equipment for percutaneous biliary calculi removal. *A*, 11-mm and 15-mm stone baskets. *B*, Curved distal tip catheter. *C*, Guide wire and holder. *D*, Fogarty balloon catheter. *E*, Syringe.

The equipment necessary for this type of study is minimal: a steerable catheter system, stone baskets, syringe, guide wire, and suitable contrast agent. Figure 19-14 shows some basic equipment used during postoperative biliary calculi removal.

Procedure. The procedure begins with a T-tube cholangiogram to determine the location and number of calculi, as well as to provide the necessary contrast during the procedure (Fig. 19-15, *A*). On completion of the cholangiogram, a guide wire is inserted through the T-tube, the T-tube is removed, and the guide wire is left in the biliary tract at the lower end of the duct (Fig. 19-15, *B*). The steerable catheter is inserted over the guide wire and positioned close to the calculus to be removed, and the guide wire is removed (Fig. 19-15, *C*). The stone basket is then advanced to the tip of the catheter (Fig. 19-15, *D*). Several positioning methods can be used to ensnare the calculus in the stone basket (Fig. 19-15, *E* and *F*). The steerable catheter and stone basket are removed, extracting the calculus (Fig. 19-15, *G*).

When multiple calculi are encountered, the steerable catheter must be reinserted and manipulated to remove subsequent stones. In such cases, the physician may insert multiple guide wires into the biliary tract through the T-tube, which makes reinsertion of the steerable catheter and stone basket easier to accomplish. Occasionally, a small stone in the lower duct can be maneuvered into the duodenum with a Fogarty balloon catheter.

In uncomplicated single calculus removal, the catheter is removed after a repeat cholangiogram. However, in cases of multiple stone removal or if a complication arises, the catheter should be left in the tract to facilitate drainage until a follow-up study is performed.

Complications. The risks associated with postoperative biliary calculi removal are minimal. Most problems occur because of improper catheter advancement that results in hemorrhage, periductal leaks, duct perforations, or pancreatitis.

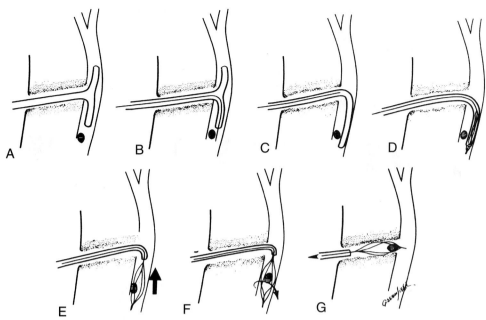

FIGURE 19-15. Schematic of the stepwise postoperative removal of a biliary calculus by a stone basket.

Nonoperative Percutaneous Biliary Calculi Removal

The method of percutaneous biliary calculi removal was developed as a modification of percutaneous transhepatic cholangiography. With angiographic methodology, catheter introduction into the biliary tree became possible. One risk of this procedure is the possibility of peritonitis as a result of the puncture; thus, a prerequisite to its use is antibiotic treatment initiated at least 1 day before the procedure and continued for 2 to 3 days after the puncture. Another means of reducing the incidence of peritonitis is by using a catheter–sheathed needle.

Procedure. When the patient has been prepared, the biliary tract must be opacified by using the fine needle transhepatic cholangiography technique. This procedure involves the percutaneous puncture of the lining with a small-gauge needle. When puncture of the lining has been confirmed, a contrast agent is injected to provide the necessary contrast for visualization of the biliary tree. Percutaneous biliary catheterization can then be done using the opacified biliary tract and fine needle system as reference points. The catheter-sheathed needle is guided by direct radiography or fluoroscopy. When the catheter-needle system has entered the biliary tract, the needle is removed, and a syringe is attached to the catheter sheath. The catheter is manipulated until bile is aspirated, and a small amount of contrast agent is injected to confirm successful intubation. The catheter is then positioned close to the hilum of the lining, and the bile is drained. Figure 19-16 shows the puncture of the lining, followed by guide wire and catheter insertion.

The removal of biliary calculi is usually done several days after the initial intubation to provide adequate drainage for patient stabilization. When this has been determined, the biliary calculi are then removed. The originally placed catheter is exchanged for a nontapered variety, and two guide wires are inserted into the biliary tree. The catheter is removed, and a steerable catheter-stone basket system is introduced over one guide wire. The calculus is removed as described (see Postoperative Biliary Calculi Removal). Another drainage catheter can then be inserted over the second guide wire, if necessary.

The basic procedure for percutaneous transhepatic biliary drainage allows other interventional procedures to be performed on the biliary tract, including percutaneous transhepatic biliary drainage,

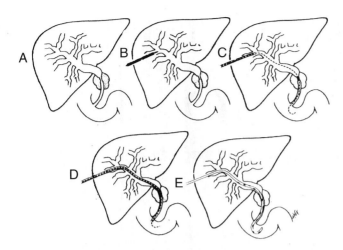

FIGURE 19-16. Schematic of the percutaneous transhepatic puncture procedure. **A**, Obstructed biliary tract. **B**, Catheter-sheathed needle insertion. **C**, Needle removed and guide wire inserted through sheath. **D**, Sheath removed and dilation catheter inserted. **E**, Dilation catheter replaced by drainage catheter with curved tip.

fine needle transhepatic cholangiography, percutaneous transhepatic biopsy, percutaneous transhepatic stone extraction, percutaneous transhepatic choledochoplasty, and percutaneous transhepatic stent insertion.

Complications. Percutaneous transhepatic biliary calculi removal, in addition to complications similar to those of postoperative biliary calculi removal (see preceding discussion), has the added risk of infection caused by the insertion and removal of needles, guide wires, and catheters. Most of these problems can be successfully treated with antibiotic therapy and usually have no long-term effects.

Endoscopic Retrograde Cholangiopancreatography

Endoscopic retrograde cholangiopancreatography (ERCP) has become a commonly practiced procedure for biliary pathologic diagnosis, biliary intervention for stone removal, and biliary drainage. Although the removal of biliary calculi is the primary indication for the procedure, it is also indicated in a number of different biliary and pancreatic disease processes such as cholangitis, obstructive jaundice, acute biliary pancreatitis, evaluation of pancreatic trauma, and suspected pancreatic cancer.

It has in most cases replaced percutaneous biliary drainage and percutaneous transhepatic cholangiography as a diagnostic and interventional tool. Imaging of the biliary system primarily for diagnosis can also be accomplished noninvasively through the use of magnetic resonance cholangiopancreatography.

Endoscopic retrograde cholangiopancreatography involves passing an endoscope through the mouth to the duodenum and into the biliary tree by catheterization through the sphincter of Oddi. The procedure is used to diagnose and treat various pathologic conditions of the gallbladder, liver, and pancreas. Once the diagnosis is made, treatment can be given to correct the problem.

Procedure

The procedure is explained to the patient, and a consent form is negotiated. Conscious sedation is applied using intravenous midazolam and meperidine or fentanyl. The endoscope is passed through the mouth, esophagus, and stomach and into the duodenum. Using the endoscope the opening of the bile duct and pancreas is located. A catheter is passed into the duct, and contrast agent is administered to determine the nature of the pathologic process (Fig. 19-17). The procedure is followed fluoroscopically, and spot films are taken to record the images. It is essential that the entire biliary tree be visualized. This may require the use of a balloon catheter if the sphincter is not well sealed. If a blockage is noted, treatment may be administered. Stents or drainage tubes can be used to traverse tumor-blocked ducts. If stones are present, the physician may elect to perform an endoscopic retrograde sphincterotomy (ERS),

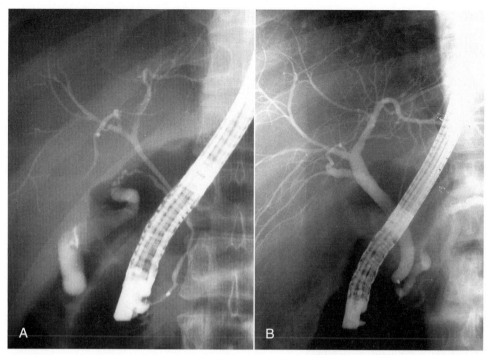

FIGURE 19-17. Examples of normal cholangiograms performed during endoscopic retrograde cholangiopancreatography. **A,** The catheter was placed in the common bile duct for opacification in a young patient. **B,** An elderly patient demonstrating a fuller appearance of the biliary ducts.

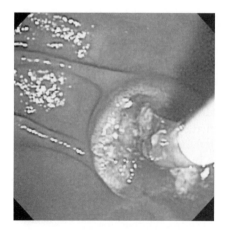

FIGURE 19-18. Photograph of an endoscopic sphincterotomy procedure.

making a cut into the papilla to enlarge the opening at the papilla (Fig. 19-18). This allows for the placement of various instruments to remove the blockage.

A basket catheter can be used to remove any stones that are found in the biliary ducts (Fig. 19-19). Occasionally the physician may find stones that are too large to be extracted easily. These stones can be fragmented using mechanical lithotripsy. This process utilizes a specialized catheter basket. Once the stone is captured the basket is retracted against a metal sheath. The pressure of the basket on the stone fractures it into manageable pieces that can be removed easily.

If the treatment is successful, the endoscope and other instruments are removed. The patient should be monitored for signs of apnea, diaphoresis, cardiac changes, respiratory complications, laryngospasm, and

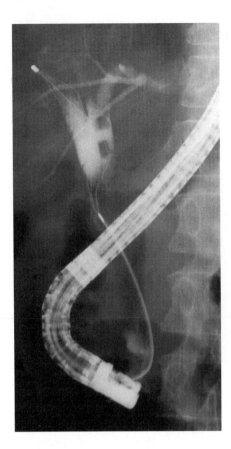

FIGURE 19-19. Stone removal during an endoscopic retrograde cholangiopancreatography (ERCP) procedure using a basket catheter.

hypotension. Once the patient is stable, the intravenous line is removed and the patient can be discharged.

Complications

A number of complications can occur as a result of ERCP. These can be classified into three areas: medication reactions, complications relating to the diagnostic portion of the procedure, and those resulting from the interventional portion of the procedure. Medication-related complications can be attributed to allergic reactions to the contrast agent used and the risks of decreased cardiac and respiratory function resulting from the use of sedatives. Although the procedure can be relatively risk-free, commonly experienced minor complications such as nausea, vomiting, and sore throat can occur.

If the physician chooses to perform an interventional procedure, the potential for complication increases. There is a possibility of perforation of the duodenum, bacteremia, hemorrhage, or infection (cholangitis or pancreatitis). Complication rates for the procedure range from 5 to 10% and are operator dependent. Occasionally surgical intervention is required to treat complications.

Extracorporeal Shock Wave Lithotripsy

Extracorporeal shock wave lithotripsy is a noninvasive method that is used therapeutically for both urolithiasis and cholelithiasis. Extracorporeal shock wave lithotripsy has been applied to the fragmentation of uroliths since 1980. It has become the method of choice for treatment of most upper tract urinary stones. Recently, the technique has been investigated in the treatment of patients with biliary calculi. It has also been shown to be cytotoxic to certain forms of tumors.[4]

Extracorporeal shock wave lithotripsy is based on the use of high-energy shock waves to fragment the stones without causing significant damage to the normal surrounding structures. The shock waves can be generated by electromagnetic, mechanical, or piezoelectric techniques. The smaller fragments resulting from the procedure can be dissolved by orally administered drugs, can be removed mechanically, or can be passed from the organ physiologically.

Specialized equipment is necessary for performance of the procedure. The equipment is manufactured by several companies, and the designs vary with the method used to produce the shock waves. Depending on the design, the patient is immersed in a water bath (first-generation) or placed in intimate contact with some sort of flexible water-containing device (second-generation), which provides the path for the shock waves to reach the site of the calculus. It has evolved into a relatively safe procedure that can be performed on an outpatient basis without the use of anesthesia.

SUMMARY

Nonvascular interventional radiography has advanced to provide a broad spectrum of diagnostic as well as therapeutic procedures. These methods have proved to be more cost effective than their corresponding surgical interventional procedures, with a considerably lower risk factor.

The use of ultrasonography and CT as guidance systems has allowed more precise percutaneous studies to be done, with lower complication rates. Magnetic resonance imaging and CT have been used to great advantage in the noninvasive diagnosis of various pathologic conditions. Fluoroscopic guidance is also used to a great extent as a guidance mechanism for cannula insertion.

Percutaneous needle biopsy can be performed in almost all areas of the body and is a safe and efficient means of acquiring samples for pathologic study. This is also true for percutaneous puncture and drainage techniques, which have the added benefit of playing both diagnostic and therapeutic roles.

The techniques involved in the extraction of calculi have been expanded to include the reestablishment of ductal patency and the placement of endoprosthetic devices, such as stents. ERCP has become a commonly performed procedure for both the diagnosis and treatment of a variety of pathologic conditions in the hepatobiliary system. Extracorporeal shock wave lithotripsy, the technique of fragmenting kidney stones and gallstones with high-energy shock waves, has gained acceptance as a therapeutic procedure in lieu of surgical intervention.

Although the contraindications for any of these procedures are minimal in most cases, percutaneous interventional studies can be carried out on patients who are very poor surgical risks, thus greatly increasing the chance for successful treatment. Many of the procedures do have the potential for major complications such as infection, perforation, and severe allergic reactions.

REFERENCES

1. Sutherland F, Harris J: Claude Couinaud: a passion for the liver. *Arch Surg* 137(11):1305–1310, 2002.
2. Chen X, Lehman CD, Dee KE: MRI-guided breast biopsy: clinical experience with 14-gauge stainless steel core biopsy needle. *AJR Am J Roentgenol* 182(4):1075–1080, 2004.
3. Rausch P, Nowels K, Jeffrey RB: Ultrasonographically guided thyroid biopsy: a review with emphasis on technique. *J Ultrasound Med* 20(1):79–85, 2001.
4. Kohri K, Uemura T, Iguchi M, Kurita T: Effect of high energy shock waves on tumor cells. *Urol Res* 18:101–105, 1990.

SUGGESTED READINGS

Anatomy

Chmielewski C: Renal anatomy and overview of nephron function. *Nephrol Nurs J* 30(2):185–190, 2003.
Gazelle G, Lee MJ, Mueller PR: Cholangiographic segmental anatomy of the liver. *Radiographics* 14(5):1005–1013, 1994.

Geboes K, Geboes KP, Maleux G: Vascular anatomy of the gastrointestinal tract. *Best Pract Res Clin Gastroenterol* 15(1):1–14, 2001.

Sampaio FJ: Renal anatomy. Endourologic considerations. *Urol Clin North Am* 27(4):585–607, vii, 2000.

Zakim D, Boyer TD (eds): *Hepatology: A Textbook of Liver Disease*, 4th ed. Philadelphia, 2003, WB Saunders.

Needle Biopsy

Baloch ZW, Li Volsi VA: Fine-needle aspiration of thyroid nodules: past, present, and future. *Endocr Pract* 10(3):234–241, 2004.

Issakov J, Flusser G, Kollender Y, et al: Computed tomography-guided core needle biopsy for bone and soft tissue tumors. *Isr Med Assoc J* 5(1):28–30, 2003.

Shankar S, van Sonnenberg E, Silverman SG, et al: Interventional radiology procedures in the liver. Biopsy, drainage, and ablation. *Clin Liver Dis* 6(1):91–118, 2002.

Sze DY: Use of curved needles to perform biopsies and drainages of inaccessible targets. *J Vasc Interv Radiol* 12(12):1441–1444, 2001.

Wu M, Burstein DE: Fine needle aspiration. *Cancer Invest* 22(4):620–628, 2004.

Puncture and Drainage Procedures

Deveney CW, Lurie K, Deveney KE: Improved treatment of intra-abdominal abscess: a result of improved localization, drainage, and patient care, not technique. *Arch Surg* 123:1126, 1988.

Gervais DA, Hahn PF, O'Neill MJ, et al: Percutaneous abscess drainage in Crohn disease: technical success and short- and long-term outcomes during 14 years. *Radiology* 222(3):645–651, 2002.

Hsu LF, Scavee C, Jais P, et al: Transcardiac pericardiocentesis: an emergency life-saving technique for cardiac tamponade. *J Cardiovasc Electrophysiol* 14(9):1001–1003, 2003.

Percutaneous Nephrostomy

Dyer RB, Regan JD, Kavanagh PV, et al: Percutaneous nephrostomy with extensions of the technique: step by step. *Radiographics* 22(3):503–525, 2002.

Funaki B, Vatakencherry G: Comparison of single-stick and double-stick techniques for percutaneous nephrostomy. *Cardiovasc Intervent Radiol* 27(1):35–37, 2004.

Kandarpa K, Aruny JE: *Percutaneous Nephrostomy and Antegrade Ureteral Stenting: Handbook of Interventional Radiologic Procedures*, 3rd ed. Philadelphia, 2002, Lippincott Williams & Wilkins.

Patel RD, Newland C, Rees Y: Major complications after percutaneous nephrostomy—lessons from a department audit. *Clin Radiol* 59(8):766, 2004.

Radecka E, Magnusson A: Complications associated with percutaneous nephrostomies. A retrospective study. *Acta Radiol* 45(2):184–188, 2004.

Wilson JR, Urwin GH, Stower MJ: The role of percutaneous nephrostomy in malignant ureteric obstruction. *Ann R Coll Surg Engl* 87(1):21–24, 2005.

Extracorporeal Shock Wave Lithotripsy

Brownlee N, Foster M, Griffith DP, Carlton CE Jr: Controlled inversion therapy: an adjunct to the elimination of gravity dependent fragments following extracorporeal shock wave lithotripsy. *J Urol* 143:1096, 1990.

Dretler SP: CT and stone fragility. *J Endourol* 15(1):31–36, 2001.

Dretler SP: Variability of renal stone fragility in shock wave lithotripsy [editorial]. *Urology* 61(6):1092–1097, 2003.

Greiner L, Munks C, Heil W, Jakobeit C: Gallbladder stone fragments in feces after biliary extracorporeal shock wave lithotripsy. *Gastroenterology* 98:1620, 1990.

Kim SC, Kuo RL, Tinmouth WW, et al: Percutaneous nephrolithotomy for caliceal diverticular calculi: a novel single stage approach. *J Urol* 173(4):1194–1198, 2005.

Rothschild JG, Holbrook RF, Reinhold RB: Gallstone lithotripsy vs cholecystectomy: a preliminary cost-benefit analysis. *Arch Surg* 125:710, 1990.

General

De Simone P, Urbani L, Morelli L, et al: The T-tube approach to biliary strictures in liver transplant recipients. *Transplantation* 79(2):254–255, 2005.

Tanrikut C, Sahani D, Dretler SP: Distinguishing stent from stone: use of bone windows. *Urology* 63(5):823–827, 2004.

Wills VL, Gibson K, Karihaloot C, et al: Complications of biliary T-tubes after choledochotomy. *ANZ J Surg* 72(3):177–180, 2002.

STUDY QUESTIONS

1. One of the interventional procedures for the treatment of chronic mesenteric ischemia is:
   a. Gelfoam embolization
   b. stent placement
   c. percutaneous gastroscopy
   d. suprapubic cystoscopy

2. Malignant ureteral strictures require the treatment with _____.
   a. percutaneous lithotomy
   b. endopyelotomy
   c. ureteral occlusion
   d. percutaneous cecostomy

3. According to research done by Claude Couinaud the liver is composed of _____ separate segments.
   a. 2
   b. 3
   c. 4
   d. 8

4. Which of the following is *not* a function of the kidneys?
   i. regulation of blood pressure
   ii. stimulation of red blood cell production
   iii. regulation of production of bilirubin
   a. i only
   b. ii only
   c. iii only
   d. i and ii only

5. Which of the following would be considered as contraindications for the use of ultrasound during needle guidance in a procedure?
   i. extremely obese patient
   ii. necessity for three-dimensional resolution
   iii. presence of overlying bone
   a. i only
   b. ii only
   c. i and iii only
   d. i, ii, and iii

6. Renal cyst puncture requires that the patient be placed in the _____ position for preparation and needle insertions.
   a. prone
   b. supine
   c. supine oblique
   d. lateral

7. The percutaneous removal of renal calculi can be accomplished through all of the following procedures except:
   a. percutaneous ultrasonic lithotripsy
   b. electrohydraulic lithotripsy
   c. endoscopic retrograde cholangiopancreatography
   d. percutaneous catheter nephrostomy

8. Which of the following would be used to facilitate the postoperative removal of biliary calculi?
   i. steerable catheter system
   ii. contrast agent
   iii. stone basket
   a. iii only
   b. i and ii only
   c. i and iii only
   d. i, ii, and iii

9. The range of catheter sizes used during percutaneous nephrostomy is between _____ French.
   a. 4 and 8
   b. 6 and 10
   c. 8 and 12
   d. 12 and 14

10. Complication rates for endoscopic retrograde cholangiopancreatography range between _____ percent.
   a. 0 and 1
   b. 1 and 3
   c. 3 and 5
   d. 5 and 10

20 *Hysterosalpingography*

Hysterosalpingography involves radiography of the female reproductive system after instillation of a contrast agent. This procedure requires sterile technique, and it is usually performed in a room equipped for specialized genitourinary radiography. Physicians as well as ancillary personnel are required to wear sterile gowns and operating room caps during the procedure. Hysterosalpingography (HSG) is of value in infertility studies and is considered a safe and painless procedure. "Radiation risks from a typical HSG are low, but they may be elevated if fluoroscopic and/or radiographic exposures are prolonged for any reason."[1]

ANATOMIC CONSIDERATIONS

The female reproductive organs are divided into external and internal groups. Hysterosalpingography involves mainly the internal group of reproductive organs—the ovaries, uterine tubes, uterus, and vagina (Fig. 20-1).

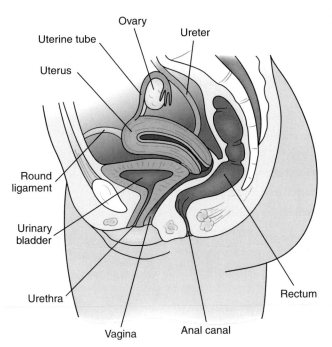

FIGURE 20-1. Schematic of the internal group of female organs.

Ovaries

The ovaries are almond-shaped, slightly flattened structures. Their size fluctuates, depending on patient age and stage of ovarian cycle. The average size is approximately 2.5 to 5 cm long, 2 cm wide, and 1 cm thick. They are located near the lateral walls of the pelvis. Before pregnancy, the ovaries are approximately at the level of the anterior superior iliac spine lying lateral to the uterus. During pregnancy, however, the uterus rises into the abdomen, pulling the ovaries away from this general location. After pregnancy, they usually assume their original position.

The ovaries are attached to the uterus by the ovarian ligament, which passes from the uterine end of the ovary to the body of the uterus.

The function of the ovaries is to produce the ova and the female sex hormones.

Uterine Tubes

The uterine tubes, or oviducts, provide the path for the ova into the uterus. The spermatozoa travel into the uterine tubes from the uterus after intercourse. Fertilization of the ovum usually occurs in the oviducts.

The oviducts can be subdivided into three parts—the isthmus, ampulla, and infundibulum.[1] The **isthmus** is thick-walled and narrow and is attached to the uterine wall. The **ampulla** is the longest and widest part of the oviduct. Its walls are relatively thin. The funnel-shaped **infundibulum** terminates in finger-like structures called fimbriae. At this point, the oviduct is opened to the peritoneal cavity. There is, however, one finger of the fimbriae that makes a physical connection with the ovary.

Uterus

The **uterus** is a thick-walled, muscular organ lying within the pelvis. Its position changes with the degree of fullness of the bladder and rectum. It can also be subdivided into several parts—the fundus, body, isthmus, and cervix (Fig. 20-2). The fundus is the rounded upper portion of the uterus. It is found above the line joining the entrance of the uterine tubes. The body of the uterus, a small triangular area between the

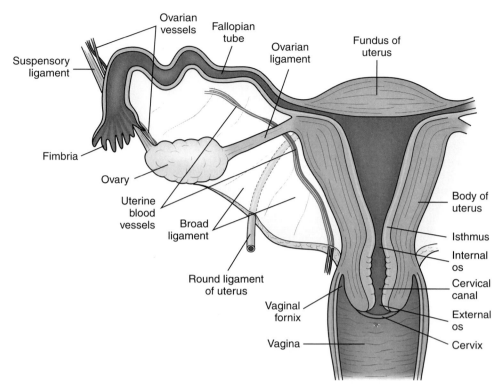

FIGURE 20-2.   Schematic cross section of the uterus.

uterine walls, extends down toward the isthmus. The body is the main portion of the uterus. Between the cervix and the body of the uterus lies the isthmus, a narrow, constricted, very short segment about 1 cm long. The cervix communicates with the vagina, and can be divided into a supravaginal and a vaginal part. The vaginal portion extends into the vagina, whereas the supravaginal part extends up to the isthmus.

Vagina

The vagina is a muscular tube about 3 in (7.6 cm) long that forms the lower portion of the birth canal. The vagina extends upward and posteriorly into the pelvic cavity lying posterior to the urinary bladder. The cervix extends into the upper portion of the vagina, providing a connection between these two structures. The vagina extends from the uterus to the outside of the body and functions to allow intercourse and a path for the fetus to exit the body.

INDICATIONS AND CONTRAINDICATIONS

Hysterosalpingography is a safe diagnostic and therapeutic tool in the diagnosis and treatment of the female genital organs. It has been used in the study of infertility to determine possible structural or functional defects not obvious by clinical examination. Many other abnormal gynecologic conditions have also been demonstrated by this procedure.

As a therapeutic tool, hysterosalpingography has been shown to be effective in some cases of infertility. The procedure has had success in restoring patency to occluded tubes, straightening kinks, stretching adhesions, and dilating narrowed tubes.

Other uses for the procedure are preoperative and postoperative evaluations of the genital organs; determination and location of ectopic, misplaced, or lost contraceptive devices; and determination of the cause for dysmenorrhea.

Ultrasound is commonly performed for diagnosis of pathologic processes of the female reproductive system; hysterosalpingography also plays a part as a diagnostic tool. The following list is a summary of the indications for hysterosalpingography and hysterosonography:

Diagnosis
- Abnormal uterine bleeding
- Patency of uterine tubes
- Congenital uterine anomalies
- Habitual abortion
- Amenorrhea
- Preoperative evaluation for localization
- Postoperative evaluation
- Location of ectopic pregnancy or lost contraceptive devices
- Dysmenorrhea
- Pelvic masses
- Fistulas
- Cervical stenosis
- Malignancy
- Endometrial polyps
- Leiomyoma

Therapy
- Restore patency of uterine tubes
- Stretch tubal adhesions
- Straighten kinks
- Dilate tubes

This list is by no means complete. The indications for any specialized procedure increase as its possibilities and limitations are evaluated.

Hysterosalpingography is contraindicated when an acute or subacute pelvic inflammation exists. In cases of vaginal or cervical infection accompanied by purulent discharge, the procedure is also contraindicated. The procedure is not advised during the immediate premenstrual or postmenstrual phase.

Active uterine bleeding also contraindicates hysterosalpingography. If the study were performed under these conditions, it would not be of diagnostic value, and there would always be the danger of seepage of the contrast medium into the general circulation.

Pregnancy is usually considered an absolute contraindication.

CONTRAST AGENTS

The contrast agents used to delineate anatomic structures during hysterosalpingography are divided into two groups—water-soluble and oily. All are organic iodine compounds, and each group has its advantages. The water-soluble contrast agents are absorbed quickly and do not leave a residue within the genital tract[2]; the ethiodized oils are extremely opaque and are well tolerated by the structures under study. The low-osmolality contrast agents offer a reduction in the burning sensation and pain experienced with the ionic water-soluble contrast agents. The choice of contrast agent is governed by physician preference and institutional protocol. The oily contrast agents are almost never used today because the water-soluble organic iodides have proved their effectiveness for this procedure. Reference to the oily contrast agents is included because they are still manufactured and occasionally used. Table 20-1 is a comparison of oily contrast media with water-soluble media.

TABLE 20-1 *Comparison of Oily and Water-Soluble Contrast Media*

Characteristic	Oil-Based Contrast Media*	Water-Soluble Media
Viscosity	High	Low to moderate
Radiopacity	Very good	Moderate to satisfactory
Absorption rate	Very slow; delayed for many months when large amounts are injected	Prompt excretion through kidneys after 20–60 minutes; this can be a desirable trait In cases of hydrosalpinx, absorption is slower; contrast may persist for 24–48 hours
Toxicity	Not observed unless decomposed oil is used.	Rare
Allergic reactions	Not observed	Occasionally observed
Peritoneal reactions	Only when large amounts are injected; not observed when small amounts are used	Observed, mostly transient
Pain	Not observed when small amounts are injected under low pressure; few complaints when pressures <200 mm Hg are used	Nearly always present; may be transient or persist for several hours post procedure
Dangers	Intravasation, pulmonary embolism	None

From Rozin S: *Uterosalpingography in gynecology*, Springfield, Ill, 1965, Charles C Thomas.
*May provide an enhanced therapeutic effect in infertility by improving the potential for normal pregnancy.

TABLE 20-2 *Contrast Media for Hysterosalpingography*

Trade Name	Iodine Content (%)	Water-Soluble	Oily
Ethiodol	37		X
Hypaque 50%	30	X	
Hypaque-m 90%	46	X	
Lipiodol 40%	38–42		X
Lipiodol 28%	26.5–29.5		
Salpix	27	X	
Sinografin	38	X	
Renografin-60	28	X	
Hexabrix	32	X	

The ideal contrast medium possesses the following characteristics:
1. Rapid absorption and excretion rates
2. Sufficient radiographic density*
3. Adequate viscosity
4. Does not cause general or local reactions
5. Ability to delineate anatomic structures

In general, when iodized oils are used, 24-hour delayed films are taken to demonstrate tubal patency. Table 20-2 is a summary of contrast media available for hysterosalpingography.

The total amount of contrast agent introduced is variable. Approximately 4 ml is required to fill a normal uterine cavity. An additional 4 ml may be required to visualize the uterine tubes, and larger amounts may be used in some disease conditions.

The negative contrast medium, carbon dioxide, can be used after positive contrast hysterosalpingography to diagnose many gynecologic problems. Approximately 100 ml of carbon dioxide is

*The opacity of the water-soluble organic iodine compounds is improved when used with digital imaging equipment.

introduced into the uterus after the removal of the positive-contrast agent. The carbon dioxide is usually absorbed within 25 to 30 minutes and causes a minimal amount of patient discomfort.

PATIENT PREPARATION

Before the day of the examination, the patient is instructed in the protocol for proper bowel cleansing. This includes taking a non–gas-forming laxative on the evening before the study. In some cases, restriction of intake is recommended.

The procedure is explained to the patient, and she is instructed to empty her bladder to prevent possible displacement of the uterus and uterine tubes. The patient is requested to irrigate the vagina and cleanse the perineal region at this time.

Unless the patient is unusually apprehensive, premedication is not required. As with all contrast examinations, a history is taken and the procedure and complications are explained to the patient. As with all invasive procedures, a consent form must be completed and signed by the patient.

If the patient indicates an allergic history, the physician performing the study should be notified because premedication with steroids, an antihistamine, or both is indicated. The history should contain the date of the last menses. Hysterosalpingography should be done toward the end of the first week after menstruation and before the twelfth day of the menstrual cycle to avoid radiation exposure to the oocyte, which becomes radiosensitive at this time. The patient's menstrual flow should have been completed for at least 3 days before the study.

Hysterosalpingography is normally done as an outpatient procedure, and follow-up care is limited. Sometimes, the patient experiences some subjective transitory aftereffects and requires bed rest before leaving the department.

PROCEDURE

Hysterosalpingography can be performed in a radiographic/fluorographic room or a radiographic room equipped with a urologic table like that used for cystoscopy and retrograde pyelography. The patient assumes the lithotomy position, and the table is adjusted to a slight Trendelenburg position.

The cervix is exposed with a bivalve speculum, a specialized catheter equipped with a balloon tip to lock the catheter in place to provide a leak-free seal and to allow transcervical access to the uterus. The contrast agent is then slowly injected and radiographs are taken. Fractional injection of the contrast agent is practiced. There are no standard routines for fractional injections as they vary with the individual patient. Images are taken and evaluated throughout the procedure.

The transcervical access catheter also provides a route for the introduction of uterine catheters for selective salpingography. Catheter size is 5 French, designed to be advanced over an appropriate guide wire. These catheters are supplied with preshaped curves and are inserted through the cervical access catheter. The tip of the catheter is placed at the uterine ostia, allowing the direct injection of contrast medium into the proximal uterine tube. This type of study is useful for differentiating between spasm and true obstruction and may serve as a therapeutic measure to dislodge any intraluminal blockage and reestablish tubal patency.

With introduction of a guide wire and coaxial catheter system through the transcervical access catheter, the proximal uterine tube can be negotiated to image the distal portion of the uterine tube. The use of selective catheterization has reduced the need for laparoscopic surgery to establish tubal patency. The transcervical catheter remains in place throughout the entire procedure to prevent the backflow of contrast medium into the vagina.

It is important to follow strict aseptic technique throughout the procedure to avoid the possibility of introducing infection into the peritoneal cavity.

If an oily contrast medium is used, the patient is required to return in 24 hours for a delayed radiograph to show whether the contrast medium has reached the free peritoneal cavity or has been trapped by pathologic uterine tubes.

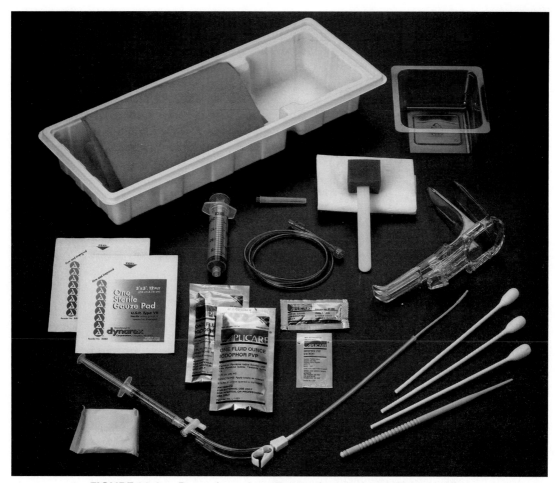

FIGURE 20-3.   Prepackaged sterile tray for hysterosalpingography.

EQUIPMENT

Hysterosalpingography requires a minimum of specialized equipment. The room must be equipped with a urology table to enable the patient to comfortably assume the lithotomy position. In some institutions, fluoroscopic control of hysterosalpingography is practiced. When fluoroscopy is used, it may be adapted for cineradiography to facilitate serial filming of the procedure. When an oil-soluble contrast medium is used, fluoroscopy can reduce the incidence of contrast medium intravasation into veins and lymph vessels, resulting in fewer cases of oil embolization.

A sterile tray should be prepared and available for the procedure. Prepackaged complete sterile disposable trays are available for the procedure (Fig. 20-3). Items recommended for inclusion include a vaginal speculum, dilators, sponge-holding forceps, tenacula, uterine cannula, sterile towels and drapes, small sterile containers, and a sanitary napkin. Additional items may be added, depending upon the specific technique used. Box 20-1 describes the contents of the prepackaged sterile tray from Cooper Surgical.

Many cannulas are available for hysterosalpingography, including the Malmstrom Westerman vacuum uterine cannula, the Leech-Wilkinson, Jarcho, and Hayes-Provis cannulae. A No. 16 or 18 Foley catheter can also be used. The cannula seals the cervical os to prevent leakage of the contrast medium during the procedure (Fig. 20-4). Cannulas differ only in their specific method of sealing the cervical os. Figure 20-5 shows the Ackrad H/S catheter set, which uses a 1.5- to 4-ml balloon to occlude the cervix.

Fundamentals of Special Radiographic Procedures

BOX 20-1	*Contents of Prepackaged Sterile Tray for Hysterosalpingography*★
Quantity	**Item**
1	5 French catheter in sterile pouch
1	Fenestrated drape
1	Disposable speculum
1	Disposable cervical dilator
2	3 × 3-in gauze pads
3	Swab sticks
1	Wide swab
1	Sterile wrap
1	Inner tray for povidone-iodine solution
1	Povidone-iodine ointment
1	Lubricating jelly packet
2	Povidone-iodine solution
1	36in extension tube
1	20-ml syringe with 18 gauge needle
1	Sanitary napkin

★Courtesy CooperSurgical, Inc., Trumbull, Ct.

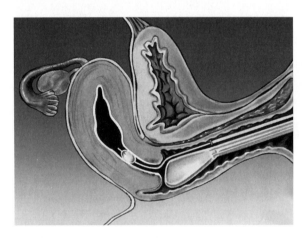

FIGURE 20-4. The balloon catheter occlusion technique for hysterosalpingography using the Elliptosphere H/S catheter.

Other items necessary for the examination include sterile gloves (various sizes), antiseptic cleansing solution for the outer vaginal area, contrast medium, and face masks.

PATIENT POSITIONING

Almost all filming during hysterosalpingography is done with the patient in the anteroposterior position (Fig. 20-6). Occasionally, other positions such as prone, oblique, and lateral may be requested if indicated by specific pathology.

The necessary anatomy can be easily recorded on a 10- × 12-in (25- × 30-cm) image receptor. The patient should be in the supine position and adjusted so that a point approximately 2 in (5 cm) superior to the symphysis pubis is centered to the image receptor. The central ray should be directed perpendicular to the midpoint of the image receptor.

If oblique views are required, the physician usually specifies the amount of obliquity necessary. The filming procedure varies with each patient, ranging from one anteroposterior view to a sequential

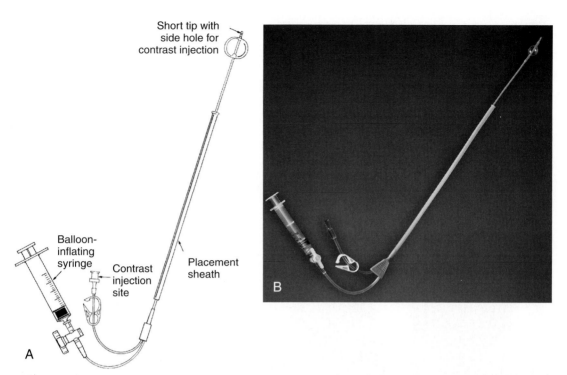

Short tip with side hole for contrast injection

Balloon-inflating syringe

Contrast injection site

Placement sheath

A

B

FIGURE 20-5. **A,** Schematic illustration of the H/S catheter set. The unit allows easier examination for both the patient and the physician and eliminates the need for a tenaculum. It is available as a basic set or in a complete procedural tray. **B,** Photograph of the H/S catheter set.

series attempting to demonstrate tubal patency by the spill of contrast medium into the peritoneal cavity (see Fig. 20-6). Accuracy is stressed because unnecessary radiation exposure to the gonads due to technical error is inexcusable.

Table 20-3 is a summary of positioning for hysterosalpingography.

OTHER MODALITIES

Hysterosonography and Contrast Hysterosalpingosonography

These studies can be performed as a screening procedure. They do not require the use of x-radiation and can be performed as the initial study in cases of infertility, dysfunctional uterine bleeding, tubal patency, and evaluation of the endometrium. The procedure can be performed with a saline infusion with or without air or with a suitable contrast agent. Hysterosonography with or without the use of contrast is accomplished as a real-time study. It is usually accomplished between the third and seventh day of the female cycle toward the end of the menstrual flow.

Patient preparation consists of the following steps:

- Take the patient's history
- Ask if the patient has any allergies (remember to check for latex allergies)
- Explain the procedure to ensure the cooperation of the patient
- Have the patient empty her bladder before the procedure
- Check if the patient has taken the recommended dose of ibuprofen
- Be sure the patient understands the benefits and risks associated with the procedure
- Have the patient sign a consent form that follows the protocol of the institution

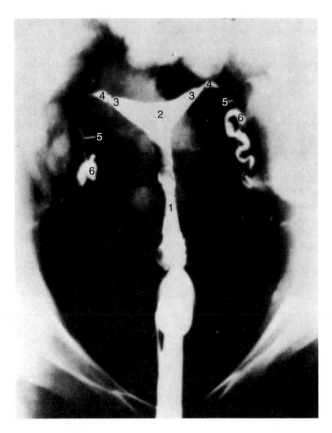

FIGURE 20-6. Radiograph of a normal hysterosalpingogram following pneumoperitoneum. *1*, Cervical canal; *2*, uterine cavity; *3*, cornua; *4*, intramural portion of the uterine tubes; *5*, uterine tubes; *6*, fimbriae.

The patient should be placed in the anteroposterior position on the lithotomy table for the procedure. Saline solution or contrast material is injected and the anatomic structures are observed and recorded using a vaginal transducer. The use of air during the procedure will enhance the demonstration of tubal patency.

After the procedure explain to the patient that there will be some cramping and the possibility of a watery discharge. This will be the result of the saline solution and Betadine that is used to sterilize the site. Provide the patient with several sanitary napkins prior to leaving the site. The physician may discuss the results at the conclusion of the procedure with the patient and in some cases prescribe an antibiotic.

SUMMARY

Hysterosalpingography is used to diagnose and treat the female reproductive system. The anatomy investigated includes the ovaries, uterine tubes, uterus, and vagina. The procedure is indicated for infertility studies and has been used to diagnose and treat a number of different structural and functional pathologic conditions. The contrast media available for use in this study include both water-soluble iodine compounds and iodized oil-based substances. In most cases the water-soluble media are preferred. Patient preparation is minimal and includes cleansing enemas and a non–gas-forming laxative. As in all contrast agent studies, the potential for allergic reactions exists. A detailed history concerning allergies, medications, and the date of last menses should be taken.

The procedure is performed transvaginally and requires a minimum of specialized equipment. Prepackaged kits are available that include all the necessary equipment for the procedure. The procedure is normally done with the patient in the supine lithotomy position. It

TABLE 20-3 *Positions for Hysterosalpingography*

Projection	Patient Position	Central Ray	Anatomy
Anteroposterior	Patient in dorsal lithotomy position, centered to table; point approximately 2 in (5 cm) superior to symphysis pubis is centered to a transverse 10- × 12-in (25- × 30-cm) cassette	Directed at a right angle to film	Speculum in vagina, cannula inserted in cervix, uterine body cavity, uterine horns, uterine tubes; spill of contrast medium into peritoneal cavity
Oblique (optional iew)	Patient rotated into either right or left posterior oblique position; cassette centered to same location as above	Directed at a right angle to film	Oblique view of above anatomy used to demonstrate pathology not otherwise well shown
Lateral (optional view)	Patient in right or left lateral position; cassette centered to same location as above	Directed at a right angle to film	Lateral view of above anatomy used to demonstrate pathology not otherwise well shown, very rarely done
Prone (optional view)	Patient rotated into the prone position, centered to the table; point approximately 2 in (5 cm) superior to the symphysis pubis centered to a transverse 10- × 12-in (25- × 30-cm) cassette	Directed at a right angle to film	Differentiates free peritoneal spill from loculated collections related to peritubal adhesions

is a sterile procedure, and good aseptic technique should be practiced. Hysterosalpingography has proved to be a safe and effective procedure in cases of infertility.

Hysterosonography is also used to diagnose pathology in the female reproductive tract. Contrast hysterosalpingosonograpy is a safe procedure performed with ultrasound that can provide a real-time functional study.

REFERENCES

1. Perisinakis K, Damilakis J, Grammatikakis K, Theocharopoulos N, Gourtsoviannis N: Radiogenic risks from hysterosalpingography. *Eur Radiol* 13(7):1522–1528, 2003.
2. Winfield AC: Contrast media for hysterosalpingography: water soluble materials are preferred. *Radiol. Rep* 2:208, 1990.

SUGGESTED READINGS

Boudghène FP, Bazot M, Robert Y, Perrot N, Rocourt N, Antoine J, Morris H, Leroy J, Uzan S, Bigot J-M: Assessment of uterine tube patency by HyCoSy: comparison of a positive contrast agent with saline solution. *Ultrasound Obstet Gynecol* 18(5):525, 2001.

Chen MY, et al: Comparison of patient reactions and diagnostic quality for hysterosalpingography using ionic and nonionic contrast media. *Acad Radiol* 2:123, 1995.

Dessole S, Farina M, Rubattu G, Cosmi E, Ambrosini G, Battista Nardelli G: Side effects and complications of sonohysterosalpingography. *Fertil Steril* 80(3):620–624, 2003.

Exacoustos C, Zupi E, Carusotti C, Lanzi G, Marconi D, Arduini D: Hysterosalpingo–contrast sonography compared with hysterosalpingography and laparoscopic dye pertubation to evaluate tubal patency. *J Am Assoc Gynecol Laparosc* 10(3):367–372, 2003.

Goldberg JM, Falcone T, Attaran M:: Sonohysterographic evaluation of uterine abnormalities noted on hysterosalpingography. *Hum Reprod* 12:2151, 1997.

Kafali H, Cengiz M, Demir N: Intrauterine lidocaine gel application for pain relief during and after hysterosalpingography. *Int J Gynaecol Obstet* 83(1):65–67, 2003.

Lang EK, Dunaway HE Jr: Salpingographic demonstration of "cobblestone" mucosa of the distal tubes is indicative of irreversible mucosal damage. *Fertil Steril* 76(2):342–345, 2001.

Papaioannou S, Afnan M, Girling AJ, Ola B, Olufowobi O, Coomarasamy A, Sharif K: Diagnostic and therapeutic value of selective salpingography and tubal catheterization in an unselected infertile population. *Fertil Steril* 79(3):613–617, 2003.

Sawada T, Kuroki J, Yoshimura Y, Kawakami S: "Crushed glass" appearance of particles observed in roentgenograms after hysterosalpingography as an indicator of pelvic abnormalities. *Fertil Steril* 68:1075, 1997.

Steiner AZ, Meyer WR, Clark RL, Hartmann KE: Oil-soluble contrast during hysterosalpingography in women with proven tubal patency. *Obstet Gynecol* 101(1):109–113, 2003.

Thurmond AS: Imaging of female infertility. *Radiol Clin North Am* 41(4):757–767, vi. Review, July 2003.

Unterweger M, De Geyter C, Frohlich JM, Bongartz G, Wiesner W: Three-dimensional dynamic MR-hysterosalpingography; a new, low invasive, radiation-free and less painful radiological approach to female infertility. *Hum Reprod* 17(12):3138–3141, 2002.

Yun AJ, Lee PY: Enhanced fertility after diagnostic hysterosalpingography using oil-based contrast agents may be attributable to immunomodulation. *AJR Am J Roentgenol* 183(6):1725–1727, 2004.

STUDY QUESTIONS

1. Which of the following is (are) not a part of the (uterine tube) oviduct?
   a. infundibulum
   b. ampulla
   c. fimbriae
   d. isthmus

2. When used in hysterosalpingography, the low osmolality contrast agents can:
   a. reduce the cost of the procedure
   b. provide a greater amount of contrast than the ionic contrast agents
   c. reduce the burning sensation felt by the patient during the procedure
   d. allow the use of half the normal quantity to produce the same amount of contrast

3. Which of the following is not a therapeutic use of hysterosalpingography?
   a. treat cystic stenosis
   b. stretch tubal adhesions
   c. dilate tubes
   d. straighten kinks

4. The procedure that is currently used as a screening procedure for female reproductive pathology is:
   a. hysterosalpingography
   b. computed tomography
   c. magnetic resonance imaging
   d. hysterosalpingosonography

5. Which of the following positions is used most frequently during hysterosalpingography?
   a. right anterior oblique
   b. prone
   c. anteroposterior
   d. lateral

STUDY QUESTIONS (*cont'd*)

6. The patient is asked to empty her bladder prior to hysterosalpingography in order to:
   a. avoid interrupting the procedure to void
   b. eliminate the possibility that the bladder would displace the uterus or uterine tubes
   c. minimize the dilution of contrast medium used during the procedure
   d. avoid compression of the vagina during the procedure

7. At which point in the female menstrual cycle is hysterosonography usually performed?
   a. during menstruation
   b. between the third to seventh day of the cycle
   c. between the tenth to thirteenth day of the cycle
   d. between the fifteenth to twentieth day of the cycle

8. The patient would be required to return for a 24-hour film when the following type of contrast agent is used:
   a. ionic organic iodide compounds
   b. nonionic organic iodide compounds
   c. oil-based compounds
   d. infused saline solution

9. The lower portion of the birth canal is formed by the :
   a. uterus
   b. cervix
   c. uterine tubes
   d. vagina

10. Which of the following would be a contraindication to hysterosalpingography?
    a. excessive gas in the abdominal cavity
    b. active uterine bleeding
    c. distended and full bladder
    d. premedication with steroids or antihistamines

CHAPTER OBJECTIVES

After completing this chapter, the reader will be able to perform the following:

- Identify the anatomy of the brain, ventricular system, and spinal cord
- List the indications and contraindications for the procedure
- Describe the patient preparation for the procedure
- Identify the type of contrast media used for the procedure
- Describe the two major puncture methods for myelography
- Describe the needle placements for lumbar, thoracic, and cervical myelography
- Describe computed tomography myelography
- Explain magnetic resonance myelography
- List the specialized equipment necessary for the procedure
- Describe the patient positioning for the procedure
- Describe the other modalities used to evaluate the central nervous system

CHAPTER OUTLINE

R adiography of the structures of the central nervous system has undergone a number of major changes in recent years. Newer modalities such as computed tomography (CT) and magnetic resonance imaging (MRI) have completely replaced invasive studies such as pneumoencephalography, ventriculography, and, to some extent, myelography.

Myelography is the radiographic demonstration of the central nervous system structures located within the spinal canal. The procedure is accomplished easily through direct instillation of a contrast agent into the subarachnoid space. This technique can demonstrate various abnormalities of the spinal cord and spinal canal.

ANATOMIC CONSIDERATIONS

The nervous system can be separated into two major divisions—the peripheral and the central nervous systems. The central nervous system consists of the brain and the spinal cord. The central nervous system processes information to and from the peripheral nervous system and is the control center for the body.

Brain

The brain is the portion of the central nervous system found in the cranial cavity. The brain comprises the pons, medulla, mesencephalon, diencephalon, cerebellum, and cerebrum.

The pons, medulla, mesencephalon, and diencephalon are the components of the brain stem. The function of the brain stem is to provide some motor, sensory, and reflex functions. The spinal cord extends from the medulla oblongata and is considered to begin at the level of the foramen magnum.

The cerebellum is also called the hindbrain and is located in the posterior cranial fossa behind the brain stem. The cerebellum consists of two hemispheres separated by a groove. The middle section of the cerebellum, the vermis, is the connection between its hemispheres. The main function of the cerebellum is to coordinate voluntary muscular activity.

The cerebrum is the largest and uppermost portion of the brain. It is divided into right and left hemispheres by a central groove, the sulcus, and is connected at the bottom of the groove by the corpus callosum. The surface of the cerebrum is convoluted and lobed. The cerebrum is composed of an outer cerebral cortex (gray matter) and an inner portion, or semiovale (white matter). The cerebrum provides the sensory, motor, and integrative functions associated with the body's mental and physical activities. This portion of the brain generates the electric waves that are monitored and recorded with an electroencephalograph.

Ventricular System

The brain, like the spinal cord, is covered by three membranes, or **meninges**; the **pia mater** (the inner layer of the meninges) and **arachnoid** (the middle layer of the meninges) are called the **leptomeninges**. The **subarachnoid space** is found between these two membranes. The arachnoid membrane follows the contour of the **dura mater** (the tough outer layer of the meninges), whereas the pia mater follows the surface contours of the brain. The cerebrospinal fluid circulates through the ventricles and subarachnoid space surrounding the brain and spinal cord.

Subarachnoid Cisternae

In some areas of the brain, the subarachnoid space enlarges to form the subarachnoid cisternae (Fig. 21-1). The cisterna magna extends down to merge with the spinal subarachnoid space. It is triangular and contains approximately 5 to 10 ml of cerebrospinal fluid. The apex of the cisterna magna points toward the vallecula. This is the portion of the subarachnoid space that lies between the fourth ventricle and cisterna magna. When air is injected into the spinal subarachnoid space it must pass through the cisterna magna and vallecula before entering the ventricular system. The flexion of the head must be accurately maintained to prevent air from entering other subarachnoid spaces rather than the ventricular system.

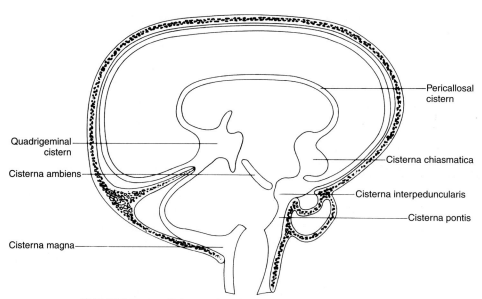

FIGURE 21-1. Schematic of the subarachnoid cisternae.

The ventricular system is a series of spaces or cavities located within the hemispheres of the brain. The system consists of four cerebral ventricles—two lateral ventricles and two other ventricles called the third and the fourth ventricles. Cerebrospinal fluid circulates in the ventricles and subarachnoid space surrounding the brain and spinal cord. The term "circulate" when applied to cerebrospinal fluid should not be compared with "circulation" as it applies to the blood. Cerebrospinal fluid is a complex substance containing various components, including water, electrolytes, and proteins. These substances are produced or absorbed in varying amounts throughout the subarachnoid space. This is the basis for the circulation of the spinal fluid. The cerebrospinal fluid flows from areas of greatest production to areas of greatest absorption, but it is not true circulation. However, the spinal fluid does move through the subarachnoid system by this production–absorption process.

Lateral Ventricles. There are two lateral ventricles, each located within one cerebral hemisphere. Each lateral ventricle has five divisions (Fig. 21-2): (1) the anterior (frontal) horn; (2) the body; (3) the trigone (isthmus or atrium); (4) the posterior (occipital) horn; and (5) the inferior (temporal) horn. Each lateral ventricle connects on each side with the third ventricle by a narrow channel known as the interventricular foramen of Monro. The anterior (frontal) horns are usually found in the frontal lobes of the brain hemispheres.

Third Ventricle. The third ventricle is bounded by the thalami superiorly and laterally and by the hypothalamus inferiorly and anteriorly. The superoanterior portion of the third ventricle supports the interventricular foramen of Monro, which connects to the lateral ventricles. In the posteroinferior portion of the third ventricle is found the aqueduct of Sylvius, by which the third ventricle communicates with the fourth ventricle below. The third ventricle is a narrow slitlike cavity located in the midline of the skull.

Fourth Ventricle. The aqueduct of Sylvius is located in the midbrain. The "aqueduct" begins at the third ventricle and extends downward, where it widens posteriorly and laterally to form the fourth ventricle. This cavity narrows below to become contiguous with the central canal of the spinal cord.

The lateral portions of the fourth ventricle are extended on each side for a variable distance, forming the lateral recesses. These open by means of the foramina of Luschka into the pontine and anterior portion of the cerebellomedullary cisternae. The fourth ventricle also connects with the

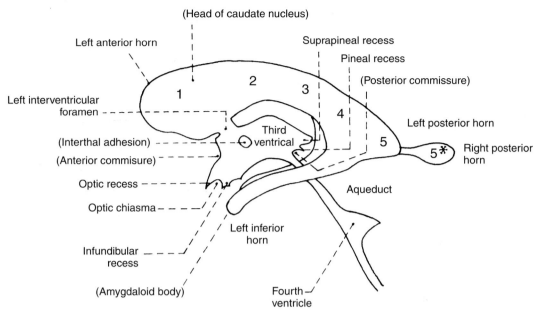

FIGURE 21-2. Schematic drawing of the ventricles of the brain in the left lateral aspect.

subarachnoid space of the cisterna magna (cerebellomedullary cisterna) through an opening called the foramen of Magendie.

Spinal Cord

The vertebral canal tends to be triangular, relatively large in the cervical and lumbar regions, and small and ovoid in the thoracic region (Fig. 21-3). The structures contained in the vertebral canal are the spinal cord and its meninges, spinal nerves and vessels, and the epidural space, which is located between the wall of the vertebral canal and the dura mater. The epidural space contains fat, venous plexuses, and nerves that supply the meninges, intervertebral disks, and ligaments.

All of these structures are important in that any aberrations may cause encroachment on the vertebral canal. The spinal cord lies loosely within the vertebral canal and extends from the foramen magnum to the lower border of the first lumbar vertebra. At this point, the spinal cord tapers into the conus medullaris, from which the filum terminale extends to the coccyx. The spinal cord averages 45 cm (18 in) in length.

The three layers—the dura mater, or outer covering; the arachnoid, middle layer; and the pia mater, the inner layer—also enclose the spinal cord and are continuous with the layers surrounding the brain (Fig. 21-4).

The spinal **dura mater** is a heavy sheath extending from its attachments with the margins of the foramen magnum to the level of the second sacral vertebra. At this point, the dura mater tapers into a covering for the filum terminale of the spinal cord. A space exists between the wall of the vertebral canal and the dura mater; this is called the epidural space. This space contains semifluid fat and many small veins. Between the dura mater and arachnoid layers is a potential subdural space. The meningeal layers contact each other, with a film of fluid separating them.

The spinal arachnoid is continuous with the cerebral arachnoid layer that covers the brain. It is a delicate membrane that follows the dura mater to its termination at the second sacral vertebra. Between the arachnoid and pia mater is the **subarachnoid space**. This space is bathed in spinal fluid and is in direct communication with the ventricles of the brain and its surrounding spaces. The

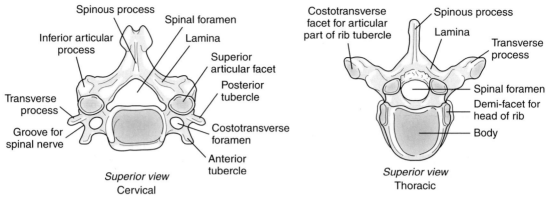

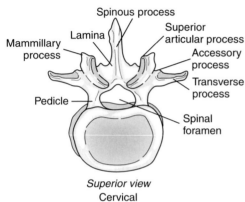

FIGURE 21-3. Representative individual vertebrae from the cervical, thoracic, and lumbar regions showing the differences in the size and shape of the vertebral canal.

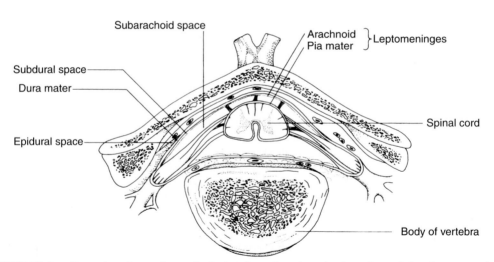

FIGURE 21-4. Superior view of a typical vertebra showing the location of the three meningeal layers.

subarachnoid space is larger around the spinal cord than in the brain. It extends to the level of the second sacral vertebra. The spinal cord ends at the upper level of the lumbar spine and the subarachnoid space continues to the second sacral segment, making an ideal location for spinal fluid withdrawal or contrast medium injection. The nerve roots are seldom damaged because of their flexibility in this area.

The spinal pia mater is the innermost membrane that invests the spinal cord. It is a thin layer that contains some blood vessels. The pia mater extends into the filum terminale and terminates within it, blending into the periosteum at the posterior of the first coccygeal segment. The pia mater and arachnoid are occasionally referred to as one layer. When this is the case, they are called the pia arachnoid layer, or the leptomeninges.

INDICATIONS AND CONTRAINDICATIONS

Subarachnoid myelography is a safe procedure that can be used to visualize the subarachnoid space around the spinal cord. It is indicated when accurate diagnosis of anatomic abnormalities or pathologic processes of the spinal cord and spinal canal is required. Some specific indications for subarachnoid myelography are as follows:

- Encroachment of intervertebral disks
- A tumor or infection, space-occupying lesions
- Abnormalities of the blood supply to the spinal cord
- Degenerative diseases of the central nervous system
- Inflammation of the membrane that covers the brain and spinal cord (arachnoid)
- Malformation of the spinal cord
- Syringomyelia

Epidural myelography is indicated when a demonstration of encroachment defects caused by tumors or herniated intervertebral disks into the lower thoracic and lumbar regions of the spinal canal is necessary.

Myelography is contraindicated when the patient exhibits signs of increased intracranial pressure.

PATIENT PREPARATION

In many cases, myelography can be done as an ambulatory procedure. When the examination is scheduled, patients should be instructed not to take medication for at least 24 hours and to increase fluid intake before the examination. It is also recommended that they not eat solid food before the study; the length of the fast is variable depending on the protocol of the institution.

When the patient arrives, the procedure should be explained and a consent form negotiated. The patient should be questioned concerning allergies, prior contrast agent reactions, results of any recent myelograms, and history of seizures. Vital signs should be taken at this time to establish a baseline for monitoring during the procedure. The information from the history should be transmitted to the physician before the study begins. If the patient is to receive any medication before the examination, it should be administered by the physician or the special procedure nurse.

The radiographic room should be set up before the patient is brought in. All equipment should be tested, and the supplies necessary for the injection should be placed within easy reach. The patient should be gowned in preparation for the study. The injection site should be shaved; when the physician arrives, the site should be surgically prepared.

During the procedure, the patient should be monitored for changes and any unusual symptoms or complaints. If specimen samples are required, care must be taken to preserve the sterile environment. Samples should be readied for laboratory analysis as soon as possible. The procedure will be determined by the protocols developed by the medical laboratory department and must be carefully followed. Any complications or reactions should be noted on the patient's chart; the individual responsible for the charting will vary depending on the hospital protocol.

At the end of the myelogram, the patient should be told of the objective symptoms resulting from the procedure, which can include headache and pain at the injection site or in the lumbar area. The patient should be instructed to remain on bed rest for 8 to 24 hours with the head slightly elevated. The patient should be instructed to alert the physician to any unusual symptoms that may occur, such as stiff neck, fever, seizures, or paralysis. If the patient appears normal, he or she may be released upon the physician's order.

CONTRAST AGENTS

Myelography can be done with either positive or negative contrast agents. The procedural differences are in manipulating the contrast agent within the subarachnoid space. Negative contrast agents are lighter than spinal fluid and will rise to the highest available portion of the spinal canal. Positive contrast agents are heavier than spinal fluid and will flow with the effect of gravity; that is, if the patient is raised to a standing position, the contrast agent will flow toward the lower spine, or if the patient is placed in the Trendelenburg position, the contrast agent will flow toward the cervical region.

The negative contrast material most often used is air. When a myelogram is done with a negative contrast agent, it is usually called a pneumomyelogram. Negative contrast agents are readily absorbed by body tissues, so their removal is unnecessary. They have found widespread usage for cervical and thoracic myelography.

The positive contrast agents used are the water-soluble organic iodides. These can be subdivided into ionic and nonionic types. Water-soluble agents give excellent visualization of the nerve roots and have the advantage of being rapidly absorbed from the subarachnoid space into the bloodstream. One major disadvantage of the ionic contrast agents is the pain caused by the intrathecal injection during the procedure. Spinal anesthesia must be given when using this type of medium, thus limiting the procedure to the lumbar area.

The most commonly used contrast agents for myelography are the nonionic water-soluble organic iodine compounds. These agents are generally administered to patients without any premedication and usually do not produce the type or degree of irritation caused by the ionic water-soluble media.

The nonionic contrast agents generally have an osmolarity similar to that of cerebrospinal fluid. They are somewhat hyperbaric and can be positioned by gravity. They have the same advantages of the other ionic water-soluble contrast media and can reveal much diagnostic information regarding the nerve roots. Once the contrast agent is introduced, any movement of the patient should be minimized to prevent its dilution. The patient should be fully hydrated before its administration to minimize the possibility of side effects. One disadvantage to the use of water-soluble contrast agents is their rapid reabsorption rate. This process begins within 30 minutes of the injection, and the radiographs should be taken quickly to avoid loss of radiopacity.

In the past Pantopaque, an ethyl-ester derivative, was commonly employed as a contrast medium in myelography. Pantopaque exhibited very slow absorption by the body tissues and was demonstrated to persist years after the procedure was done. The material was not soluble in the cerebrospinal fluid and needed to be removed after the examination was completed.

PROCEDURE

The two principal methods by which contrast medium may be injected into the subarachnoid space are lumbar puncture and cisternal puncture. The former is used most often, whereas the latter is reserved for use when complete obstruction of the subarachnoid space has been determined.

Lumbar Puncture Method

This method provides a satisfactory injection point for most forms of subarachnoid myelography—cervical, thoracic, and lumbar. Various postural maneuvers are required to distribute the material along the areas of interest.

The patient is placed in either a seated or lateral decubitus position for the injection. The skin is prepared and infiltrated with a suitable anesthetic agent. The needle and stylet are then inserted into the

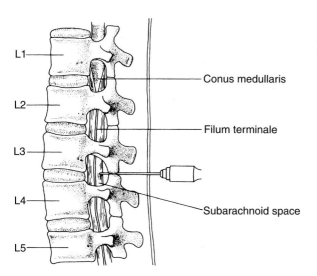

FIGURE 21-5. Lumbar region of the spine showing the location of the spinal structure. Spinal cord trauma is avoided at this level.

L1

Conus medullaris

L2

Filum terminale

L3

L4

Subarachnoid space

L5

subarachnoid space. The stylet is removed, and an indication of successful entry is the free flow of spinal fluid from the needle.

The site of injection is the lower lumbar region, because this area reduces the possibility of trauma to the spinal cord (Fig. 21-5). The injection site for lumbar myelography is usually in the interspace between the second and third lumbar vertebrae (L2–L3), whereas for cervical and thoracic myelography the injection can be made lower (at the level of the L3–L4 or L4–L5 interspace). The lower lumbar region is usually the site of disease, and the higher injection point is required to minimize the possibility of needle deformities becoming confused with pathology.

When a successful lumbar puncture is made, a small sample of spinal fluid is collected for laboratory analysis. At this time, manometric pressure measurements may be made, and injection of the contrast medium can proceed. This is usually accomplished by withdrawing a small amount of spinal fluid and replacing it with an equal amount of contrast agent, with the total amount being dependent on the area of the spine under examination and the type of contrast agent used (positive or negative).

After instillation of the contrast agent, the stylet is replaced and the examination can proceed. The patient is rotated into the prone position and secured by means of a foot platform and shoulder harness; through the use of a tilting radiographic table, the contrast agent is distributed over the area of interest.

During myelography with a water-soluble contrast agent, the first radiograph is usually taken with the needle still in place. This is done to ensure that the needle is in the subarachnoid space and to record the puncture site radiographically to confirm or exclude the possibility of localized puncture bleeding. Once the initial radiograph has been completed satisfactorily, the needle is removed. Because the water-soluble iodine compounds are readily absorbed by the body, there is no need to remove the contrast agent after the examination is complete.

Cisternal Puncture Method

When it is impossible to perform a lumbar puncture for the injection of contrast material, a cisternal puncture can be performed. The injection is made into the cisterna magna or cerebellomedullary cisterna (Fig. 21-6). The injection site is shaved, prepared surgically, and a local anesthetic is given. A special needle is then inserted between the occipital bone and the atlas, passing through the atlanto-occipital membrane and advancing about 1 to 2 cm until spinal fluid appears. This procedure must be carefully performed to avoid trauma to the medulla. It is generally reserved for

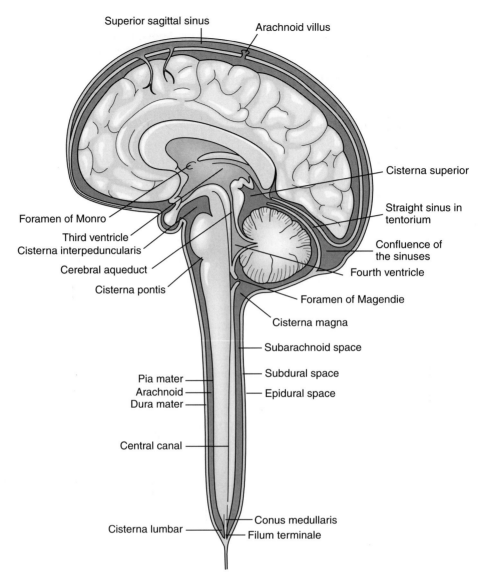

Superior sagittal sinus

Arachnoid villus

Cisterna superior

Straight sinus in tentorium

Foramen of Monro

Third ventricle

Cisterna interpeduncularis

Cerebral aqueduct

Cisterna pontis

Confluence of the sinuses

Fourth ventricle

Foramen of Magendie

Cisterna magna

Subarachnoid space

Subdural space

Pia mater

Arachnoid

Epidural space

Dura mater

Central canal

Conus medullaris

Cisterna lumbar

Filum terminale

FIGURE 21-6. A schematic illustration showing the relationship of the cerebellomedullary cisterna (cisterna magna) with the other structures within the skull.

use when there is obstruction of the lumbar region of the spinal canal. Other indications for use of this method include lumbar epidural abscess, spondylitis, and infection of the dermal tissue of the lumbar region.

Sacral Hiatus Puncture Method for Epidural Myelography

The preceding injection methods may be used for all forms of subarachnoid myelography. Epidural myelography, however, requires a special injection method for introducing the contrast agent into the extradural space. This is sometimes called the sacral hiatus puncture method because of the location of needle insertion (Fig. 21-7). The procedure may be performed on an outpatient basis and has the added advantage that the contrast medium is readily absorbed and excreted by the kidneys.

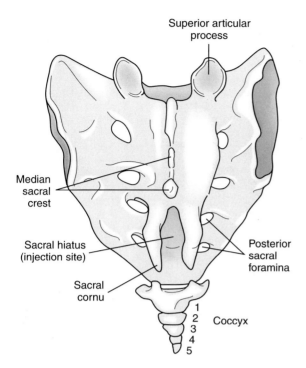

Superior articular process

Median sacral crest

Sacral hiatus (injection site)

Posterior sacral foramina

Sacral cornu

1
2
3
4
5
Coccyx

FIGURE 21-7. Illustration of the sacrum showing the sacral hiatus.

The patient is placed in the prone position between a footrest and shoulder harness. A small pad is placed under the lower abdomen to present the sacrum at the proper angle for needle insertion. The area is surgically prepared and infiltrated with local anesthetic. The needle is then inserted into the epidural space through the sacral hiatus. The needle position is confirmed radiographically, and 5 ml of anesthetic solution is injected. The angiographic table is then placed in a 30-degree Trendelenburg position, 20 ml of contrast agent is injected, the needle is withdrawn, and the puncture site is covered. Finally, the table is returned to its original position, and radiographs are made.

Computed Tomography of the Spine

CT is an important adjunct to the diagnosis of spinal cord pathology. The study is generally used to confirm a localized pathologic process that may or may not have been demonstrated by large-field myelography. If follow-up CT is indicated, the myelogram is usually obtained with a water-soluble iodinated contrast medium. This type of contrast agent provides improved resolution of the structures within the spinal canal. Figure 21-8 illustrates the images of the spinal cord and subarachnoid space as demonstrated by CT. Computed tomography is commonly used as a screening examination for patients with head trauma. The primary uses for CT in neuroradiology include the diagnosis of spinal stenosis, subarachnoid hemorrhage, acute head trauma, and cases in which metallic hardware would preclude the use of MRI. CT is still the study of choice when attempting to differentiate calcifications, especially those appearing in certain lesions such as chondrosarcoma, craniopharyngioma, and tuberous sclerosis.

Magnetic Resonance Imaging of the Spine

MRI is also used to image abnormalities of the spine and spinal cord. The development of surface coils that increase the signal-to-noise ratio and the use of various motion-compensating techniques to

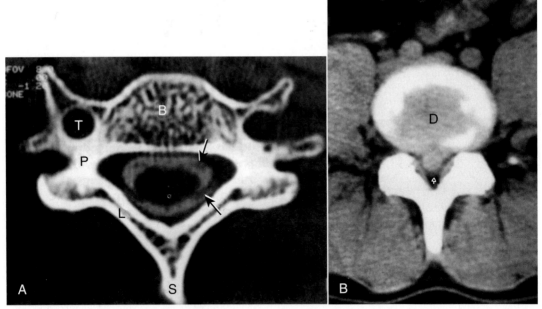

FIGURE 21-8. **A,** Axial computed tomographic (CT) image of a typical cervical vertebra showing the dorsal and ventral nerve rootlet *(arrows)* emerging from the spinal cord, body (*B*), transverse foramen (*T*), pedicle (*P*), lamina (*L*), and spinous process (*S*). **B,** Unenhanced CT of vertebra with central herniated disk (see *white arrow*). *D* refers to the appearance of both the disk and vertebral body with same density.

overcome the artifacts produced by the motion of the cerebrospinal fluid have made possible higher-quality images of vertebral anatomy. MRI is becoming the primary imaging modality for diagnosis of thoracic and lumbar spine pathology. The procedure is noninvasive and provides excellent soft tissue detail. Figure 21-9 shows some MR images of the cervical spine.

Historically, both pneumoencephalography and ventriculography were used to image pathology in the brain, but these studies are now obsolete, and the diagnosis of brain pathology has been replaced by MRI. MRI has also become the primary means of diagnosing a diverse group of intracranial abnormalities, including congenital anomalies as well as a variety of neoplastic disease processes and white matter lesions, especially in patients with multiple sclerosis. CT is frequently used for this procedure. MRI is also useful in the diagnosis of hemorrhage, vascular anomalies, and cerebral infarction.

EQUIPMENT

Myelography can be performed in any diagnostic radiographic room equipped with a tilting radiographic table and fluoroscopic unit. The radiographic table should be able to tilt in both directions to provide the positions required to move the contrast agent within the subarachnoid space. It should also be equipped with a footrest and shoulder harness to support the patient during the movement of the contrast material. Image intensification with monitoring facilitates the fluoroscopic portion of the examination.

A sterile spinal puncture tray should be available for use during myelography. Box 21-1 lists the equipment found in a typical sterile spinal myelography tray.

Because cross-table lateral views with a horizontal beam are usually made, some type of support should be available to hold the grid cassette at right angles to the x-ray beam.

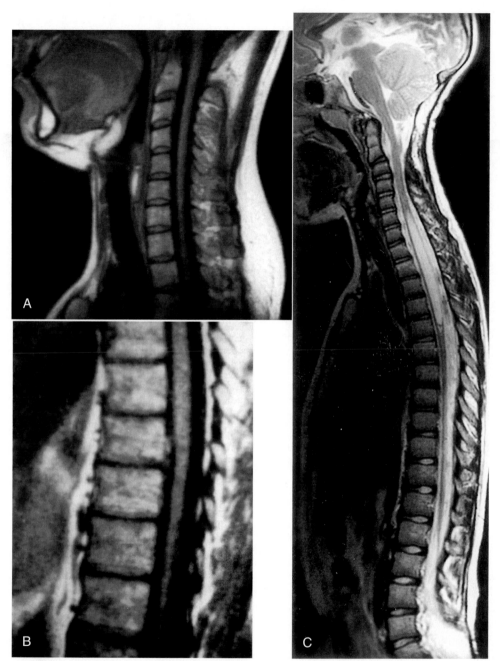

FIGURE 21-9. **A,** Magnetic resonance imaging of the normal cervical spine. **B,** T1 image of the thoracic spine showing herniation of the intervertebral disk. **C,** 48 FOV T2W1 MR image showing a Chiari II malformation.

PATIENT POSITIONING

After injection of the contrast agent, the radiographic table is moved through various positions while the flow of contrast material is monitored fluoroscopically. Spot films may be performed during this portion of the examination. Because myelography can be performed with either positive or negative contrast agents, the various postural maneuvers necessary for the distribution of the

BOX 21-1	*Equipment in a Typical Sterile Myelography Tray*
Equipment	**Amount and Size**
Spinal manometer	1
Three-way stopcock (not Luer-Lok)	1
Luer-Lok syringe	1 (2 ml)
Luer-Lok syringe	1 (5 ml)
Luer-Lok syringe	1 (10 ml)
Medicine glass	1
Hemostat	1
Towel	1
Applicators	3 (6 in)
Gauge needles	1 each (18 and 22 gauge)
Needle	1 (^{5}/$_8$ in, 25 gauge)
Topper sponges	12 (3 × 3 in)
Specimen tubes with black rubber corks	3
Surgical drape	1

contrast agent will differ. Of course, this is a result of the physical properties of the contrast agent. Both the postural maneuvers and fluoroscopic portion of the procedure vary considerably with the type of contrast agent (positive or negative) used and with the area of the spinal cord under examination; because they are under the direct control of the radiographer performing the procedure, a detailed description is not given in this text. However, the various radiographic positions required at the conclusion of the fluoroscopic portion of the procedure are discussed. Because positive contrast myelography is performed more often, positioning relevant to this method is presented.

In general, most radiographs are taken with a horizontal beam directed across the table at a grid cassette. Occasionally, the vertical beam projections may be requested by the physician. The anatomy demonstrated will vary with the region under examination.

Lumbar Myelography

In this region, four views may be taken, three of which are performed with a horizontal beam.

Cross-Table Lateral Projection

In this view, the patient is prone. A 10- × 12-in (25-× 30-cm) grid cassette is supported on the side of the patient opposite the table. The exact level of the image receptor is determined by the radiographer performing the examination. The central ray is directed across the table to the midpoint of the image receptor. The structures demonstrated are lateral views of the vertebral bodies, intervertebral spaces of the lumbar vertebrae, and lumbar subarachnoid space (Fig. 21-10).

A variation of this basic position can be done to demonstrate the lowest portion of the lumbar subarachnoid space. The patient is in the same position as in the previous view; however, the radiographic table is raised into a semiupright position that allows the positive contrast agent to drop to the lowest portion of the subarachnoid space. A cross-table lateral view is performed, with the image receptor centered to the level of the L5–S1 interspace.

Cross-Table Oblique Projection

The patient is placed in a 45-degree right or left anterior oblique position. A 10- × 12-in (25- × 30-cm) grid cassette is supported next to the patient, centered at about the level of the L4–L5 interspace (Fig. 21-11). The central ray is directed horizontally (across the table) at a right angle to the midpoint of the image receptor. Collimation to the field size or area of interest is essential for good detail. This view demonstrates the lumbar subarachnoid space in an oblique projection.

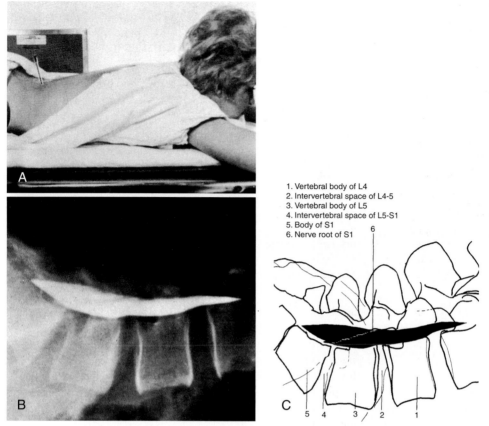

1. Vertebral body of L4
2. Intervertebral space of L4-5
3. Vertebral body of L5
4. Intervertebral space of L5-S1
5. Body of S1
6. Nerve root of S1

FIGURE 21-10. The cross-table lateral projection. **A,** The cross-table lateral projection. **B,** Radiograph. **C,** Labeled tracing showing the contrast column in the lumbar region.

Cross-Table Lateral Decubitus Projection

The patient is turned into a true lateral position with the knees and hips flexed (Fig. 21-12). A 14- × 17-in (35- × 42.5-cm) grid cassette is placed against the patient's abdomen to include the entire lumbar area. (If the needle has been removed, the image receptor may be placed against the patient's back.) The central ray is directed at a right angle to the midpoint of the image receptor. Collimation of the beam ensures maximum detail.

Posteroanterior Projection with Vertical Beam

For the frontal view, the patient is placed in the prone position and centered to the midline of the table. An 11- × 14-in (27.5- × 35-cm) image receptor may be used, centered to the L4–L5 interspace. The central ray is directed at a right angle to the film. The Bucky should be used to maximize detail, and collimation should be to field size.

Thoracic Myelography

The additional overhead tube views required for thoracic myelography are essentially the same as for lumbar myelography. The major difference is in the image receptor size used. For all views in the thoracic region, a 14- × 17-in (35- × 42.5-cm) image receptor should be used. As in lumbar myelography, collimation is critical to maximize detail.

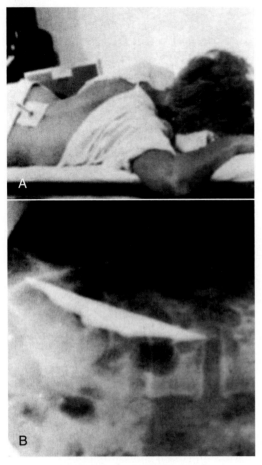

FIGURE 21-11. The cross-table oblique projection. **A**, The cross-table oblique projection. **B**, Radiograph. **C**, Labeled tracing showing an oblique view of the lumbar region with the contrast column.

1. Axillary pouch of nerve root of L5
2. Nerve root of S1
3. Axillary pouch of nerve root of S1

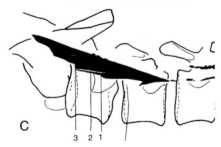

Cervical Myelography

In general, only cross-table lateral views with the overhead tube are taken during cervical myelography. Frontal views are usually not requested because the patient's head must remain hyperextended. This is required to prevent the contrast material from entering the skull, because it cannot return to the cervical region.

In the routine cross-table lateral view, the lower cervical and upper thoracic regions are not well demonstrated. A specialized view is required to eliminate the superimposition of the shoulders—Twining's view or the swimmer's view.

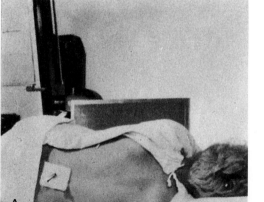

FIGURE 21-12. The cross-table lateral decubitus projection. **A,** The cross-table lateral decubitus projection position. **B,** Radiograph. **C,** Labeled tracing depicting the lumbar region with the needle in situ.

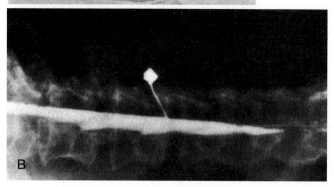

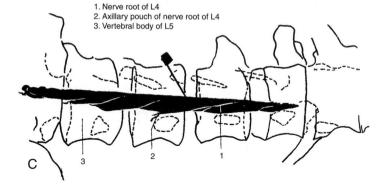

1. Nerve root of L4
2. Axillary pouch of nerve root of L4
3. Vertebral body of L5

Swimmer's View

The patient is placed in the prone position with the head hyperextended and the median sagittal plane perpendicular to the table. The arm closest to the tube is placed next to the patient, and the opposite hand is placed above the patient's head. This position is comparable to the body's position while swimming (Fig. 21-13). A 10- × 12-in (25- × 27.5-cm) grid is supported next to the patient, centered at the level of the seventh cervical vertebra. The central ray is directed at a right angle to the cassette. The radiographic table should be tilted up slightly to pool the contrast agent in the desired area. Detail is maximized by collimating the field size.

A summary of the overhead tube positions for opaque myelography is presented in Table 21-1.

TABLE 21-1 *Positioning for Opaque Myelography*

Region Examined	Projection	Patient Position	Central Ray	Anatomy
Cervical	Cross-table lateral	Patient prone, midsagittal plane perpendicular to table, head hyperextended, arms at side	Horizontal cross-table to enter at C3, perpendicular to center of image receptor*	C1–C6, posterior margin of foramen magnum, clivus, cervical subarachnoid space
	Swimmer's	Patient prone, midsagittal plane perpendicular to table, head hyperextended, one arm at side, other arm above head	Horizontal cross-table to enter at C7, perpendicular to center of image receptor*	Lower cervical and upper thoracic regions
Thoracic	Cross-table lateral	Patient prone, arms raised	Horizontal transtable to enter at T7, perpendicular to center of image receptor*	Lateral view of thoracic subarachnoid space
	Cross-table lateral decubitus	Patient in right or left lateral position, arms raised	Horizontal cross-table to enter at T7, perpendicular to center of image receptor*	Lateral decubitus view of thoracic subarachnoid space
Lumbar	Cross-table lateral	Patient prone, arms raised, table either horizontal or slightly upright	Horizontal cross-table, perpendicular to center of image receptor*	Lateral lumbosacral region from L3–S1; with horizontal table, lateral view of lowest portion of subarachnoid space, vertebral bodies from L4 to coccyx
	Cross-table oblique	Right or left anterior oblique, arms raised	Horizontal cross-table, perpendicular to midpoint of image receptor*	Oblique view of lumbar subarachnoid space
	Cross-table lateral	Right or left lateral position, arms raised, knees and hips flexed	Horizontal cross-table, perpendicular to midpoint of image receptor*	Lateral decubitus view of lumbar subarachnoid space
	Posteroanterior	Prone position, arms flexed	Vertical beam to enter at L4–L5 interspace at right angles to image receptor*	Frontal view of lumbar subarachnoid space

*Conventional film/screen systems require a grid.

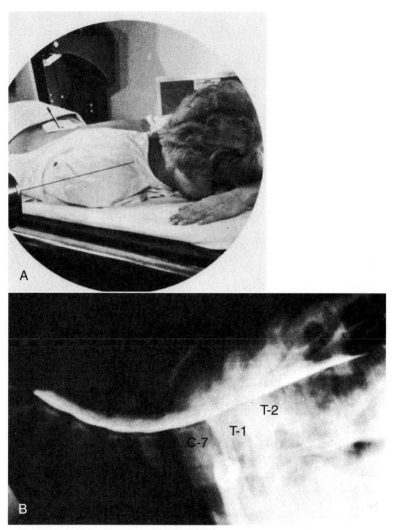

FIGURE 21-13. Swimmer's projection. **A,** The patient positioned for the swimmer's projection. **B,** Radiograph of the cervical region showing the contrast column.

SUMMARY

Myelography is used to provide an accurate diagnosis of structural abnormalities of the spinal cord and spinal canal. The nervous system consists of the brain ventricular system and spinal cord. Three layers of tissue enclose the spinal cord and brain. These are the dura mater, pia mater, and arachnoid. The space between the pia mater and arachnoid layers is referred to as the subarachnoid space. The injection of contrast medium into this space is the basic premise for myelography. Water-soluble organic iodine compounds are used to provide the necessary contrast to visualize the structures of the nervous system. The contrast agent readily mixes with the cerebrospinal fluid and can be positioned at the three levels of the spine: cervical, thoracic, and lumbar.

The procedure can be done as an ambulatory outpatient study. Because it is an invasive study, an informed consent document must be negotiated with the patient or the legal guardian. Medications should be suspended for at least 24 hours prior to the procedure. The patient should also be instructed to increase the intake of fluid to reduce the potential for contrast medium reactions. The injection site for lumbar myelography is between the L2–L3 interspace. Thoracic and cervical myelography can use a lower position for the needle insertion, often between L3–L4 or L4–L5.

CT and MRI are being used as alternative diagnostic methods for this study. Each of the modalities has advantages and disadvantages that dictate when each should be used.

The patient positioning varies with the area being studied and the preference of the physician performing the procedure. Myelography is a safe procedure for the demonstration of the structures located in the nervous system.

SUGGESTED READINGS

Botwin KP, Skene G, Tourres-Ramos FM, et al: Role of weight-bearing flexion and extension myelography in evaluating the intervertebral disc. *Am J Phys Med Rehabil* 80(4):289–295, 2001.

Cissoko H, Lemesle F, Jonville-Bera AP, et al: Aseptic meningitis after iohexol myelography. *Ann Pharmacother* 34(6):812–813, 2000.

Eames FA, Cloft HJ: Discontinuing patient medications prior to myelography. *AJR Am J Roentgenol* 184(2):695, 2005.

Hayman LA, Fuller GN, Cavazos JE, et al: The hippocampus; normal anatomy and pathology. *AJR AM J Roentgenol* 171:1139–1146, 1998.

Herzog RJ: Radiologic imaging in spinal stenosis. *Instr Course Lect* 50:137–144, 2001.

Katayama H, Heneine N, van Gessel R, et al: Clinical experience with iomeprol in myelography and myelo-CT: clinical pharmacology and double-blind comparisons with iopamidol, iohexol, and iotrolan. *Invest Radiol* 36(1):22–32, 2001.

Klein KM, Shiratori K, Knake S, et al: Status epilepticus and seizures induced by iopamidol myelography. *Seizure* 13(3):196–199, 2004.

Kufeld M, Claus B, Campi A, et al: Three-dimensional rotational myelography. *AJNR Am J Neuroradiol* 24(7):1290–1293, 2003.

Maly P, Sundgren P, Baath L, et al: Adverse reactions in myelography. *Acta Radiol* (suppl) 399:230–237, 1995.

Miller GM, Krauss WE: Myelography: still the gold standard. *AJNR Am J Neuroradiol* 24(3):298, 2003.

Murata Y, Yamagata M, Ogata S, et al: The influence of early ambulation and other factors on headache after lumbar myelography. *J Bone Joint Surg Br* 85(4):531–534, 2003.

Ruberu NN, Saito Y, Honma N, et al: Granulomatous meningitis as a late complication of iodized oil myelography. *Neuropathology* 24(2):144–148, 2004.

Smith RR: Myelographic complications associated with drug interactions. *AJR Am J Roentgenol* 177(3):713, 2001.

STUDY QUESTIONS

1. When using the sacral hiatus puncture method for myelography the contrast material is injected into the:
   a. left ventricle
   b. extradural space
   c. subarachnoid space
   d. cisterna magna

2. The injection site for lumbar myelography is usually between:
   a. L1–L2
   b. L2– L3
   c. L4–L5
   d. T12–L1

3. The leptomeninges are composed of the:
   a. arachnoid and pia mater
   b. pia mater and dura mater
   c. dura mater and arachnoid
   d. spinal cord and dura mater

STUDY QUESTIONS (*cont'd*)

4. The movement of certain contrast agents by gravity is because the agents are:
   a. hyperbaric
   b. hypobaric
   c. equal to the consistency of cerebrospinal fluid
   d. less viscous than cerebrospinal fluid

5. When the lower cervical and upper thoracic regions are not well demonstrated the _____ should be used.
   a. left lateral decubitus position
   b. anteroposterior view
   c. right internal oblique view
   d. swimmer's view

6. The cisternal puncture method is used when:
   a. the patient is extremely obese
   b. the lower extremities cannot be flexed
   c. the lumbar puncture approach is impossible
   d. contrast agent is required to flow into the ventricles

7. Which of the following is not considered to be a part of the brain?
   a. pons
   b. medulla oblongata
   c. filum terminale
   d. mesencephalon

8. The largest and uppermost portion of the brain is called the:
   a. pons
   b. hindbrain
   c. cerebrum
   d. filum terminale

9. Which of the following pieces of equipment is not necessary for myelography?
   a. footrest
   b. fluoroscope
   c. shoulder harness
   d. catheter

10. A disadvantage to the use of the oily contrast agents is:
    a. their higher cost
    b. that they are absorbed slowly and must be removed from the patient
    c. that they do not provide sufficient contrast
    d. that patients tend to have more reactions to the substance

22 *Sialography*

The radiographic visualization of the salivary glands and ducts is called sialography. The evaluation of the salivary glands is most often accomplished with computed tomography or magnetic resonance imaging; however, sialography becomes the method of choice when a definitive diagnosis is required for pathology such as sialadenitis (inflammation of the salivary glands) and the oral component of 'Sjögren's syndrome (an autoimmune disease process that causes dry eyes and dry mouth). Sialography involves the introduction of a water-soluble contrast agent into the orifices of the salivary ducts. In most cases, this procedure requires a minimum of specialized equipment and can be performed in a regular radiographic or fluoroscopic room.

ANATOMIC CONSIDERATIONS

The salivary glands secrete saliva into the mouth. Saliva is a liquid that is approximately 99% water. The salivary glands secrete between 1000 and 2000 ml of saliva every day. Found in the saliva are basically

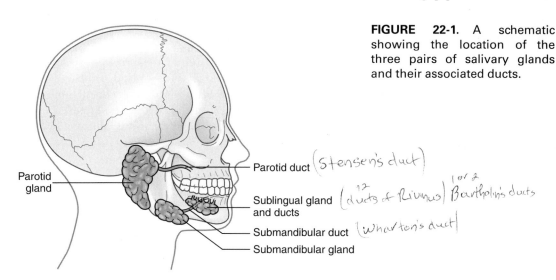

FIGURE 22-1. A schematic showing the location of the three pairs of salivary glands and their associated ducts.

Parotid duct (Stensen's duct)

Parotid gland

Sublingual gland and ducts (12 ducts of Rivinus) Bartholin's ducts 1 or 2

Submandibular duct (Wharton's duct)

Submandibular gland

two types of materials secreted by the salivary glands—**mucus**, a combination of mucin and water that is a very viscous substance used to lubricate food particles and maintain oral hygiene, and **serous fluid**, which contains the enzyme amylase, a substance that begins the digestive process of starches.

There are three pairs of salivary glands—the **parotid** glands, **submandibular** glands, and **sublingual** glands (Fig. 22-1).

Parotid Glands

These are the largest of the salivary glands, with each consisting of a superficial and a deep portion. The parotid glands lie anterior and somewhat inferior to the ear. The deep portion of the parotid gland extends into the neck approximately 0.75 in below and behind the angle of the mandible. The **parotid duct**, also called **Stensen's duct**, is between 5 and 7 cm long. It courses across and to the anterior margin of the masseter muscle, where it turns medially, opening into the mouth opposite the second upper molar tooth. Occasionally, a small accessory lobe may be found, the socia parotidis.

Submandibular Glands

The submandibular glands, also called the submaxillary glands, lie medial to the body of the mandible, with each gland also composed of a superficial and a deep portion. The superficial portion is inferior and anterior to the angle of the mandible, where its posterior portion can be found next to the apex of the parotid gland. It extends anteriorly along the mandibular body. A small, deep portion of the gland curves around the posterior border of the mylohyoid muscle and extends into it. The **submandibular duct**, also called **Wharton's duct**, arises from this deep portion. It averages approximately 5 cm in length, passing anteriorly and medially to the mandible and opening at the sides of the base of the frenulum.

Sublingual Glands

These are the smallest of the three pairs of salivary glands. They are located under the mucosa of the mouth and form a longitudinal ridge at either side of the base of the tongue, the sublingual fold. The sublingual glands, unlike the parotid or submandibular glands, do not have a single duct. There are approximately 12 smaller **sublingual ducts**, the **ducts of Rivinus**, coming from the superior border of the gland to open at the sublingual fold. One or two of these ducts, Bartholin's ducts, may open into the submaxillary duct.

INDICATIONS AND CONTRAINDICATIONS

Sialography is used to demonstrate the relation of the salivary glands to their adjacent structures. It provides both diagnostic and preoperative information in cases of salivary gland pathology. Other indications for sialography are calculi, strictures of the ducts, sialectasia (dilation of a duct), fistulas, and demonstration of pleomorphic salivary gland tumors, commonly called mixed parotid tumors.

Contraindications for this procedure include severe inflammation of the salivary ducts and history of sensitivity to iodinated contrast media.

CONTRAST AGENTS

Two types of contrast media—water-soluble and oily—are used to opacify the salivary glands. The final choice remains with the physician performing the procedure. Certain factors govern the use of a specific type of contrast medium for a particular procedure. Contrast media, such as Ethiodol, have a very slow excretion rate and can cause granulomatous tissue formation, which can be disadvantageous in cases in which complete removal of the contrast medium is impossible. It contains 37% iodine (475 mg/ml) combined with *ethyl* esters of the fatty acids of poppyseed oil. This type of contrast medium provides a greater density in the ducts and parenchyma when tomography is used. For routine sialography, a water-soluble contrast medium is usually used.

PATIENT PREPARATION

Sialography does not require specific preprocedural preparation by the patient. A history should be taken before the study to determine if the patient has allergies or has had prior reactions to iodinated contrast media. It is important to have the patient remove any radiopaque materials such as false teeth or removable bridgework prior to the examination. The patient should be monitored for signs of reaction during the examination. At the conclusion of the study, the patient is usually given a secretory stimulant to clear the contrast medium from the gland and ducts.

PROCEDURE

Scout films of the area of interest may or may not be taken. In cases of suspected **sialolithiasis** (salivary gland or salivary duct calculi), scout films are mandatory. In cases in which scout films are not taken, stones may be obliterated by the contrast medium, causing an inaccurate diagnosis to be made. The study may be performed with fluoroscopic visualization and spot filming as well as with overhead radiographic projections. Computed tomography, ultrasonography, and magnetic resonance imaging are replacing conventional sialography. Although the primary means of diagnosis has been ultrasonography, conventional sialography still has a place in the realm of interventional radiography for the treatment of pathology of the salivary glands.

After scout films have been taken, the radiologist locates the orifices of the salivary ducts by having the patient express some saliva. The physician can either palpate the salivary gland or have the patient suck on a lemon slice. When the salivary duct is located, it is dilated with standard double-ended blunt dilators or with silver lacrimal probes. After dilation of the orifice, the duct is cannulated. Several types of cannulas are available, but the use of a modified Abbott butterfly set has proved successful in most cases, especially if the patient has to be moved to another location for additional study. The modification is accomplished by filing the beveled tip of the needle flat and smooth with a medium-fine metal file. The wings of the butterfly are then secured with a hemostat. This allows for ease of insertion of the cannula into the duct. The cannula should be prefilled with the contrast medium to avoid injection of air bubbles.

After the duct has been successfully cannulated, the cannula is immobilized. When the modified butterfly setup is used, the patient is instructed to close the mouth. When a blunt-tipped or other type of cannula is used, a folded piece of sterile gauze is placed between the cannula and the tongue; the tubing is held in place by closing the mouth and lips around it. The tubing and syringe are taped to the shoulder or chest, and the contrast medium is then slowly injected. This is usually done with fluoroscopy and spot films. Overhead films or tomography may also be done at this time. Occasionally, delayed films may be requested to determine functional emptying of the gland. There are two major methods of injecting the contrast agent—manual and hydrostatic. Manual injection is accomplished as described previously. The hydrostatic method uses gravity to introduce the contrast agent. The syringe barrel, with the plunger removed, is secured to an intravenous pole about 25 to 30 cm above the level of the salivary duct. Filling is accomplished slowly and is usually monitored with fluoroscopy.

This procedure may be used for parotid and submandibular sialography. Once Wharton's duct has been entered for sublingual sialography, the cannula should not be advanced too far. This allows the sublingual ducts located just behind the orifice to be filled. Sublingual sialography is not usually feasible because of the anatomic structure of the sublingual ductal system. In some patients, however, because of anatomic variations that provide access through Wharton's duct or, in rare cases, through a single sublingual duct anomaly, retrograde filling of the sublingual duct system is possible.

EQUIPMENT

Sialography can be performed in any radiographic or fluoroscopic room. Most supplies needed for this study can be found in any radiology department and assembled just before the examination or in the form of a prepackaged sialography setup. The system used will depend on the number of studies done.

The supplies required will vary according to the type of cannula preferred by the physician. A typical sialography setup is given in Box 22-1. Additional necessary items are sterile disposable gloves, anesthetic (topical), and contrast agent of choice. The sterile setup will vary with the preference of the radiologist performing the procedure, and it may be necessary to have two or more different types of setups to provide for the physician's preference.

PATIENT POSITIONING

In most cases, fluoroscopy is used to monitor the filling of the salivary glands with the contrast medium. The radiologist performing the procedure usually takes spot film radiographs in several different positions. Overhead radiography is then done to include lateral, anteroposterior, posteroanterior, tangential, and basal projections or specific combinations as required by the radiographer. Tomography or computed tomography may also be performed as part of the procedure. In cases of ductal obstruction or **sialectasia**, delayed films are requested to evaluate gland and duct functions.

BOX 22-1   *Contents of Typical Sialography Tray*

Equipment	Amount, Type, and Size
Syringe	1 ($2^1/_2$ or 3 ml)
Adhesive tape	1 roll ($^1/_2$ in)
Cotton swabs	2–3
Extension tubing	1 (size dependent on cannula used)
Gauze pads	10 (4 × 4 in)
Cannulas	4 (blunt-tipped, single sideport; 19, 21, 23, and 25 gauge)*
Cannulas	4 (modified butterfly setup; 19, 21, 23, and 25 gauge)*

*Size used depends on the duct size.

Anteroposterior Projections
Standard Anteroposterior Projection

In this projection, the patient is placed in either the supine recumbent or the erect position. The head is adjusted to a true anteroposterior position with the median sagittal plane perpendicular to the table. The patient's chin is depressed toward the chest to place the orbitomeatal baseline perpendicular to the film. The image receptor should be centered just below the patient's mouth. The beam is collimated to the film size, and the central ray is directed perpendicular to the midpoint of the image receptor. This projection is used primarily to demonstrate the parotid gland.

Tangential Anteroposterior Projection

The patient is placed in either the supine recumbent or the erect position. The head is adjusted so that the acanthomeatal line is at a right angle to the image receptor. The patient's head is rotated slightly toward the affected side. The amount of rotation should be just enough to place the parotid gland at a right angle to the image receptor. The angle of the mandible should be centered to the film. The central ray is directed at a right angle to the midpoint of the image receptor.

Posteroanterior Projections

The positioning techniques for these projections produce views similar to those taken in the anteroposterior projections. The parotid gland lies approximately midway between the anterior and posterior aspects of the body, allowing for either anteroposterior or posteroanterior positioning of the patient.

Standard Posteroanterior Projection

In this projection, the patient is placed in either the prone recumbent or the erect position. The nose and forehead are placed against the image receptor. The patient's head is adjusted to a true posteroanterior position, with the orbitomeatal baseline at a right angle to the film. The image receptor should be centered approximately 2½ in inferior to the gonion. The central ray should be directed at a right angle to the image receptor.

Tangential Posteroanterior Projection

The patient is placed in either the prone recumbent or the erect position with the chin and nose in contact with the image receptor. The head is rotated so that the longitudinal axis of the mandibular body is perpendicular to the film. The vertical plane is centered so that it runs through the angle of the mandible to the center of the image receptor. The central ray is directed at a right angle to the midpoint of the image receptor.

Lateral Projections
True Lateral Projection

The patient is placed in the seated, erect, or semiprone position. The head is adjusted to a true lateral position. The median sagittal plane is parallel to the image receptor. The neck should be slightly extended to prevent possible superimposition of the salivary glands with the cervical spine. The central ray is directed at a right angle to the midpoint of the image receptor, entering at a point approximately 1 in anterior to the external auditory meatus.

Modified Lateral Projection

The patient is placed in the seated, erect, or semiprone position with the affected side down. The head is adjusted to a true lateral position and rotated forward 15 degrees. The skull is centered to a point approximately 1 in anterior to the external auditory meatus. The central ray is directed at a right angle to the midpoint of the image receptor.

TABLE 22-1　*Positions for Sialography*

Projection	Patient Position	Central Ray	Image Receptor Size	Anatomy
Lateral oblique	Semiprone or seated erect; head in true lateral position (midsagittal plane parallel to image receptor)	Tube angled 25° cephalad to enter inferior to and just behind angle of upper mandible	8 × 10 in (20 × 25 cm)	Parotid gland
Lateral (true)	Seated erect or semiprone; head in true lateral position (midsagittal plane parallel to image receptor); neck slightly extended	Directed perpendicular to midpoint of image receptor	8 × 10 in (20 × 25 cm)	Submaxillary gland
Lateral (modified)	Seated erect or semiprone; head in modified lateral position (midsagittal plane rotated forward approximately 15°)	Directed perpendicular to midpoint of image receptor	8 × 10 in (20 × 25 cm)	Parotid gland
Inferosuperior occlusal	Supine with shoulders and thorax supported; head in submentovertical position (fully extended); transverse axis of body parallel to table	Directed perpendicular to plane of occlusal packet	Occlusal	Submaxillary gland, sublingual gland
Tangential posteroanterior	Prone or erect; chin and nose in contact with image receptor; longitudinal axis of mandibular body perpendicular to image receptor; center angle of mandible to the center of image receptor	Directed perpendicular to midpoint of image receptor	8 × 10 in (20 × 25 cm)	Parotid gland
Tangential anteroposterior	Supine or erect; orbitomeatal line perpendicular to image receptor; head rotated slightly toward affected side; center angle of mandible to the image receptor	Directed perpendicular to midpoint of image receptor	8 × 10 in (20 × 25 cm)	Parotid gland

Continued

Fundamentals of Special Radiographic Procedures

TABLE 22-1 *Positions for Sialography (cont'd)*

Projection	Patient Position	Central Ray	Image Receptor Size	Anatomy
Posteroanterior	Prone or erect; nose and forehead against image receptor, centered 2½ in inferior to gonion; head adjusted to true posteroanterior position; orbitomeatal baseline perpendicular to image receptor	Directed perpendicular to midpoint of image receptor	8 × 10 in (20 × 25 cm)	Parotid gland
Anteroposterior	Supine or erect; chin depressed toward chest; orbitomeatal baseline placed perpendicular to film by centering the image receptor just below the mouth	Directed perpendicular to midpoint of image receptor	8 × 10 in (20 × 25 cm)	Parotid gland

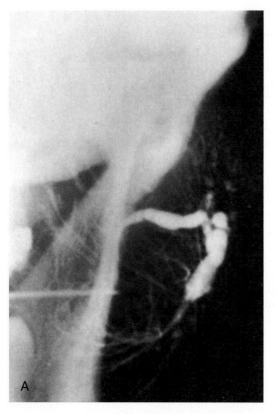

A

FIGURE 22-2. Representative sialographic radiographs. **A,** Anteroposterior projection.

Continued

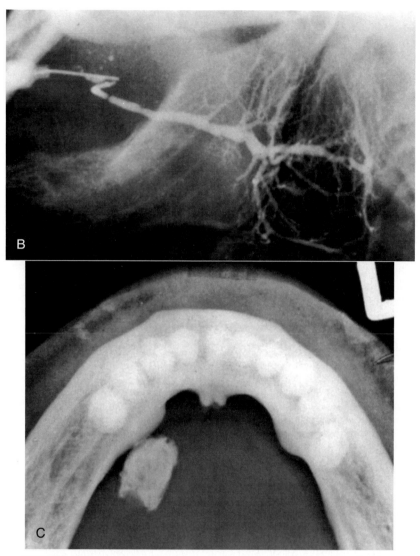

FIGURE 22-2, *cont'd.* **B**, Lateral projection. **C**, Occlusal projection.

Lateral Oblique Projection

With the patient in either an erect, seated, or semiprone position, the head is placed in a true lateral position and centered at the level of the external auditory meatus. The central ray is directed at an angle of 25 degrees cephalad to the midpoint of the image receptor.

Inferosuperior (Occlusal) Projection

The patient is placed in the supine position. The shoulders and thorax are supported by a pillow or folded sheets. The head is gently dropped into a submentovertical position, with the neck fully extended. The median sagittal plane should be perpendicular to the film. The transverse axis of the body is adjusted so that it is parallel with the table. An occlusal film is inserted into the patient's mouth. Placement of the packet depends on the gland to be radiographed. The packet should be inserted lengthwise when the submaxillary gland is opacified; when the sublingual glands are radiographed, the packet should be placed more anteriorly in the mouth and can be inserted crosswise. The central ray is directed at a right angle to the plane of the film.

Table 22-1 summarizes the positions used during sialography. Figure 22-2 illustrates some representative radiographs taken during sialography.

SUMMARY

Salivary gland pathology has been successfully diagnosed using sialography. The procedure involves the introduction of a water-soluble contrast agent into the affected salivary gland followed by imaging. There are three pairs of salivary glands: the parotid, which is the largest; the submandibular; and the sublingual glands.

Imaging of the salivary glands is most commonly accomplished using computed tomography and magnetic resonance imaging. Conventional sialography is performed in cases in which a definitive diagnosis of sialadenitis, salivary calculus, or Sjögren's syndrome is required.

The procedure is simply performed by cannulation of the specific salivary duct with a small-gauge needle. The duct is dilated, and the contrast agent is administered. Filming is then accomplished. The study carries no major complications with the exception of possible reaction to the contrast medium used.

SUGGESTED READINGS

Baurmash HD: Submandibular salivary stones: current management modalities. *J Oral Maxillofac Surg* 62(3):369–378, 2004.

Bull PD: Salivary gland stones: diagnosis and treatment. *Hosp Med* 62(7):396–399, 2001.

Drage NA, Brown JE, Escudier MP, et al: Balloon dilatation of salivary duct strictures: report on 36 treated glands. *Cardiovasc Intervent Radiol* 25(5):356–359, 2002.

Freling NJ: Imaging of salivary gland disease. *Semin Roentgenol* 35(1):12–20, 2000.

Heverhagen JT, Kalinowski M, Rehberg E, et al: Prospective comparison of magnetic resonance sialography and digital subtraction sialography. *J Magn Reson Imaging* 11(5):518–524, 2000.

Salerno S, Cannizzaro F, Lo Casto A, et al: Late allergic reaction following sialography. *Dentomaxillofac Radiol* 31(2):154, 2002.

Shojaku H, Shojaku H, Shimizu M, Seto H, Watanabe Y: MR Sialographic evaluation of sialectasia of Stensen's duct: comparison with x-ray sialography and ultrasonography. *Radiat Med* 18(2):143–145, 2000.

Thomas DV, Wolinski AP: Submandibular calculus on conventional sialography. Accessed online at URL *http//www.eurorad.org/case.cfm?UID=1446*, 2002.

Yousem DM, Kraut MA, Chalian AA: Major salivary gland imaging. *Radiology* 216(1):19–29, 2000.

Zabel K: Sialography puts recurrent parotid sialadenitis on hold, *Dermatology Times*, 1011, 1997.

STUDY QUESTIONS

1. Wharton's duct opens in the mouth:
   a. within the masseter muscle
   b. at the base of the frenulum
   c. 0.75 in below and behind the angle of the mandible
   d. at the level of the social parotidis

2. A contraindication of sialography includes:
   a. sialectasia
   b. severe inflammation of the salivary glands
   c. calculi
   d. strictures

STUDY QUESTIONS (*cont'd*)

3. The use of oily contrast agents can cause:
   a. a loss of contrast
   b. reduction in the visualization of calculi
   c. granulomatous tissue reactions
   d. pleomorphic necrosis

4. In sublingual sialography the cannula is inserted into:
   a. the masseter muscle
   b. Stensen's duct
   c. Wharton's duct
   d. mylohyoid muscle

5. At the conclusion of the study the patient:
   a. is required to have 24 hours of bed rest
   b. is sent home with the cannula in place
   c. is given a secretory stimulant to purge the salivary glands
   d. is treated with anticoagulant medication

6. The use of an intravenous setup approximately 30 cm above the duct introduces the contrast agent:
   a. rapidly
   b. by hydrostatic pressure
   c. in a greater concentration
   d. while monitored by conventional radiography filming

7. In the inferosuperior projection the occlusal film is positioned _____ when filming the submaxillary gland.
   a. crosswise
   b. lengthwise
   c. at the top of the head
   d. against the angle of the mandible

8. In the lateral oblique projection the central ray is directed at an angle of _____ to the film.
   a. 20 degrees caudad
   b. 20 degrees cephalad
   c. 25 degrees caudad
   d. 25 degrees cephalad

9. The smallest of the salivary glands are the
   a. submaxillary
   b. submandibular
   c. sublingual
   d. parotid

10. Which of the following pathologic conditions would require that a scout film be taken before the procedure begins?
    a. stenosis
    b. sialolithiasis
    c. sialectasia
    d. granulomatous tissue formation

23 *Arthrography*

Radiography of a joint space and its surrounding structures is called arthrography. The many joints in the human body vary in structure and arrangement. They are freely movable (diarthrodial), slightly movable (amphiarthrodial), or immovable (synarthrodial). All joints are junctions between bones or between cartilage and bone.

Joints can be grouped by structural feature into three groups—fibrous, cartilaginous, and synovial. Fibrous and cartilaginous joints permit very little movement, if any. Synovial joints, on the other hand, permit free movement of the articulating bones. Arthrography is exclusively concerned with this last group of joints. Figure 23-1 shows the joints exhibiting diarthrosis (free movement) and synarthrosis (fibrous and cartilaginous).

ANATOMIC CONSIDERATIONS

Synovial joints are classified according to axis of movement, as follows:

Gliding or plane joint (e.g., articular processes of the vertebrae): permits a sliding of one surface on the other. Joint motion is limited by ligaments and surrounding structures.

Hinge joint (e.g., knee): allows movement in only one plane. The movements of this joint are flexion and extension.

Pivot joint (e.g., radial head): permits rotational movement around a pivot in one axis.

Ellipsoidal or condylar joint (e.g., wrist joint): an oval head or condyle articulates with an elliptic cavity. This joint exhibits movements of flexion, extension, adduction, abduction, and circumduction. An ellipsoidal joint is incapable of axial rotation.

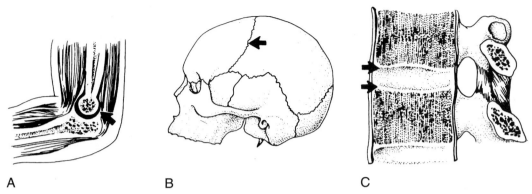

FIGURE 23-1. Diarthrotic and synarthrotic joints. **A,** Synovial joint. **B,** Fibrous joint. **C,** Cartilaginous joint.

Saddle joint (e.g., carpometacarpal joint of the thumb): similar to ellipsoidal or condyloid joints in its movements. Structurally, its articular surfaces are convex in one direction and concave in the other, at right angles to each other.

Ball-and-socket joint (e.g., hip joint): formed by a concave socket that receives a ball-shaped head. It permits movement in three axes—flexion, extension, adduction, abduction, and rotation.

A summary of the various individual synovial joints and their types and movements is presented in Table 23-1.

Synovial joints take their name from the fluid contained within the joint space (Fig. 23-2). **Synovial fluid** is a clear viscous fluid that serves primarily as a lubricant to facilitate joint movement. This fluid, along with the specialized articular surfaces and intra-articular structures (the menisci, disks, and fat pads), allows for almost frictionless movement of the joint surfaces.

Synovial fluid resembles the white of an egg in consistency, and it nourishes the hyaline cartilage lining the articular surfaces. The synovial fluid is produced by the synovial membrane, the inner lining of the joint capsule.

The synovial joint space is enclosed in a fibrous layer called the joint capsule. The fibers composing the joint capsule are arranged in irregular bundles that make them sensitive to any tension from the joint. Nerve endings are also located within the joint capsule; they pass impulses to the spinal cord and brain to transmit information regarding position and movement of the joint. The joint capsule attaches to the articulating bones just beyond the joint space uniting the bones of the joint.

The inner surface of the fibrous joint capsule is lined with a connective tissue called the synovial membrane. This membrane covers all the structures within the joint except the hyaline articular cartilage, menisci, and intra-articular disks. It produces the synovial fluid that lubricates the joint surfaces.

Hyaline articular cartilage is located on the bearing surfaces of the bones composing the joint. It does not contain nerve endings or blood vessels.

The intra-articular joint structures include the menisci, fat pads, synovial folds, and intra-articular disks. These intra-articular structures aid in providing efficient lubrication of the articular surfaces.

Ligaments may be present within the joint space as well as in the joint capsule. The accessory ligaments limit motion in undesirable directions and function as sense organs of motion and position.

Because joints constitute a mechanical system, wear and tear can be expected even though friction has been greatly reduced, and this usually results in the destruction of the hyaline articular cartilage. Other factors culminating in deterioration of the joints are trauma and disease.

TABLE 23-1   *Description of Individual Joints*

Joint	Articulating Bones	Type	Movement
Atlantoepistropheal	Anterior arch of atlas rotates about dens of axis (epistropheus)	Diarthrotic (pivot type)	Pivoting or partial rotation of head
Vertebral*	Between bodies of vertebrae	Synarthrotic cartilaginous; amphiarthrotic by other system of classification	Slight movement between any two vertebrae but considerable motility for column as whole
	Between articular processes	Diarthrotic (gliding)	
Clavicular			
Sternoclavicular	Medial end of clavicle with manubrium of sternum; only joint between upper extremity and trunk	Diarthrotic (gliding)	Gliding; weak joint that may be injured comparatively easily
Acromioclavicular	Distal end of clavicle with acromion of scapula	Diarthrotic (gliding)	Gliding; elevation, depression, protraction, and retraction
Thoracic	Heads of ribs with bodies of vertebrae	Diarthrotic (gliding)	Gliding
	Tubercles of ribs with transverse processes of vertebrae	Diarthrotic (gliding)	Gliding
Shoulder	Head of humerus in glenoid cavity of scapula	Diarthrotic (ball-and-socket type)	Flexion, extension, abduction, adduction, rotation, and circumduction of upper arm; one of most freely movable of joints
Elbow	Trochlea of humerus with semilunar notch of ulna; head of radius with capitulum of humerus	Diarthrotic (hinge type)	Flexion and extension
	Head of radius in radial notch of ulna	Diarthrotic (pivot type)	Supination and pronation of lower arm and hand; rotation of lower arm on upper, as in using screwdriver
Wrist	Scaphoid, lunate, and triquetral bones articulate with radius and articular disk	Diarthrotic (condyloid)	Flexion, extension, abduction, and adduction of hand
Carpal	Between various carpals	Diarthrotic (gliding)	Gliding
Hand	Proximal end of first metacarpal with trapezium	Diarthrotic (saddle)	Flexion, extension, abduction, adduction, and circumduction of thumb and opposition to fingers; motility of this joint accounts for dexterity of human hand compared with animal forepaw

Continued

TABLE 23-1   *Description of Individual Joints (cont'd)*

Joint	Articulating Bones	Type	Movement
	Distal end of metacarpals with proximal end of phalanges	Diarthrotic (hinge)	Flexion, extension, limited abduction, and adduction of finger
	Between phalanges	Diarthrotic (hinge)	Flexion and extension of finger sections
Sacroiliac	Between sacrum and two ilia	Diarthrotic (gliding); joint cavity mostly obliterated after middle life	None or slight (e.g., during late months of pregnancy and during delivery)
Symphysis pubis	Between two pubic bones	Synarthrotic (or amphiarthrotic), cartilaginous	Slight, particularly during pregnancy and delivery
Hip	Head of femur in acetabulum of os coxa	Diarthrotic (ball-and-socket type)	Flexion, extension, abduction, adduction, rotation, and circumduction
Knee	Between distal end of femur and proximal end of tibia; largest joint in body	Diarthrotic (hinge type)	Flexion and extension; slight rotation of tibia
Tibiofibular	Head of fibula with lateral condyle tibia	Diarthrotic (gliding type)	Gliding
Ankle	Distal ends of tibia and fibula with talus	Diarthrotic (hinge type)	Flexion (dorsiflexion) and extension (plantar flexion)
Foot	Between tarsals	Diarthrotic (gliding)	Gliding; inversion and eversion
	Between metatarsals and phalanges	Diarthrotic (hinge type)	Flexion, extension, slight abduction, and adduction
	Between phalanges	Diarthrotic (hinge type)	Flexion and extension

*Vertebrae are not easily dislocated. They are securely held by the following ligaments—anterior and posterior longitudinal ligaments (between anterior and posterior surfaces of bodies of vertebrae); supraspinous ligaments, called ligamentum nuchae in cervical region (between tops of spinous processes); interspinous ligaments (between sides of spinous processes); and ligamentum flavum (between laminae).

INDICATIONS AND CONTRAINDICATIONS

This procedure is used to obtain diagnostic information regarding the joints and surrounding soft tissues or cartilage. It has been used primarily in the investigation of the knee and shoulder joints; it has also shown its diagnostic value by demonstrating various diseases of the hip, elbow, ankle, and temporomandibular joints. Magnetic resonance imaging (MRI) has become the method of choice in the evaluation of many arthrographic disorders. The use of surface coils has improved the signal-to-noise ratio, which has had a profound effect on image resolution. MRI is used to study abnormalities in the knee, temporomandibular joint, hip, shoulder, wrist, and ankle.

Arthrography is a safe procedure that can be used to delineate the joint space and its surrounding structures, providing accurate diagnostic information concerning lesions of the menisci and other soft

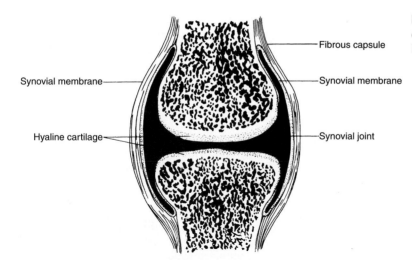

FIGURE 23-2. Schematic of a synovial joint, showing its major features.

Labels: Fibrous capsule, Synovial membrane, Synovial membrane, Synovial joint, Hyaline cartilage

tissue structures of the joint. It is indicated in cases of suspected injury to the meniscus of the joint, particularly tears. The procedure is also advised for the diagnosis of suspected capsular damage, rupture of the articular ligaments, cartilaginous defects, arthritic deformities (specifically of the temporo-mandibular joint), congenital luxation (dislocation) of the hip joint, and the extent of damage resulting from traumatic injuries of the joint. Subtalar arthrography is valuable in making the diagnosis of calcaneofibular ligament injury in recurrent instability of the ankle.[1]

There are relatively few absolute contraindications to arthrography. Hypersensitivity to iodine is a relative contraindication to positive contrast arthrography.

CONTRAST AGENTS

Arthrography can be performed with a negative contrast agent, positive contrast agent, or both.

Pneumoarthrography uses air or other easily absorbed gases. One disadvantage to the use of negative contrast agents is that large amounts are usually necessary (i.e., 100 to 150 ml), and this produces a somewhat painful distention of the joint. The diagnostic accuracy of the "air" study is considerably less than that when the other two contrast methods are used. This diminished diagnostic accuracy results because there is relatively little difference in density between the joint anatomy and the contrast medium. A possible hazard of pneumoarthrography is air embolism, which occurs rarely but cannot be totally disregarded.

Positive contrast arthrography is performed with nonionic, water-soluble contrast media because they are readily absorbed, are usually well tolerated, and are easily excreted by the body. They also produce arthrograms of greater diagnostic accuracy. The concentration of the positive contrast medium should be no more than 30%.

The double-contrast arthrogram combines the best of both methods to produce a highly accurate diagnostic study. With the use of both types of contrast medium, smaller amounts of each can be used, thus providing a more comfortable study for the patient and reducing the possibility of air embolism. The negative contrast agent provides a background for the small amount (approximately 5 to 10 ml) of positive contrast medium. The positive contrast agent coats the joint space, outlining the anatomy without the disadvantage of obscuring any small pathologic structures such as small bone fragments.

Magnetic resonance arthrography is performed using gadolinium as the contrast medium. Gadolinium is a clear substance that when injected into a vein accumulates in abnormal tissue. In its elemental state gadolinium (Gd) is considered to be highly toxic; however, as an injectable contrast agent for patients undergoing MRI the element is combined with ~~EDTA~~, rendering it safe.

DTPA : Diethylene Triamine Penta-acetic acid

Gadolinium can reduce relaxation times and thereby enhance signal intensity, making the tissue appear brighter. The safety of the substance has been proved, and the side effects are minimal. These can include mild headache, nausea and local pain, low blood pressure, allergic reactions, urticaria, and shortness of breath. Several companies manufacture the contrast medium, and it is sold under the trade names Magnevist (Berlex Laboratories), ProHance (Bracco Diagnostics), and Omniscan (Nycomed Amersham).

PROCEDURE

The arthrographic procedure varies with the site to be studied. It is a simple procedure and is useful for the investigation of all encapsulated joints. Arthrography, however, is an invasive procedure and can pose certain risks for the patient. Among these risks is the potential for reaction to the contrast agent. This type of reaction is relatively uncommon, but its occurrence should not be discounted. The most common type of reaction to the procedure is the vasovagal reaction, which can be triggered by fright, pain, or trauma. It is usually accompanied by nausea, perspiration, and pallor. Other possible reactions include allergy to the anesthetic agent and inflammatory synovitis.

MRI is becoming the modality of choice for evaluation of the various joint spaces, all but replacing the invasive procedures. The use of an intravenous gadolinium contrast agent can be used to enhance the joint and its fluid. Because this is the case, a discussion of the procedure as it applies to all possible joint spaces is not warranted. However, the presentation of the procedure as it applies to the knee should give the reader an idea of the process. There would necessarily be different requirements for arthrography of the other joints, as mentioned in the indications and contraindications section.

Radiographs may be taken by using either a vertical or horizontal x-ray beam or with the use of fluoroscopy and spot films. The horizontal beam method is generally used during double-contrast arthrography. With the use of a horizontal beam, smaller amounts of contrast agent can be used to produce a study that is more accurate and less uncomfortable to the patient. Arthrography should be carried out under strict aseptic conditions because infection of the joint can be a serious complication of the procedure. In single-contrast arthrography, the patient is placed in the supine position. Other positions for the injection may be used, depending on the physician's preference. The extremity under investigation can be placed in a special frame that widens the intrastructural spaces and allows the contrast agent to be distributed freely around the meniscus.

Because of the introduction of the contrast agent into the joint space the patient may experience a sensation of tightness in the joint. This could last as long as 24 hours after the procedure. Some additional pain can also be associated with the procedure but can easily be treated with analgesics. This should dissipate within 24 to 48 hours after the procedure.

When the knee has been properly positioned to permit easy entrance into the joint cavity, the needle is inserted behind the patella (retropatellar) with the tip directed toward its articular surface. Approximately 2 to 4 ml of anesthetic agent is then introduced. Synovial fluid is withdrawn, followed by injection of the contrast agent. When this has been completed, the joint is actively moved to spread the contrast medium into the articular surface of the joint. On completion of this maneuver, radiographs are taken of each side of the joint to demonstrate the anterior, middle, and posterior portions of the menisci.

Fluoroscopy is used extensively throughout the procedure, and spot films are taken to document any pathology. Fluoroscopy can also be used to localize the landmarks in the joint space. The radiographer draws a line on each side of the laterally placed knee to topographically locate each aspect of the tibial plateau. The extremity must be in maximal extension while this is being done. The identification of the landmarks is important for the closely coned radiographs that follow.

Double-contrast arthrography demonstrates the menisci to best advantage and is useful when injured menisci or articular ligament damage is suspected. With this method, the positive contrast medium coats the meniscus and then drains to the lowest point of the knee while the air rises,

TABLE 23-2 *Contrast Media Injection Sites*

Joint	Injection Site	Amount of Contrast Medium (ml)
Lower Extremity		
Ankle	Insertion made from ventral surface of ankle toward medial malleolus in the area of the upper medial corner of the talus.	6–8 ml (single contrast)
Hip	Insertion made approximately 4 cm below inguinal ligament, avoiding the femoral artery	8–10 ml
Upper Extremity		
Elbow	Insertion made from the lateral side to enter the joint space between the radial head and capitulum. Elbow flexed 90°	5–6 ml (single contrast)
Shoulder	Insertion made approximately 2 cm lateral from acromioclavicular joint toward humerus	6–8 ml and 12 ml air (double contrast)
Temporomandibular joint	Two injections necessary because intra-articular disk separates joint into upper and lower parts; insertion made at point anterior to tragus directed toward the face to puncture upper cavity; lower cavity cannulated by directing needle caudally	0.5–1.0 ml

offering a contrast similar to that seen during a double-contrast study of the colon. In cases in which the meniscus is torn, a single-contrast study may obscure the pathology or fail to demonstrate it. Single-contrast studies are usually reserved for demonstrating loose particles in the joint.

On completion of the fluoroscopic identification of landmarks, the patient is placed in the supine position. The knee is washed and swabbed with an antiseptic solution. Under local anesthesia, the needle is introduced into the joint between the patella and the medial femoral condyle. Some synovial fluid is aspirated; then, both air and the positive contrast medium are introduced. As before, the knee must be moved to properly distribute the contrast medium within the joint. The patient is then placed in the prone position, with a small support located under the distal femur and a small sandbag placed over the ankle to provide the necessary widening of the joint space. The radiographic recording begins.

The fluoroscopic method is the simplest method. The positioning for spot films is accomplished under direct fluoroscopy. Scout films and additional overhead radiographs are usually required to complete the fluoroscopic study; these additional projections are usually specified by the physician. Occasionally, a view of the intercondyloid fossa is requested; however, a true lateral with 90-degree flexion of the knee for the cruciate ligaments is a standard view for this procedure.

Table 23-2 is a summary of the injection sites for some other joints usually studied by arthrography.

EQUIPMENT

The equipment necessary for arthrography is minimal. The procedure itself, especially the double-contrast technique, depends on the use of a fluoroscopic unit. Therefore, the radiographic room should be equipped with an image-intensified fluoroscopic unit. Filming can be accomplished using a well-collimated beam, and additional equipment is not a requirement.

BOX 23-1	*Contents of Typical Arthrogram Tray*
Equipment	**Amount, Type, and Size**
Medicine cup	1 (2 oz)
Basins (small)	1
Forceps	1
Syringe	1 (5 cc, Luer-Lok)
Syringes	2 (20 cc, Luer-Lok)
Syringe	1 (30 cc, Luer-Lok)
Needle	1 (25 gauge, $5/8$ inch)
Needle	1 (20 gauge, $1^1/_2$ inch)
Needle	1 (18 gauge, $1^1/_4$ inch)
Connector tube	1 (10 inch)
Sterile towels	3
Sterile drape	1
Gauze pads	5 (4 in × 4 in)
Prep sponges	2
Adhesive tape	1

Because the injection must be carried out under aseptic conditions, a sterile tray is required. In addition to the items listed in Box 23-1, the special procedure room should have available sterile disposable gloves, antiseptic solution, anesthetic, and contrast agents.

PATIENT POSITIONING

Regardless of the method chosen, scout films should always be taken. Four projections—anteroposterior, internal and external 45-degree obliques, and true lateral—should be taken.

With the vertical beam method, five projections are usually also required. These are listed in the order in which they are taken—anteroposterior, supine external 45-degree oblique, supine internal 45-degree oblique, posteroanterior with knee flexed approximately 30 degrees, and mediolateral with knee flexed 90 degrees. These must be taken accurately and quickly, especially during positive contrast arthrography, because of the rapid absorption of the contrast agent.

The double-contrast arthrogram requires that two sets of six radiographs be made tangentially to the meniscus. After each exposure, the patient is rotated 25 to 30 degrees from the prone through the lateral and finally to the supine position. Both the lateral and medial menisci are radiographed in this manner. If the series is begun with the patient in the prone position and the leg in a lateral anterior oblique position, the first two exposures will demonstrate the posterior portion of the medial meniscus, the third and fourth exposures will demonstrate the middle portion of the medial meniscus, and the last two exposures will demonstrate the anterior portion of the medial meniscus. At this point, the patient is in the supine position. The patient is then placed in the prone position again. The same six exposures are made at 30-degree intervals from the prone to the supine. This set of radiographs demonstrates the posterior, middle, and anterior portions of the lateral meniscus.

The projections taken during double-contrast arthrography should be closely but accurately collimated. Exposure times should be short, and the kVp should be as low as possible to produce good short scale contrast. Because positive contrast media are used, the radiographs must be completed rapidly as a result of the rapid absorption of the contrast medium and the subsequent loss of contrast.

Table 23-3 is a summary of the arthrographic positions for knee arthrography. Figure 23-3 shows some joint images that illustrate the results of both conventional arthrography and MRI techniques.

TABLE 23-3 *Positions for Knee Arthrography*

Projection	Patient Position	Central Ray	Anatomy
	Scout Films		
Anteroposterior	Patient supine, knee maximally extended and centered to an 8- × 10-in (20- × 25-cm) image receptor	Angled approximately 6° caudad, to enter slightly below tip of patella	Preliminary views of knee joint before instillation of contrast medium show distal femur, proximal tibia and fibula, and patellar shadow
Internal oblique	Patient supine, knee joint extended, extremity rotated internally 45° and knee centered to an 8- × 10-in (20- × 25-cm) image receptor	Angled approximately 6° caudad	
External oblique	Patient supine, knee joint extended, extremity rotated externally 45° and knee centered to an 8- × 10-in (20- × 25-cm) image receptor	Angled approximately 3° cephalad	
Lateral	Patient comfortably positioned so that knee is in "true" lateral position in 90° flexion	Angled 3° cephalad	
	Vertical Beam Technique		
Anteroposterior	Patient supine, knee maximally extended and centered to an 8- × 10-in (20- × 25-cm) image receptor	Angled approximately 6–9° toward ankle	Anteroposterior view of contrast-filled knee joint
Supine external oblique	Patient supine, leg rotated 45° externally, knee centered to an 8- × 10-in (20- × 25-cm) image receptor	Angled approximately 6° toward ankle	External oblique view of contrast-filled knee joint
Supine internal oblique	Patient supine, leg rotated 45° internally, knee centered to an 8- × 10-in (20- × 25-cm) image receptor	Angled approximately 9° toward ankle	External oblique view of contrast-filled knee joint
Posteroanterior	Patient prone, knee flexed approximately 30° and centered to an 8- × 10-in (20- × 25-cm) image receptor	Angled approximately 6° cephalad	Posteroanterior view of contrast-filled knee joint
Mediolateral	Patient supine and rotated toward affected side, knee flexed 90° and centered to an 8- × 10-in (20- × 25-cm) image receptor	Angled 3–5° cephalad	Lateral view of contrast-filled knee joint

Continued

TABLE 23-3   *Positions for Knee Arthrography (cont'd)*

Projection	Patient Position	Central Ray	Anatomy
	Horizontal Beam Technique		
Tangential	Medial meniscus: patient initially in prone position, extremity positioned in lateral anterior oblique position, six exposures made; after each exposure, patient rotated 30° until supine position achieved	Directed horizontally at right angles to a lead-shielded 7- × 17-in (17.5- × 42.5-cm) cassette; field size 2.5 × 7 in (6.25 × 17.5 cm)	Tangential views of medial meniscus
	Lateral meniscus; patient in prone position, extremity placed on tunnel table in anterior medial oblique position, six exposures made; after each exposure, patient rotated 30° until supine position achieved		Tangential views of lateral meniscus

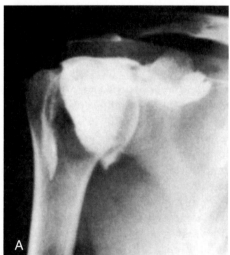

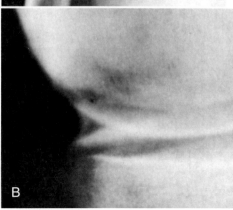

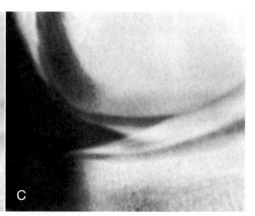

FIGURE 23-3.   **A,** Conventional shoulder arthrographic image. **B** and **C,** Selected images from a conventional knee arthrogram showing a normal **(B)** and abnormal **(C)** meniscus.

Continued

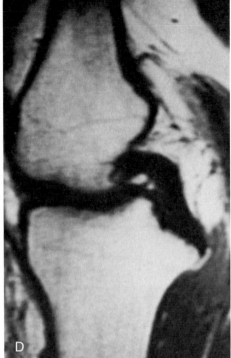

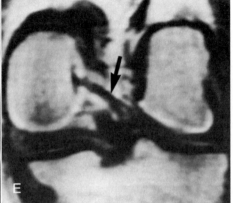

FIGURE 23-3, *cont'd*. **D** and **E,** Magnetic resonance images of the normal knee in a lateral projection **(D)** and frontal projection **(E).** The arrow denotes a normal right anterior cruciate ligament as it appears in the frontal projection.

SUMMARY

Arthrography is the imaging of a joint space and its surrounding structures. The study can be accomplished with conventional radiography; however, MRI is currently the method used to evaluate pathology in the joint space.

The contrast agent used for conventional arthrography is the water-soluble iodide variety. A single- or double-contrast study can be performed when using this technique. MRI utilizes gadolinium as the contrast agent. Gadolinium is a relatively safe material when complexed with EDTA. The structures imaged with the substance have a brighter appearance on the image.

Arthrography can be applied to any joint; some of the more common sites are the knee and shoulder. The study is considered to be invasive and can result in some complications. These are generally related to the type of contrast agent administered.

During conventional arthrography fluoroscopy is often used to follow the contrast and perform the imaging. The needle entry site and positioning are dependent upon the joint being imaged. The injection sites for several joints are summarized in the chapter. Specific positioning is determined by the physician and facilities at the institution.

REFERENCE

1. Sugimoto K, Takakura Y, Samoto N, et al: Subtalar arthrography in recurrent instability of the ankle. *Clin Orthop* 394:169–176, 2002.

SUGGESTED READINGS

Blum A, Loeuille D, Iochum S, et al: MR-arthrography: general principles and applications. *J Radiol* 84(6):39–57, 2003.

Chung CB, Corrente L, Resnick D: MR arthrography of the shoulder. *Magn Reson Imaging Clin North Am* 12(1):25–38, 2004.

Ehara S, Itoi E, Sashi R: Injection of rotator interval for shoulder arthrography. *AJR Am J Roentgenol* 183(4):1172–1173, 2004.

Jackson JL, O'Malley PG, Kroenke K: Evaluation of acute knee pain in primary care. *Ann Intern Med* 139(7):575–588, 2003.

Kieser CW, Jackson RW: Eugen Bircher (1882–1956), the first knee surgeon to use diagnostic arthroscopy. *Arthroscopy* 19(7):771–776, 2003.

Morag Y, Jacobson JA, Shields G, et al: MR arthrography of rotator interval, long head of the biceps brachii, and biceps pulley of the shoulder. *Radiology* 235(1):21–30, 2005.

Schneider TL, Schmidt-Wiethoff R, Drescher W, Fink B, Schmidt J, Appell HJ: The significance of subacromial arthrography to verify partial bursal-side rotator cuff ruptures. *Arch Orthop Trauma Surg* 123(9):481–484, 2003.

STUDY QUESTIONS

1. The type of joint that permits the sliding of one surface on another is called a _____ joint.
   - **a.** hinge
   - **b.** synovial
   - **c.** gliding
   - **d.** synarthrodial

2. The clear viscous fluid that serves as the joints' lubricant is:
   - **a.** water
   - **b.** synovial fluid
   - **c.** gadolinium
   - **d.** interstitial solution

3. The site of needle insertion in knee arthrography is the:
   - **a.** retropatellar space
   - **b.** popliteal vein
   - **c.** anterior to the patella
   - **d.** one half inch above the apex of the patella

4. When nonionic contrast agents are used in arthrography the concentration should be no greater than:
   - **a.** 20%
   - **b.** 30%
   - **c.** 40%
   - **d.** 50%

5. Double-contrast arthrography of the knee demonstrates the:
   - **a.** menisci to best advantage
   - **b.** retropatellar apace
   - **c.** intercondylar fossa
   - **d.** loose particles over the joint

6. Which of the following is not an indication for arthrography?
   - **a.** cartilaginous defects
   - **b.** ruptures of the ligaments
   - **c.** hypersensitivity to iodine
   - **d.** arthritic deformities

7. Normal wear and tear on the joint surfaces results in:
   - **a.** trauma
   - **b.** hyaline articular cartilage damage
   - **c.** elimination of synovial fluid from the joint
   - **d.** ligament tears

8. The shoulder is an example of a _____ joint.
   - **a.** hinge
   - **b.** sliding
   - **c.** pivot
   - **d.** ball-and-socket

9. Ligaments serve the purpose of:
   - **a.** limiting the motion of the joint in undesirable directions
   - **b.** capturing the contrast agent for excretion
   - **c.** supporting the synovial membrane
   - **d.** providing the synovial fluid to the joint

10. The most common reaction to the contrast agent used during arthrography is:
    - **a.** cardiac arrest
    - **b.** respiratory distress
    - **c.** anaphylactic response
    - **d.** vasovagal response

1 *Custom Formation of Catheters*

CUSTOM SHAPING

Catheters supplied today are preshaped and molded. Institutions and physicians who perform research on new techniques and procedures may require catheters that are designed to specifications or shapes that are not commercially available. In these cases, catheters may need to be custom shaped. Bulk thermoplastic catheter materials are available from several companies for this purpose.

The equipment necessary for the process includes a guide wire matching the inside diameter of the catheter tubing, an alcohol burner, a scalpel handle and blade, a hole punching tool, a hot water bath, and a flanging tool. Figure A-1, *A* through *F*, illustrates the process of custom shaping. There are six steps in the process: preparation of the catheter tip, cutting the catheter tip, cutting the catheter length, shaping the distal end of the catheter, inserting side holes (if needed), and forming the proximal end. The catheters prepared by this method are used only for research purposes. Once the procedure becomes accepted in clinical practice, the catheter can be commercially manufactured for general use. Custom-shaped catheters are rarely needed today; however, a discussion of the process is presented for historical as well as informational purposes.

Preparation of Catheter Tip

Insert the guide wire into the lumen of the catheter tubing approximately 20 cm. Heat the tubing over the alcohol burner while pulling the tubing in opposite directions (Fig. A-1, *A*). The tubing will soften, and the lumen will conform to the diameter of the guide wire and form an even taper. Immerse the catheter in cold water to fix the shape.

Another method of forming the distal end of the catheter is shown in Figure A-1, *B*. There is no need for heat because the tubing will stretch to conform to the tip of the guide wire in the lumen of the tubing. This method is used with catheter tubing other than radiopaque polyethylene tubing. When the tubing is sufficiently stretched around the guide wire, the unfilled portion should be cut off close to the tip of the guide wire to form a rounded catheter tip.

Cutting the Catheter Tip

After the tip has been tapered and while the guide wire is still in the lumen of the tubing, the free end of the tubing should be cut with a sharp scalpel. The guide wire used to prepare the catheter tip should never be used in a procedure. The catheter material should be cut at the point that best approximates the diameter of the guide wire used. The tubing should be rolled on a flat surface while slight pressure is applied on the scalpel blade (Fig. A-1, *C*).[1] It is essential that the cut tip be smooth to avoid vascular trauma.

Cutting the Catheter Length

When the tip of the catheter has been prepared, the tubing should be cut to the proper length.

Custom Shaping the Distal End

With the guide wire still in place, bend the catheter into the shape required for the procedure, and immerse it in hot water. It is important that the thinner walls of the tapered tip *not* be placed in the hot water because of possible deformation of the walls and end holes (Fig. A-1, *D*). When the entire wall of the tubing has been heated and the catheter has softened, transfer the tubing to a cool water bath to fix the desired shape.

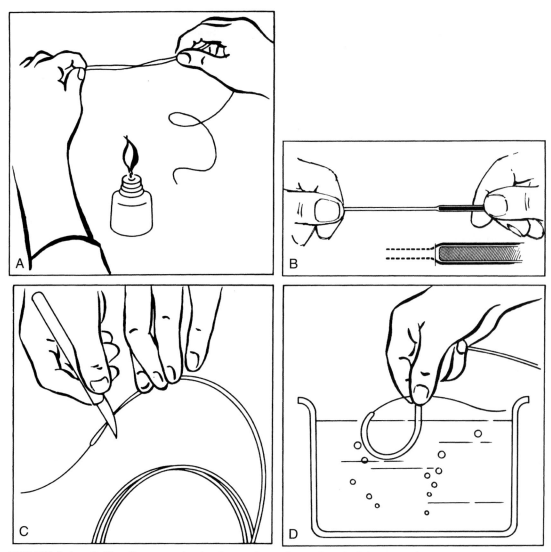

FIGURE A-1. **A,** The first step in the formation of a catheter. A length of catheter tubing with a guide wire inserted is heated over an alcohol burner. It is gently stretched to adapt to the diameter of the guide wire. The guide wire used in this procedure should not be used during a special procedure. **B,** The cold formation is used primarily with radiopaque Teflon, radioparent polyethylene, radioparent Teflon, and radiolucent vinyl tubings. After being stretched, the catheter tubing will conform to the guide wire insert and should be cut off close to it to form a rounded catheter tip. **C,** Cutting the catheter tip after stretching. The catheter should be rolled on a flat surface while gentle pressure is applied on the knife blade. **D,** Shaping the distal end of the catheter. The catheter–guide wire combination is placed in hot water. As the catheter softens, it can be formed into the desired shape. The combination is then transferred to a cold water bath to fix the position of the tip. *Continued*

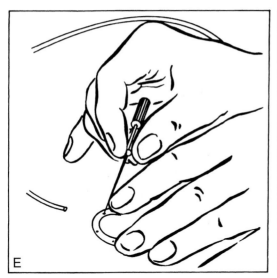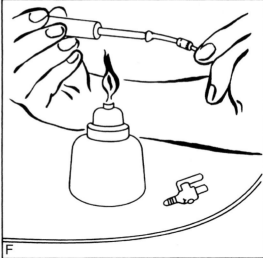

FIGURE A-1, *cont'd.* **E,** The procedure for punching holes in the distal tip of the catheter. **F,** The formation of the proximal end of a catheter. The adapter cap is placed on the tubing, which is heated over an alcohol burner. When it has softened, the flanging tool is used to form the cone-shaped proximal end. The shape is fixed under cold water with the flanging tool in place.

Placement of Side Holes

Placing side holes in the distal end of the catheter reduces the whiplash effect created by injection of contrast medium through a single end hole and increases the delivery rate of the catheter. Side holes should be placed so that the catheter wall is not weakened; they should not be placed in areas in which the guide wire could lodge as catheters are being exchanged. Therefore, holes should never be placed in the thin walls of the tapered tip or in direct opposition to each other.

Side holes are made with a punching tool that is a hollow cannula with a sharp cutting edge. Rotate the punching tool while applying slight pressure to it (Fig. A-1, *E*). A stylet longer than the cannula is used to remove the plugs of tubing from inside the cannula. It is important that the piece of catheter wall not be left in the lumen of the catheter to avoid its introduction into the patient's vascular system.

Forming the Proximal End

An adapter must be fitted to the proximal end of the catheter tubing to connect it to the injection device. A catheter flanging tool can be used to shape the proximal end of the tubing to fit the adapter cone (Fig. A-1, *F*). Place the adapter cap on the tubing with the opening facing the proximal end. Heat the flanging tool, and then carefully press it to the end of the catheter tubing. With the tool in place, fix the flange under cold water. The connection should be tested for leakage before use.[1]

A second method of forming the flange in the end of the catheter tubing is to rotate it slowly over an alcohol burner while holding the tubing horizontally. Fix the shape in the usual manner under cool water.

REFERENCE

1. *Instruments and Catheters for Radiography.* Solna, Sweden, 1970, Firma AB Kifa.

2 *Reference Sources for Pharmaceutical Information*

Each advanced procedure department should have at least one source of information about the various pharmaceuticals that can and are used before, during, and after the procedures. Pharmacology is a field in itself, and it would be impossible for any one textbook to present in-depth coverage on all the possible medications that are used in all of the institutions performing advanced procedures.

The following represent some of the possible references textbooks that can give the members of the diagnostic/interventional team a ready source of information concerning the drugs specific to that department.

Handbook on Injectable Drugs, 2004
Lawrence A. Trissel
Macmillan Publishers, Ltd
ISBN: 1585280410

Teddy Bear Book, Pediatric Injectable Drugs, 7th edition, 2003
American Society of Health Systems Pharmacists
ISBN: 1-58528-054-2

AHFS Dosing Companion, 2004
American Hospital Formulary Service
ISBN: 1-58528-028-3

Drug Interaction Facts, 2004
David Tatro
Facts and Comparisons (Drugfacts.com)
ISBN: 1-57439-180-1

Institute for Safe Medication Practices
http://www.ismp.org

Physician's Desk Reference, 58th edition 2004
Thompson PDK
ISBN: 1-56363-471-6

Answers to Study Questions

CHAPTER 1
1. d   2. b   3. c   4. d   5. a   6. b   7. b   8. d   9. b   10. d

CHAPTER 2
1. b   2. c   3. a   4. d   5. a   6. c   7. d   8. c   9. a   10. c

CHAPTER 3
1. d   2. b   3. d   4. c   5. a   6. a   7. d   8. c   9. a   10. c

CHAPTER 4
1. b   2. b   3. c   4. b   5. c   6. b   7. d   8. b   9. a   10. b

CHAPTER 5
1. c   2. b   3. c   4. a   5. c   6. d   7. c   8. d   9. b   10. c

CHAPTER 6
1. c   2. c   3. c   4. c   5. c   6. d   7. c   8. b   9. a   10. d

CHAPTER 7
1. b   2. c   3. c   4. b   5. c   6. d   7. c   8. b   9. c   10. d

CHAPTER 8
1. d   2. c   3. b   4. a   5. d   6. d   7. b   8. c   9. a   10. a

CHAPTER 9
1. c   2. c   3. b   4. a   5. b   6. c   7. d   8. a   9. c   10. b

CHAPTER 10
1. b   2. c   3. a   4. a   5. d   6. a   7. b   8. b   9. c   10. b

CHAPTER 11
1. d   2. b   3. b   4. d   5. c   6. a   7. b   8. a   9. d   10. b

CHAPTER 12

1. a   2. b   3. b   4. a   5. d   6. c   7. b   8. b   9. a   10. c

CHAPTER 13

1. b   2. c   3. a   4. a   5. d   6. a   7. d   8. d   9. c   10. b

CHAPTER 14

1. b   2. d   3. a   4. b   5. b   6. d   7. d   8. b   9. b   10. b

CHAPTER 15

1. b   2. b   3. c   4. b   5. a   6. b   7. d   8. b   9. c   10. b

CHAPTER 16

1. a   2. b   3. c   4. d   5. a   6. c   7. c   8. b   9. a   10. c

CHAPTER 17

1. b   2. d   3. b   4. a   5. c   6. b   7. a   8. c   9. d   10. c

CHAPTER 18

1. d   2. c   3. a   4. c   5. c   6. b   7. d   8. a   9. d   10. b

CHAPTER 19

1. b   2. c   3. d   4. c   5. d   6. a   7. c   8. d   9. c   10. d

CHAPTER 20

1. d   2. c   3. a   4. d   5. c   6. b   7. c   8. c   9. d   10. b

CHAPTER 21

1. b   2. b   3. a   4. a   5. d   6. c   7. c   8. d   9. d   10. b

CHAPTER 22

1. b   2. b   3. c   4. c   5. c   6. b   7. a   8. d   9. c   10. b

CHAPTER 23

1. c   2. b   3. a   4. d   5. d   6. c   7. b   8. d   9. a   10. d

Glossary

aberration   A departure from the norm.

ablation   The destruction or removal of tissue.

aerial image   The image that is formed in the air by the remnant radiation that exits the object or patient.

agonist   A drug or chemical that has a specific affinity to certain cells and that will produce a predictable response.

ambient   Refers to the surrounding area or room.

amplitude   Refers to the range or width.

analgesic   A substance that is used to reduce pain.

analog   A continuous representation in which both measurement and reproducibility are imprecise.

anaphylactic   Pertaining to the hypersensitivity response to a substance.

anastomose   To join two blood vessels.

aneurysm   A localized dilation in the wall of a blood vessel.

angioplasty   An interventional technique used to restore the opening in a stenosed vessel.

angular momentum   A measure of the amount of spin or orbital motion of an object. When the atomic nuclei spin in the presence of a gravitational field the nucleus will wobble because of the effect of gravity. This wobble is referred to as precession. The action is similar to a spinning top; when it begins to slow down, it continues to spin on its axis, but it also tends to cause the entire spinning top to wobble.

anion   A negatively charged ion.

antagonist   A drug or chemical that will oppose or counteract the action of another drug or chemical substance by binding to a receptor site in a cell without producing a biologic response. It is the opposite of an agonist.

anticholinergic   A substance that inhibits the transmission of parasympathetic nerve impulses, which results in the reduction of spasm in smooth muscle.

antiemetic   Refers to a substance that relieves nausea and vomiting.

antitussive   Substance that reduces or inhibits the cough reflex.

arteriotomy   Cutting into an artery to gain access.

atherectomy   The procedure used to scrape away plaque from the lumen walls of an artery using a special catheter.

atherosclerosis   The formation of plaque in the lumen of blood vessels, causing a narrowing of the channel, resulting in a decreased blood supply to structures supplied by the vessel.

attenuation   The reduction in intensity of an x-ray beam due to its interaction with matter.

autoclaving   The sterilization of implements using steam under pressure.

becquerel (Bq)   Unit named after Henri Becquerel, the discoverer of radioactivity. One becquerel is equal to 1 disintegration per second or 27.03×10^{-11} Ci.

bifurcation   A splitting into two channels or branches.

biopsy   Excision of a piece of tissue for microscopic examination.

biphasic   Pertaining to two separate injection phases during a single radiographic study.

biplane   The use of two separate image recording devices in opposite planes to simultaneously record the images produced during a procedure.

blood urea nitrogen (BUN)   The level of nitrogen in the blood in the form of urea, the chief nitrogenous component of urine. The normal levels are 9 to 25 mg/ml. This value gives the technologist a rough estimate of kidney function.

bolus   A dose of contrast material that is intravenously injected all at once.

bradycardia   An abnormally slow heart rate of less than 60 pulses per minute.

bronchography   Radiography of the bronchi using a contrast agent to coat the walls of the airway.

cannula   A small flexible tube with a removable pointed rod that can be inserted into a blood vessel.

cardiovascular   Pertaining to the circulatory system.

cardioversion   When there is an irregular heartbeat, the application of a high-energy current can cause the heart to return to a normal or regular beat.

catheterization   The process of passing a catheter into a vessel during a radiographic procedure.

cation   A positively charged ion.

CCD (charge-coupled device)   A light-sensitive computer chip that can store and display the data collected about an image. CCDs are commonly found in digital video and digital still cameras.

Charrière   A gauge scale for measurement of the diameter of catheters: 1 Charrière = 1 French = $\frac{1}{3}$ mm.

chelate   A ringlike complex with a metal ion firmly bound and isolated.

chemotoxicity   Pertaining to poisoning from chemical substances.

cisterna   Cavity or dilation that serves as reservoir for body fluids such as cerebrospinal fluid or lymph (e.g., the cisterna magna and cisterna chyli, respectively).

collateral   Refers to a small branch vessel that is considered to be secondary or accessory.

commissure   The place where the leaflets of a cardiac valve fuse. The procedure for opening of the orifice of the valve is called a commissurotomy.

concentric   Describes two or more circles having a common center.

concomitant   Occurring at the same time.

contiguous   In physical contact with or touching.

curie (Ci)   Unit named after Marie Curie, one of the pioneers in the field of radioactivity. One Curie represents radioactivity equal to 3.7×10^{10} disintegrations per second (dps).

cytologic   Pertaining to the cells.

diapositive image   A reverse image that is used to superimpose over an angiogram film to remove the extraneous anatomic structures, allowing a clear picture of the contrast agent–filled vessels.

diastole   The period of relaxation of the chambers of the heart during which blood enters.

DICOM standard   A standard file format that can be interpreted by equipment from many different companies. The acronym DICOM stands for the digital imaging and communications in medicine.

digital data   Values represented by a table of numbers. The data has no meaning until it is manipulated by a computer program.

dimer	A molecule formed by joining two molecules of a simpler compound.
dysmenorrhea	Painful menstruation.
embolization	An interventional radiographic procedure that creates an artificial clot to reduce or stop bleeding.
embolus	A foreign object that can circulate in the bloodstream, potentially becoming lodged in a vessel.
extracorporeal	Outside the body.
fibrinolysis	The normal physiologic mechanism that removes small clots by dissolving them with an enzyme called fibrinolysin.
flanging tool	An implement used to create a collarlike flare at the end of tubing.
flow rate	The amount of material delivered in a specific amount of time.
gauss	A unit of magnetic field strength equal to 1/10,000 tesla (see also *tesla*).
half-life	The time interval for a specific number of unstable nuclei to decay (disintegrate) to one half their original number.
hemodynamic	Pertaining to the physiology of blood circulation.
hemolysis	The breakdown of red blood cells with the release of hemoglobin.
hemostasis	The cessation of blood flow.
histamine	A substance found in all cells that is released in allergic or inflammatory reactions.
homozygous	Having a 100% chance of inheriting a particular disease.
hyperosmolality	Pertaining to an increase in the concentration of osmotically active components.
hypertonic	Having a greater concentration of solute than another solution.
hypokalemia	A condition in which an insufficient amount of potassium is detected in the systemic bloodstream.
hypotonic	Having less of a concentration of solute than another solution.
immiscibility	The inability of a substance to mix with another substance, such as oil and water.
in situ	In the correct or natural place.
in vivo	In a living organism.
incipient	Beginning to appear or show itself.
interventional	Refers to treatment of conditions that were previously managed surgically utilizing radiographic techniques.
interventional radiography	Procedures used to improve the physical function of a patient using radiologic monitoring.
intracranial	Within or inside the bony skull.
intradermal wheal	An eruption within the dermis caused by the subcutaneous injection of a substance.
intralymphatic	Within the lymphatic vessels.
intrinsic	Pertaining to an inherent part or quality of a substance.
ionic	Pertaining to an electrically charged particle. Describes the ability to separate into ions.
ischemia	The decrease of blood flow to a body structure characterized by pain in the area.

isotonic — Having the same concentration of solute as another solution.

iterative — A technique used to reconstruct data that is characterized by repetitions.

Larmour frequency — The type of atom reflects the rate of the frequency of the precession to the strength of the external magnetic field. It is expressed by the formula $\omega_0 = \gamma B_0$.

lattice — A three-dimensional cross-linked structure.

leptomeninges — A term used to collectively describe the pia mater and arachnoid membranes that surround the brain and spinal cord.

lithotomy position — Lying supine with the knees and hips flexed and raised. The feet are usually supported in stirrups.

lithotripsy — The breaking up of stones in the urinary and biliary systems using high-energy shock waves.

Luer-Lok — That portion of the syringe or connector that holds the needle securely in place.

lumen — A channel or cavity within an organ or structure.

lymphangiography — Radiography of the lymph nodes and lymph channels.

magnetic dipole — Refers to the individual magnetic properties that atoms possess. Each of these is similar to a small bar magnet and has both a north and a south pole.

magnetic gradient — The changes in strength of a magnetic field in a certain direction.

magnetic moment — Particular atoms will exhibit magnetic properties. They will have a north and south pole. These are randomly oriented in the patient, and their net magnetic field would add up to zero; however, when exposed to an external magnetic field they will orient themselves with the plane of the magnetic field creating a net magnetic moment.

meninges — The membranes that surround the spinal cord and brain.

miscibility — The ability of a substance to mix with another substance.

monochromatic — Having only one color or wavelength.

multiphasic — Pertaining to more than one injection phase within a single radiographic study.

neoplastic — Refers to the abnormal growth of new tissue.

nephrostomy — Catheter insertion into the kidney for the purpose of drainage.

neuroradiography — Radiography of the nervous system and its components.

nonionic — Refers to the inability to separate into ions.

obturator — A thin metal rod that is inserted into a needle set to block its lumen.

occlude — To obstruct or block a channel.

osmolality — The pressure a solution exerts on a semipermeable membrane, which separates a solution from a solute. Osmolality is expressed as milliosmols per kilogram of water.

osmolarity — The pressure a solution exerts on a semipermeable membrane, which separates a solution from a solute. Osmolarity is expressed as milliosmols per kilogram of solution.

osmole — The substance in solution such as molecules or ions, having the same osmotic pressure as one mole of a nonelectrolyte. Osmoles are expressed in grams.

oximetry — The measurement of the oxygen content of arterial blood using a device referred to as an oximeter.

pallor — An unnatural absence of color in the skin.

PCN — Percutaneous catheter nephrostomy.

Fundamentals of Special Radiographic Procedures

percent duty factor	The amount of time that an x-ray tube can be used under certain operating conditions. These are usually expressed as percent duty factor curves.
percutaneous	Refers to a procedure that is performed through the skin, such as the placement of a catheter into a blood vessel (percutaneous catheterization).
peripheral	Pertaining to the outside of an area surrounding an organ or structure.
pharmacologic	Refers to the properties, actions, origins, or uses of drugs.
photoemissive	Refers to a substance that will produce an electron flow when stimulated by visible light.
popliteal	Refers to the blood vessel that is an extension of the femoral artery.
porphyria	An inherited disease characterized by an abnormal increase in the production of porphyrins, substances that occur naturally in many compounds in the body.
precession	The motion of a spinning object that appears as a wobble around a vertical axis.
pseudoaneurysm	Refers to a vessel that is torturous or has damaged layers, giving the impression of a true aneurysm.
psychogenic	Pertaining to a physical symptom or sign or that originates in the mind or has an emotional component.
PTA	Percutaneous transluminal angioplasty.
radiolucent	A property of low–atomic number substances that decreases attenuation, producing relatively dark images on the radiographic film.
radiopaque	A property of high–atomic number substances that increases attenuation, producing relatively light images on radiographic film.
reactive hyperemia	The increase in blood flow in response to some sort of mechanical intervention such as the creation of an artificial ischemia (reduction in blood supply) by using a mechanical device to restrict the flow of blood. Once the device has been removed the blood will flow rapidly through the site, markedly increasing the amount of blood supply to the part.
renin	An enzyme that is produced when the blood pressure is low. This substance initiates a series of reactions that ultimately result in the production of angiotensin II, which is a vasoconstrictor causing the blood volume and pressure to increase.
resonance	The process of the absorption of energy by an object tuned to a specific frequency.
restenosis	The abnormal closure of a vessel lumen following an interventional procedure.
retroperitoneal	Pertaining to those organs that are attached to the abdominal wall and partly covered by the peritoneum, the serous membrane that covers the entire abdominal wall.
ripple	Also known as voltage ripple. It represents the variation in the peak voltage supplied to the x-ray tube. Single-phase power has 100% voltage ripple; three phase, six pulse produces voltage with only 13% ripple; three phase twelve pulse results in a 4% voltage ripple while high-frequency generators will have less than 1% voltage ripple.
sequester	To isolate.
shunt	An abnormal connection between the chambers of the heart.
stenosis	The abnormal narrowing of an opening, channel, or passageway.
stent	A device used to support the walls of blood vessels, cavities, or body openings.
Stubbs needle gauge	Relates the outside diameter of a needle to a whole number. The larger the number, the smaller the outside diameter of the needle.
stylet	A thin metal rod that can be inserted into a needle. Used to clean the lumen of the needle.

systole	The contraction of the heart muscle that drives the blood through the circulatory system.
tachycardia	Abnormal contraction of the heart muscle in excess of 100 beats per minute.
tesla	The unit of magnetic flux density equal to 1 volt per second per square meter.
thrombolysis	Chemically dissolving a clot.
thrombosis	Refers to the abnormal formation of clots in the blood vessels.
thrombus	A collection of platelets, fibrin, and cellular elements attached to the interior wall of a blood vessel.
tomography	The radiographic technique that produces an image of a structure at a predetermined depth without the superimposition of structures that lie above or below the specified depth.
torque	A twisting force.
trackball	A peripheral computer device that moves the cursor around the screen.
transjugular intrahepatic portosystemic shunting (TIPS)	The percutaneous method of creating an artificial connection between the portal and hepatic venous systems to reduce portal hypertension.
Trendelenburg position	A position in which the head is lower than the legs and the body is inclined.
Valsalva maneuver	Forced expiration against a voluntarily closed airway.
vasa recta	Small blood vessels that provide a blood supply to the small intestine.
vascular	Pertaining to blood vessels.
vasoconstriction	The narrowing of the lumen of a vessel.
vasodilation	The widening of the lumen of a vessel.
vector	Refers to the direction and magnitude of a force.
venipuncture	The puncture of a blood vessel through the skin for the purpose of withdrawing a sample of fluid.
Vieussens' ring	An important means of collateral circulation around the heart formed by smaller branches of the artery that supplies the right ventricle.
viscosity	The quality of a fluid caused by the adhesion of its molecules by which it resists shape change or relative motion within itself.

Illustration Credits

CHAPTER 1

Figures 1-1 and 1-2 courtesy Siemens Medical Solutions, Malvern, Pa.

Figures 1-3 to 1-6, 1-8, and 1-9 courtesy Varian Medical, Salt Lake City, Utah.

Figures 1-7 from Fauber T: *Radiographic imaging and exposure,* ed 2, St Louis, 2004, Mosby.

CHAPTER 2

Figures 2-2 to 2-4, 2-7, 2-8, and 2-13 courtesy Siemens Medical Solutions, Malvern, Pa.

Figure 2-5 courtesy Eastman Kodak, Rochester, NY.

Figures 2-11 and 2-12 from *Principles of subtraction in radiology,* Wilmington, Del, 1971, E I du Pont de Nemours.

CHAPTER 3

Figures 3-1 to 3-5 and 3-14, *A* courtesy Medrad, Inc., Indianola, Pa.

Figures 3-6, 3-7, and 3-9 to 3-13 courtesy E-Z-EM, Inc., Lake Success, NY.

Figures 3-8 and 3-14, *B* courtesy Tyco-Mallinckrodt, Hazelwood, Mo.

CHAPTER 4

Figures 4-1, 4-7, 4-10, and 4-12 courtesy Becton-Dickinson and Company, Franklin Lakes, NJ.

Figures 4-2, 4-3, 4-8, and 4-9 from Kaufman JA, Lee MJ: *Vascular and interventional radiology,* St Louis, 2004, Mosby.

Figure 4-4 courtesy of Medi-Tech/Boston Scientific Corporation, Natick, Mass.

Figure 4-5 from United States Catheter and Instruments Corporation, CR Bard, Inc., Murray Hill, NJ.

Figure 4-11 courtesy Baxter Healthcare, Deerfield, Ill.

CHAPTER 5

Figures 5-1 and 5-2 courtesy Baxter Healthcare, Deerfield, Ill.

CHAPTER 8

Figure 8-1 courtesy Datex-Ohmeda, Madison, Wis.

Figures 8-5, 8-6, and 8-8 from Kadir S: *Diagnostic angiography,* Philadelphia, 1986, WB Saunders.

CHAPTER 9

Figures 9-1, *A* to *D*, 9-6 to 9-8, and 9-12 from Seeram E: *Computed tomography technology,* Philadelphia, 1982, WB Saunders.

Figures 9-1, *E* and *F*, 9-13 to 9-15 courtesy GE Imatron, Inc., South San Francisco, Calif.

Figures 9-2, 9-5, and 9-9 to 9-11 courtesy Siemens Medical Solutions, Malvern, Pa.

CHAPTER 10

Figures 10-1, 10-13, and 10-14 from Picker International, Norcross, Ga.

Figures 10-2 and 10-3 from Fonar, Inc., Melville, NY.

Figures 10-7 and 10-11 from Partain CL, James AE Jr, Rollo FD, Price RR: *Nuclear magnetic resonance (NMR) imaging,* Philadelphia, 1983, WB Saunders.

CHAPTER 11

Figures 11-1, 11-2, and 11-4 courtesy Siemens Medical Solutions, Malvern, Pa.

Figure 11-3 from Thrall J, Ziessman H: *Nuclear medicine: The requisites,* ed 2, St Louis, 2001, Mosby.

Figure 11-5 from Gambhir S, Ell P: *Nuclear medicine in clinical diagnosis and treatment,* ed 3, London, 2004, Churchill Livingstone.

CHAPTER 12

Figures 12-12 and 12-13 from Gedgaudas E, Moller J, Castaneda-Zuniga E, Amplatz K: *Cardiovascular radiology,* Philadelphia, 1985, WB Saunders.

Figures 12-14, *A* and *B* courtesy RADI Medical Systems, Wilmington, Mass.

Figure 12-14, *C* courtesy Instromedix, San Diego, Calif.

CHAPTER 13

Figures 13-1, *B,* 13-5, and 13-7 from Witten MU: *Emmett's clinical urography: an atlas and textbook of roentgenologic diagnosis,* ed 4, Philadelphia, 1977, WB Saunders.

Figures 13-7, *A* and *C* from Meschan I: *Synopsis of radiologic anatomy with computed tomography,* Philadelphia, 1980, WB Saunders.

Figure 13-8, *A* from *X-Ray Focus,* vol 12, 1973. Copyright Ilford, Inc.

Figure 13-8, *B* from Winthrop Laboratories, New York, NY.

Figure 13-8, *C* from *Radiol Clin North Am* 2:426, 1963-1964.

CHAPTER 14

Figure 14-1 from Valji K: *Vascular and interventional radiology,* Philadelphia, 1999, WB Saunders.

CHAPTER 15

Figure 15-2, *B* from Juergens JL, Spitelli JA, Fairbairn JF II: *Allen-Barker-Hines, peripheral vascular disease,* ed 5, Philadelphia, 1980, WB Saunders.

Figure 15-6 from O'Rahilly R: *Anatomy,* Philadelphia, 1983, WB Saunders.

Figure 15-10 from Kadir S: *Diagnostic angiography,* Philadelphia, 1986, WB Saunders.

CHAPTER 16

Figure 16-2 from Ramsey RB: *Neuroradiology with computed tomography,* Philadelphia, 1982, WB Saunders.

Figure 16-6 from Gardner E, Gray DJ, O'Rahilly R: *Anatomy,* ed 4, Philadelphia, 1975, WB Saunders.

Figure 16-8 from Putman C, Ravin C: *Textbook of diagnostic imaging,* vol 1, Philadelphia, 1988, WB Saunders.

Figure 16-9 from Krayenbuhl H, Yasargil M: *Cerebral angiography*, ed 2, London, 1968, Butterworth.

Figures 16-10, *A*, 16-11, *A*, and 16-13 from Selman J: *Skull radiography*, Springfield Ill, 1966, Charles C Thomas.

Figures 16-10, *B*, 16-11, *B*, 16-12, *B*, and 16-12, *C* from Toole JF, Patel AN: *Cerebrovascular disorders*, ed 2, New York, 1974, McGraw-Hill.

CHAPTER 17

Figures 17-1, 17-4, and 17-6 from Kadir S, Kaufman SL, Barth KH: *Selected techniques in interventional radiology*, Philadelphia, 1982, WB Saunders.

Figure 17-2 from Medi-Tech/Boston Scientific Corporation, Natick, Mass.

Figures 17-5, 17-17, and 17-18 courtesy Cook Incorporated, Bloomington, Ind.

Figures 17-7, 17-9, and 17-13, *C* from Topol E: *Textbook of interventional cardiology*, Philadelphia, 1990, WB Saunders.

Figure 17-8 from Abela GS, Seeger JM, Pry RS, et al: Percutaneous laser recanalization of totally occluded human peripheral arteries: a technical approach, *Dynamic Cardiovasc Imag* 1:302-308, 1998.

Figure 17-10 from Simpson JB, Selmon MR, Robertson GC, et al: Transluminal atherectomy for peripheral vascular disease, *Am J Cardiol* 61:96G-101G, 1988.

Figure 17-11 courtesy Tyco-Mallinckrodt, Hazelwood, Mo.

Figure 17-13, *A, B, D, E* courtesy Interventional Technologies, Inc., San Diego. Calif.

Figure 17-13, *C* from Topol E: *Textbook of interventional cardiology*, Philadelphia, 1990, WB Saunders.

Figures 17-14, 17-16, and 17-19 courtesy Boston Scientific/Vascular Corporation, Natick, Mass.

Figure 17-15 from Kern MJ: *The cardiac catheterization handbook*, ed 4, St Louis, 1999, Mosby.

Figure 17-20 from Weissleder R, Wittenberg J, Harisinghani M: *Primer of diagnostic imaging*, ed 3, Philadelphia, 2003, Mosby.

Figures 17-21 and 17-23 from Kessel D, Robertson I: *Interventional radiology: a survival guide*, ed 2, St Louis, 2005, Elsevier.

Figure 17-22 from Valji K: *Vascular and interventional radiology*, Philadelphia, 1999, WB Saunders.

CHAPTER 18

Figures 18-1 and 18-2 from Valji K: *Vascular and interventional radiology*, Philadelphia, 1999, WB Saunders.

Figures 18-3 to 18-5, and 18-8 from Kern M: *The cardiac catheterization handbook*, ed 4, Philadelphia, 2003, WB Saunders.

Figures 18-6 and 18-7 from Kessel D, Robertson I: *Interventional radiology: a survival guide*, ed 2, St Louis, 2005, Elsevier.

CHAPTER 19

Figure 19-1, *A* and *B* from Valji K: *Vascular and interventional radiology*, Philadelphia, 1999, WB Saunders.

Figures 19-1, *C,* and 19-2 from Weissleder R, Wittenberg J, Harisinghani M: *Primer of diagnostic imaging*, 3rd ed, Philadelphia, 2003, Mosby.

Figures 19-3 to 19-7, 19-9 to 19-11, and 19-13 to 19-16 from Athanasoulis CA et al: *Interventional radiology*, Philadelphia, 1982, WB Saunders.

Figure 19-8 from Newhouse JH, Pfister RC: Percutaneous catheterization of the kidney and perirenal space, trocar technique, *Urol Radiol* 2:157, 1981.

Figure 19-12 from Pfister RC, Yoder IC, Newhouse JH: Percutaneous uroradiologic procedures, *Semin Roentgenol* 16:135, 1981.

Figures 19-17 to 19-19 from Ginsberg G, Kochman M: *Endoscopy and gastrointestinal radiology,* Philadelphia, 2004, Mosby.

CHAPTER 20

Figures 20-3, 20-4, and 20-5, *B* courtesy CooperSurgical, Inc., Trumbull, Ct.

Figure 20-6 from Potchen EJ, Koehler RP, Davis DO: *Principles of diagnostic radiology,* New York, 1971, McGraw-Hill.

CHAPTER 21

Figure 21-2 from O'Rahilly R: *Basic human anatomy: a regional study of human structure,* ed 3, Philadelphia, 1983, WB Saunders.

Figure 21-8, *A* from Putman C, Ravin C: *Textbook of diagnostic imaging,* Philadelphia, 1988, WB Saunders.

Figures 21-8, *B,* and 21-9, *C* from Grossman R, Yousem D: *Neuroradiology* ed 2, St Louis, 2003, Elsevier.

Figure 21-9, *A* and *B* from Partain CL, et al: *Magnetic resonance imaging,* ed 2, Philadelphia, 1988, WB Saunders.

Figures 21-10 to 21-13 from *Radiography of the spine,* Wilmington, Del., 1966, E I du Pont de Nemours.

CHAPTER 22

Figure 22-2 from Randow RM, Polayes IM: *Diseases of the salivary glands,* Philadelphia, 1976, WB Saunders.

CHAPTER 23

Figure 23-3 from Putman C, Ravin C: *Textbook of diagnostic imaging,* vol 1, Philadelphia, 1988, WB Saunders.

APPENDIX 1

Figure A-1 from *Instruments and Catheters for Radiography.* Solna, Sweden, 1970, Firma AB Kifa.

Index

Page numbers followed by f indicate figures; those followed by t indicate tables; those followed by b indicate boxed material.

Fundamentals of Special Radiographic Procedures